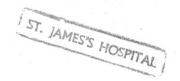
This book is to be returned on or before
the last date stamped below.

LIBREX

David Tayle

One by

ONE BY ONE

ONE BY ONE

DAVID TAYLOR

BOOK CLUB ASSOCIATES
LONDON

Zoovet first published in Great Britain
by George Allen & Unwin 1976

Doctor in the Zoo first published in Great Britain
by George Allen & Unwin 1978

Going Wild first published in Great Britain
by George Allen & Unwin 1980

This collection first published in one volume
by George Allen & Unwin 1984

This edition published in 1984 by
Book Club Associates
By arrangement with George Allen & Unwin (Publishers) Ltd.

The jacket photograph shows Rob Heyland as Don Turner in the
BBC tv production ONE BY ONE, produced by Bill Sellars and
directed by Christopher Baker and Richard Bramall.
Photograph copyright BBC Enterprises Ltd.

ISBN 0 04 925031 0

Printed in Great Britain by Hazell Watson and Viney Limited,
Member of the BPCC Group, Aylesbury, Bucks

Zoovet

The World of a Wildlife Vet

One

Slowly, painfully, Chota the elephant shuffled through the damp, grey Manchester morning towards the zoo dispensary. Her back was arched and her spine stood out like the keel of an upturned boat. Her ribs heaved distinctly under the tight dry skin where the weeks of chronic pain had stripped the flesh from her bones. Each leg was advanced reluctantly only a few inches at a time, accompanied by a low grunt and a small puff of steaming breath from the tip of her trunk. Moving for Chota was a continuing agony.

Twenty years before, as a six-month-old baby, she had been taken from her mother and put into a small stockade near Calcutta with a large number of other young elephants, most of them well under the age of weaning. Here she had waited several months for the arrival of the European animal dealers who would come to buy new stock. Tended by ragged elephantmen who fed the youngsters on watered cow's milk and balls of damp rice, some of the young elephants had died from attacks of acute enteritis or from strangulating hernias of their navels. The others, including Chota, had survived and had seemed to thrive well enough. But rice balls and watery milk are no adequate substitute for the rich sustenance that flows from the twin teats between the forelegs of a mother elephant. The balance of minerals, the content of calcium and phosphorus and vitamins, was wrong and, although nothing could be seen from the outside nor would be for many years, the delicately forming structures of the baby elephant's joints suffered serious damage. Nineteen years of careful, well-balanced feeding in the zoo at Manchester could not repair the

3

original faults in the growing tissues, and eventually the dread signs of osteoarthritis had appeared.

After all that time the rice balls of India had led to small holes appearing in the smooth, oiled bearing surfaces of Chota's fetlock joints. The holes had grown larger, the springy covering of tough cartilage had been eaten away, and the bare bones of the upper and lower parts of the joints had begun to grind remorselessly away on one another. First the elephant had shown stiffness, then lameness, and then a profound disinclination to move at all because of the pain. It was no use her shifting the weight from one leg to another: all the joints were as bad and each one was carrying around one ton of weight on its raw surfaces. Chota knew the worst pain of all was when she had to rise to her feet after reclining. Then the poor hind fetlocks had to take two tons of pressure each. It was too much. She became unwilling to lie down and because of the constant pain her standing sleep was fitful and increasingly brief. Chota became exhausted and began to lose weight.

The vet had done everything possible to relieve the pain and slow down the disease, but this was 1950 and the new range of anti-arthritic drugs, the cortico-steroids, the injectable analgesics and phenylbutazone were not readily available for veterinary use. Chota had flatly refused to eat powdered aspirin in her food for the dose was one third of a pound of the stuff and even in molasses or jam the taste could not be disguised. The elephant keeper had tried to drench the aspirin into Chota by standing on a chair and pouring the white suspension into her mouth from a watering can but to no avail. Her podgy pink tongue had curled up and blocked the narrow space at the back of her mouth and not a drop had got through. The thick skin around the inflamed joints had dispersed much of the heat from poultices which were applied and there had been no sign of any easing. So, after much discussion, the zoo director and the veterinary surgeon had decided on euthanasia.

Chota's last day of life was my introduction to zoo animal medicine as a student. Newly arrived at University, I was

4

spending my first half-term 'seeing practice' with the firm of vets who looked after Belle Vue Zoo, Manchester, and the first visit on my first day travelling round with the senior partner was to the zoo to put an end to Chota's misery. The main room of the dispensary had been cleared of everything except a small instrument table by the time we arrived. Matt Kelly, the head keeper, and his deputy were waiting for us, subdued and tense. Matt had known Chota for many years and was an expert in the handling and management of elephants. On summer days he had supervised the crowds of children who had taken rides round the grounds on Chota and her friend, Mary. Nobody said very much as we unloaded the equipment from the vet's car: syringes, needles, large bottles of barbiturate.

When everything was prepared Matt gave the order for Chota to be brought in. The elephant keeper led and coaxed her forward. The keeper had been at the zoo for over twenty years. He had taken care of the baby when she arrived shivering, hairy and wide-eyed on a cold December morning after a long sea passage from Bombay. He had slept with her in the elephant house during her first few weeks in her new home, made up her gruel, selected the best fruit for her and kept over-indulgent visitors and other members of the staff at bay. He had brushed her daily, oiled her skin once a week, cleared her of ticks and lice and seen her through bouts of colic and diarrhoea and constipation. He had manicured her toenails to stop cracking, hardened the soles of her feet with formaldehyde to avoid rot and fished irritating hay awns out of her ears. The young elephant knew that he always took the chill off her drinking water and that he kept boiled sweets, with the wrappings off, in his left-hand coat pocket. Soon after her arrival, she had burnt herself by pressing too hard against a radiator and the keeper had sat up all night with her, sponging the burn with a soothing lotion. She had learned to trust and respect him. By means of the boiled sweets he had taught her to perform some simple tricks. She could tell by the tone of his

5

voice when he was annoyed and he sometimes admonished her by slapping her or tapping her with the round end of a walking stick. The spiked elephant stick, its sharpened point and hook hidden in gaily coloured feathers, an instrument used viciously in some circus quarters, was something she knew nothing about.

Chota shambled to a stop in the middle of the dispensary. Her keeper toyed nervously with her ear and spoke quietly to her in the pidgin Indian that elephant keepers use. Looking up into her gentle grey eyes, I wondered how one could examine and treat such gigantic creatures. If I had known how many more sick and diseased elephants I was one day going to deal with, I should have found the prospect unnerving.

The vet had finished his preparations. The keeper rubbed the animal's right ear and murmured closely to her, while Matt Kelly took the left ear and flapped it forwards. With pressure from his thumb he raised one of the great blood vessels that run close to the skin along the back of the ear. With a quick jab the vet inserted a needle into the vein. Chota made a little squeal but did not move. Blood flowed from the needle and the vet attached a tube leading to a large bottle of barbiturate solution. Raising the bottle as high as he could above his head, he allowed the liquid to flow slowly in the vein. Over three pints of the anaesthetic would be required: the days when I would knock down a fully grown bull elephant with two c.c.'s of a drug simply popped under the skin were yet to come. Minutes passed and the liquid continued to flow. Chota stood quietly gazing down at us. She began to blink her eyelids and a tear ran slowly down her cheek from the corner of one eye. Then she sighed and her eyelids drooped progressively until they were almost closed.

'Don't anyone stand too close to her now,' said the vet. 'She'll go down any time.'

We backed away and the vet stood warily, the rubber tube between bottle and needle fully extended. Very gently, Chota began to sway backwards and forwards. Suddenly she buckled at the knees, pitched forwards, and with a tired groan slipped

6

over onto her side. The needle was still in the vein and the liquid flowed on. Another bottle, the fourth, was connected to the rubber tube. Now Chota was completely unconscious, free at last from the throbbing fire in her limbs. The elephant keeper, deathly pale, slipped quietly out of the door.

We stood and watched as the anaesthetised elephant continued to breathe steadily. The fifth and final pint of barbiturate was connected to the tube and I took over from the vet the strain of holding the bottle as high as possible to give maximum flow. I stood looking down at Chota's great head. More tears were trickling out of the one closed eyelid that I could see and making their way erratically across the dusty cheek. The only noise was the bubbling of air into the bottle as the syrupy liquid slowly disappeared down the tube. When all the drug had been used the needle was withdrawn from the ear and we stood round Chota's body, watching. Still the mighty chest rose and fell with a regular rhythm. The vet bent down and flicked at Chota's eyelid with his finger: the long luscious eyelashes twitched. There was still some reflex there. Crouching down he pushed his hand into her mouth and tugged at the slippery ball of her tongue. The pink ball resisted, quivering and contracting under his grasp. When he took his hand away it pulled itself back like a great pink toad retiring beneath a stone. Half an hour passed, an hour. Still Chota breathed gently on in oblivion.

The vet was talking quietly to Matt Kelly. 'This is the trouble with barbiturates. They're very slow in a big animal like this, especially with the strongest solution we've got containing only one grain in a c.c. At least it's absolutely painless. Wouldn't have fancied shooting her.' I remembered hearing that a veterinary student had recently been killed in Scotland by a bullet ricocheting from the skull of a zoo elephant that was being destroyed.

'I think we'd better try to hurry things up a bit.' The vet had other cases in the zoo to attend to. 'Let's try some carbon monoxide.'

A keeper came in through the door pushing a motor bike. Behind him two others struggled under the weight of a heavy folded tarpaulin. Chota breathed steadily on as the tarpaulin was unfolded and arranged over her body until she was completely covered by it. The black heap in the middle of the dispensary floor had none of the features of an elephant. It was more like a pile of sand sheeted as a protection against the rain. Now a tube was attached to the exhaust pipe of the motor bike which was propped up on its stand close to the invisible elephant's head. The free end of the tube was pushed under the tarpaulin and the engine of the bike was kicked into life. The metallic crackle of the machine rattled round the bare room. As a blue haze began to fill the air, we left the dispensary. Matt wedged the double doors open and arranged for a keeper to stay on guard outside so that no-one would enter while we went round other parts of the zoo.

An hour later we returned to the dispensary. Chota still breathed on, though with barely perceptible movements of her chest. Her reflexes were much weaker and her tongue was an unpleasant dark colour. It was arranged that the gassing should continue and that we should come back to the zoo in the afternoon to perform a post-mortem. The elephant keeper, utterly distraught, had been sent home.

When we had finished the day's rounds we drove back to Manchester and reached the zoo just after its closing time. The offices and animal houses were dark, the staff had left, but the dispensary was brightly lit. As we went in through the doors I stopped in astonishment. The room had been transformed into a slaughterhouse. The remains of Chota, massive pink, red and grey chunks, lay in piles on the floor or hung from hooks. The air was thick with steam and the strong, acrid smell of dead elephant. Knackermen had been called in to dismember the carcass and they were arranging the organs and limbs in ordered groups for inspection by the vet. Heart and lungs here, head there, intestines unravelled and displayed in neat zig-zags. It was an ogre's kitchen. Hosepipes swept blood and excrement continually towards the drains. The men chatted cheerfully and deftly honed their knives with steels that they carried in wooden holsters hanging from their belts. An elephant was something very unusual for them. They were used to the daily harvest of cattle carcasses, bloated through overeating new grass or withered from the tubercle bacillus. This was something out of the ordinary with lots of interest and scope for jests. It was fresh and they would be paid good overtime.

It was my first post-mortem on a large animal, and as awesome in its way as my first sight of the Jungfrau or the interior of King's College chapel. Of the indifference with which the knackermen, full of oaths and wisecracks, tossed the great floppy ears about, I did not know what to think. The vet poked and prodded around in the piles of steaming flesh. With a scalpel he sliced into organs of interest, split blood vessels and scraped away slime.

'See how the lungs are strapped to the ribs with all this white gristle?' he asked me. 'It looks like very severe pleurisy.'

At the time I had not even begun to study pathology and knew nothing of the ways in which diseased tissues change, but I saw how the lungs were indeed covered by thick fibrous bands which attached them firmly to the inside of the chest wall.

'That's where lots of people make mistakes when doing elephant p.m.'s,' he continued. 'They think they've found something and diagnose pleurisy, when in actual fact it's part of an elephant's normal architecture. Unique but normal.'

Years later I found that old records of elephant autopsies did indeed frequently report the presence of 'chronic pleurisy', and on one occasion this error led to a case of anthrax in an elephant which died in a British zoo being missed. The virulent disease spread horrifically when the carcass, apart from the 'pleurisy'-affected areas, was fed to other carnivorous inmates of the zoo.

The vet cut into the joint cavities of poor Chota's limbs.

Severing the powerful ligaments and tough capsules, he cracked open bearing surfaces and revealed their ravaged features. There it was: angry deep ulcers worming their way through the cartilage, blood and clumps of cells like rice grains mixed with the joint oil. The fetlocks of each leg showed the same degree of damage. Matt Kelly had seen many elephants develop the progressive signs of arthritis, and it had always ended this way. He shook his head grimly as he watched the vet probe into the joints with the scalpel, following the ulcers like worm holes deep into the tender bone.

'It was just as well,' he murmured. 'She must have suffered horribly.'

At the end of the post-mortem we drove silently home. I would write up the case for the report that a student had to present after seeing practice. Surely, I thought, there must be better ways of doings things for suffering elephants in the future. How many more of these magnificent creatures would I see brought down so sadly? What would it be like to handle a case of disease in a large zoo animal on one's own responsibility? But of one thing I was utterly certain: I was determined that when I had qualified I would concentrate on the health problems of exotic animals.

Two

My desire to work with animals stretches back further than my memory. As a small child I never considered for a moment becoming anything other than a veterinary surgeon. Animals rather than people interested me, and the mysteries of disease in animals were particularly fascinating. The little blobs of fluffy fungus that grew with unfailing regularity on each year's batch of tadpoles in the jam jars that I kept in my bedroom, the itchy bald patches that sometimes afflicted second-rate speci-mens of white mice begged from the testing room at the gasworks, the hedgehogs found torpid and dying for no apparent reason on the playing fields, the pathetic cast ewes inexplicably unable to struggle to their feet, so often seen during walks over the moors round my home – these were the things that fired my ambition. Animal disease seemed then, and still does, somehow 'purer' than human medicine. Matters are not complicated by the fantasies or mendacities of the patient, although I did learn in general practice that owners can exhibit hypochondria on behalf of their pets, that pet poodles or scrapyard alsatians frequently reflect the tempera-ments of their masters, that bears can develop troublesome haemorrhoids, and that goats accustomed to experiencing symptoms of the 'bends' during repeated experimental 'dives' in pressure tanks soon learn to fake the typical clinical picture in order to receive rewards of food, just like the human malingerer.

Even as a boy my fascination was more with wild animals than domestic ones. Toads, bats, hedgehogs, lizards – these creatures still interest and excite me more powerfully than

11

pedigree dogs or thoroughbred horses. I still consider it a privilege to touch and handle an undomesticated animal. Close contact with the warm hair, the skin, the chunky muscle of wild animals, even the touch of a walrus or a rhino or a lion, gives me a physical thrill. How I envied the older boys at Manchester Grammar School when I first entered the Biology Department and heard how they had been given octopus to dissect in the practical scholarship examinations for University. One bright lad had been given his oral test on a strange skull that was shaped just like a bird's but was as big as a pig's. We new boys, struggling with the innards of the frog and dogfish, marvelled at the strange object and puzzled over what it could be and what fiendish traps might lie ahead for us when it was our turn to sit the examinations. It was my first meeting with a creature that was to figure largely in my life twenty years later, for the skull was that of a bottle-nosed dolphin.

After studying veterinary medicine at Glasgow University for five years, I toyed with the idea of going to Kenya to research in sleeping sickness of animals and similar protozoal diseases. At the last minute I decided to stay in Glasgow and do a course in comparative pathology. It was a wise move, for much of the investigation of disease in exotic animals depends on the proper handling, examination and interpretation of specimens of diseased tissue, on microscopic work, and on the bacteriological testing of samples of blood, pus and other liquids. After one year of this I went back to my home town of Rochdale to join a general practice dealing with a wide range of large and small animals. Most importantly, it was the firm with which I had 'seen practice' and which had as a client the large zoo at Belle Vue in Manchester. As well as being able to work with exotic animals I would receive a sound grounding in all aspects of general veterinary work.

A young vet could not have practised anywhere better. We had everything: rugged moorland sheep farms, cattle farms, riding schools, prison farms, greyhound kennels, and all the dogs and cats and budgerigars that teem in the cobbled streets, shabby avenues and high-rise flats of the cotton towns of Greater Manchester. Stitching and cutting, injecting and lancing, struggling to replace the prolapsed womb of a cow on a Pennine farm at three o'clock on a blizzard-swept February morning, digging up rotten carcasses of pigs to obtain pancreas glands for swine fever tests, pinning stray tomcats' fractured limbs just after closing time on Saturday nights, delicately removing fatty tumours as big as plums from parrots with doting owners and beaks that could slice steel – it was the finest training.

The art of surgery is the same in a peke or a panda, a donkey or a zebra. The more I learnt about handling animal tissues, opening and closing limbs and organs, using drugs and handling violent, awkward and terrified animals and owners, the more I would be able to do for similar problems in wild animals. Surgery is after all just needlework on living, bleeding flesh. The more you learn to cut and stitch confidently and neatly, the more practice you have, the better you become. Likewise, it is by his work on the obstetric problems of cows, dogs and horses that a vet must acquire his skill in correcting the baby's position manually within the womb, and in performing Caesarean operations. There just are not enough cases of complicated birth occurring in giraffes or polar bears for him to refine his techniques by working on those species alone.

As well as the collection in the Manchester Zoo, I came across a growing number of privately owned exotica during my years in Rochdale. Knowing that I was interested in the problems of these offbeat pets, and often unable to find a vet in their locality who was willing to examine the creature or knew the first thing about treating it, the owners would bring their beloved snakes or monitor lizards or bush babies for miles. Some owners were more ambitious. There was a spinster lady in Bury who favoured slow lorises, and a family in Higher Blackley who had no televison set but sat instead at night around the built-in herpetarium in the lounge and watched their collection of diamond-backed rattlesnakes and twelve-foot boa constrictors dispose of white rats. Then there was the clumsy idiot who let a spitting cobra escape from its tank and make off angrily for the darkness of the machinery behind my surgery refrigerator.

Something Ray Legge, the director of the Manchester Zoo, once said about it being 'understandably the usual practice' for zoos to call in doctors of human medicine when their great apes were ill struck a nerve in me. Of course it was understandable in some ways. Great apes – gorillas, orang-utans and chimpanzees – do resemble man in many respects and have similar disease problems, but doctors never seemed to treat cases of disease in animals quite seriously enough. We had had lots of co-operation from medical workers at places such as Manchester University, but when it came down to it they were interested mainly in their narrow speciality, getting the specimens, the samples they could work on. The ophthalmologists were keen to get specimens for their collections of retinas or lenses, the anaesthetists were happy to try out new hypnotics, the virologists wanted blood serum and more blood serum for their comparative studies. All well and good, but none of them was interested or cared deeply enough for the animals as individuals, as patients with problems to be cured. To some vets and doctors, treating exotic animals may be a welcome change from routine work, something to tell the wife about tonight, but to me it was and is completely serious.

I decided that it was time for someone in the veterinary profession, not using animals just for research purposes, to show that the medicine of great apes was a serious veterinary field. I would study for the Fellowship of the Royal College of Veterinary Surgeons in Diseases of Zoo Primates. On my half-days off I worked at the great ape house in Belle Vue or pored over books in the Medical Library at the University. At weekends I travelled round the British zoos such as Twycross and Regent's Park which have extensive primate collections. I made the most of every photographer's monkey or circus chimp that came my way during surgery hours. Eventually,

14

after a long written examination in Glasgow and a practical and oral examination at Edinburgh Zoo, I obtained my FRCVS. To celebrate, my wife, Shelagh, and I bought a Japanese bronze of a mother tortoise and her brood and I went off to my first big international symposium on zoo animal diseases in Austria. I had made up my mind to leave general practice and see if I could earn a living purely from exotic animals.

If I was going to do it I must do it properly. No more dogs or cats or pigs or cattle. I would set up an office at my home just outside Rochdale and accept nothing but calls concerning exotic animal cases. It was a gamble. Like all vets I am bound by rules of professional conduct so it was not possible to advertise my presence, and snakes and monkeys and parrots are much, much thinner on the ground in Lancashire than are dogs and ponies. Nor is there much in the way of fees when treating sore eyes in a child's three-inch terrapin or replacing the prolapsed anus of a six-inch grass snake.

First of all I had to learn much more about zoo animals and in particular about the other side of the fence, the non-veterinary aspects. It is fine for a vet to dash into a zoo and advise on this or that problem and then disappear, but what about the many other facets of zoo keeping and maintenance? I needed to know more about the economics of purchasing, breeding and feeding stock, the education of staff, the political set-up within a zoo company, questions of transport and housing and public relations. I needed to know especially how all these things bear upon the welfare of the animal inmates. So I became curator-cum-veterinary officer for Flamingo Park Zoo in Yorkshire and the other zoos owned by the same company. Apart from handling an ever-increasing number of exotic animals, I found myself thrust into the strange new world of non-veterinary zoo work. On the one hand I was veterinary officer responsible for the health of killer whales, tigers and performing parrots and on the other hand, wearing my curator's cap, I had rapidly to master the day to day

15

problems of staff management, food buying, cleaning and sweeping and public relations. I was also in charge of first aid and the toilet block!

Most important of all, it was through Flamingo Park that I was first able to study some of the most exciting zoo exhibits. One of the first zoos to bring dolphins into Europe, Flamingo Park sent me all over the world to learn more about the habits and special requirements of sea mammals and other rare animals. I began to travel extensively – to Greenland to see musk ox and walrus (having equipped myself with the latest Arctic survival clothing from a shop behind Manchester Cathedral, I arrived in Narssarssuaq in Greenland one November day to find the Eskimos tiptoeing through the snow in winklepickers and suede jackets), to all the major zoos of Europe, to the marinelands of Canada and the United States and, most important of all, to the United States Navy base at Point Mugu in California. It was from the vets of the US Navy's undersea warfare research department that I learned the basic techniques of examining dolphins and whales and sealions, and it was at Point Mugu that I experienced the thrill of taking my first blood sample from a dolphin – a dolphin that the Americans were training to plant limpet mines on enemy submarines.

Gradually, my interest in primate diseases was overtaken by the medical problems of cetaceans, the whale and dolphin family. As with general zoo work, it was essential to learn every bit of the booming dolphinarium and marineland business. With the skilled dolphin fishermen of the Gulf of Mexico I went out hunting for the nimble and intelligent bottle-nosed dolphins. In boats that could touch 65 mph and turn on a sixpence at full speed, and with spotter planes overhead searching for suitable schools of dolphins, I learned how to handle the newly caught animals, how to stop a baby dolphin once aboard from committing suicide by literally holding its breath, and how to tell the difference between a shark and a dolphin tangled in the nets and out of sight deep beneath the ocean. The techniques of shipping these delicate animals across continents and over oceans had to be mastered, as had the problems of overheating, of cracking skin, of bed sores, of parasites, mercury poisoning and pneumonia. So much and so different from the surgery in Rochdale and the lectures and demonstrations at University.

Andrew Greenwood, my partner, joined me in 1972, having been a student seeing practice with me while still at Cambridge. Intensely interested in exotic animal diseases and particularly in marine mammals and in falconry, after qualifying he had researched for the Royal Navy in pathological problems associated with diving. Increasingly during that time he had stood in and done locums for me while I was globetrotting. We travel at the drop of a hat all over the world to wild animals in need of help. Our bags contain changes of clothes and toilet equipment, certain key drugs and medicines which might be unobtainable overseas, a few basic instruments and a selection of sample bottles, tubes and blood specimen needles. The office is full of airline timetables, lists of hotels in Timbuktu and Toronto, maps of the German autobahn system and receipts from credit card companies. Good communications are essential – each of our cars is fitted with a radio telephone linked to a private nationwide network and sometimes when out of our vehicles we carry personal radio pagers. Above all the work is satisfying and exciting and we are proud to be doing it. It is all simply summed up for me in the two words of our original telegraphic address: ZOOVET ROCHDALE.

17

Three

Right up to the beginning of the sixties exotic animal medicine was in a sorry state, lagging far behind the new developments in diagnosis and treatment that were revolutionising domestic animal practice. The key problem was the difficulty of getting to grips with dangerous and hyperexcitable animals and rendering them safely immobile or unconscious for surgery, close examination or the delivery of young. Two things were essential above all else: effective, well-tolerated anaesthetics for a vast range of species with differing anatomies and physiological functions and a good means of administering them. Of course we had the barbiturates which worked well if injected into a vein, but how to persuade a pain-wracked rhino to stand still while you raise his jugular with the pressure of one thumb and squeeze in an intravenous needle with the other? New gases such as halothane were superseding ether and chloroform, but what persuades a bolshy sealion to inhale deep of the soporific vapour in the face mask when, as an accomplished deep-sea diver, he is used to holding his breath for ten minutes at a time? Drugs which in capsule or tablet form bring speedy oblivion to a human with an empty stomach tended to get lost in the hundredweights of digesting food and churning liquid inside a hippo's or elephant's stomach. Or they produced bizarre responses, as when I tried one reliable human tranquilliser by mouth on bison. Instead of making the animals calm and sleepy, it whipped them into an amazing state of sexual frenzy, transforming even the most decrepit old males into bellowing satyrs that dashed about mounting every female they could lay their hooves on.

Quieting a dangerous or nervous patient was not the only problem in anaesthetising exotic animals. Nine years after Chota's tragic end in the dispensary at Belle Vue Zoo, I was called to attend her old friend, Mary, who had been suffering from increasingly severe attacks of toothache. Elephants have a peculiar tooth arrangement with a system of continual replacement throughout their lifetime of the grinding molars. The teeth develop from buds at one end of a groove in the jaw, move forwards into use as they grow, and then fall out to be replaced by others coming along the groove behind them. This process sometimes hits snags. A tooth jams instead of falling out cleanly and the animal shows all the signs of tenderness and irritation in the mouth that humans would associate with an impacted wisdom tooth. Mary's problem was one stage worse than this: she had developed an abscess at the base of a tooth root in the lower jaw. The abscess enlarged and caused severe pain within the unyielding confines of the bony jaw. Mary became irritable and grumpy. She ate little other than soft over-ripe bananas. She drooled saliva more than usual and would open her mouth for inspection only with great reluctance.

When I was first called to examine her I asked the keeper to persuade Mary to open her mouth. Eventually, after lots of soothing talk, I could put my hand inside. Feeling about in an elephants's mouth is not the least hazardous of veterinary procedures. There is not much room, and it is easy to find one's fingers being pushed by the strong muscular tongue between the grinding surfaces of the teeth, a most excruciating experience. When I tapped the infected molar with the back of my knuckle, Mary pulled back, beat me lustily about the head with her trunk and screeched like a pig. A root abscess: normally one would extract the tooth and all would be well. At least that was how things went in other animals, but in an elephant it was quite a different matter. The tooth in question was firmly embedded in the jaw and, like all elephant teeth, had multiple curved roots which sweep deep down into the jawbone and interweave intricately with the bony tissue around them.

Pulling, even with giant forceps, was out of the question and so was elevating, the flicking out of a tooth by means of a lever-like instrument. I decided to try medical treatment instead, to destroy the abscess by injections of antibiotics and to relieve pain by injectable analgesics.

The snag with this course is that the trouble tends to flare up again some weeks or months later. Sure enough the injections produced rapid disappearance of all symptoms and within a day Mary was her own amenable self again. Two or three weeks later the zoo rang up to say that Mary was beginning to show the same symptoms again but this time the pain was so bad that she was banging her head against the wall. I drove down at once to Manchester and sure enough a very forlorn Mary was having trouble again with an abscess under the same tooth. The drug injections quickly put matters right and the following day the elephant had stopped the head-banging.

Over the next six months Mary had four more attacks of toothache involving the same tooth root and each attack was more severe and lasted longer than the one before. The headbanging became the principal symptom. Mary would stand for hours close to the wall of the elephant house, deliberately rocking on her ankles and crashing the affected side of her head against the brickwork with a regular, dull, horrible thud that could be heard two hundred yards away. She had knocked the paint off a large area of the wall and loosened the pointing between the bricks. The last attack was the worst. Mary refused all food but stood night and day against the wall, seeking to counter the aching focus in her jaw by temporarily distracting the throbbing nerves as one ton of head jarred into the brickwork. It was terrible to listen to and unpleasant to watch: she was bruising and cutting the skin on the side of her face and she was becoming ill-tempered and unpredictable to handle. What was more, the wall was definitely no immovable object assailed by an irresistible force. It was beginning to bulge outwards, many bricks were loose, and the zoo director feared that the structure of the building was now at serious risk. We had to do something more positive. The tooth causing all the trouble would have to come out.

It was clear that the only way to remove the offending molar was to perform a major operation on the jaw. The gum along the side of the tooth root would have to be flapped up, the thick covering plate of bone would then be chipped away and the tooth with its roots intact could be teased, cajoled and manoeuvred sideways out of the jaw. This would mean a long period under general anaesthetic: a shot of local as performed by the dentist, or even a nerve block, the numbing of the nerve to the tooth by surrounding it with local anaesthetic at some point on its path back towards the brain, would not be feasible. The area of tissue involved was too large and complicated and the animal was in far too agitated a state. Anyway it would be impossible to do the necessary work unless she was lying down with her head still.

The problem was that at this time, the late fifties, there was no really suitable general anaesthetic available for the elephant. Major operations on the elephant had rarely been performed. Local anaesthetic was used for minor matters but otherwise it had been a question of tying the poor creature down with chains and hobbles and using the crudest of methods. Giving chloroform or ether was virtually impossible; barbiturates had to be given intravenously in ridiculously large doses, had a nasty knack of damaging the veins and tissues round about where they were injected and depressed breathing seriously, while chloral hydrate, the old stand-by of horse practitioners, was so disgustingly bitter when given in water that an animal would need to be stopped from drinking for three or four days before it would accept the doctored liquid. I decided to look into the possibility of using a new and promising drug which I had been using for two or three years on other exotic creatures.

Giving Mary a stiff dose of pain-killer and antibiotics to relieve the situation, I announced that we would operate on her the following day and that suitable preparations should be

21

made. Then I went home to consider further the matter of anaesthesia in this, my first case of major surgery on the elephant.

The new drug, phencyclidine, had been the first important breakthrough in modern zoo animal anaesthesia. It was highly concentrated, formed a stable solution which had no annoying tendency to go off, and could produce its effects when given by any route including by injection under the skin, by mouth or in a flying dart. Its taste was not too bitter, so that when used to spike the fruit drinks or milk of those discerning and wide-awake customers, the great apes, it usually went down un-noticed. There were disadvantages, too. The dose was calculated on body weight, and once it was administered there was no way of neutralising its effects, which wore off gradually over a number of hours. Some animals such as polar bears were easily overdosed with the stuff, and I noticed how little phencyclidine they needed to knock them flat out compared with brown or Himalayan black bears. Wolves, the first animals on which I had ever used the chemical and the tranquillising gun, frequently developed alarming convulsions when uncon-scious under phencyclidine. The drug had proved to be unsuitable for horses and I had discovered to my dismay that it had serious untoward effects in zebra: instead of anaesthetis-ing an animal which had broken out of its pen and could only be dosed by means of a flying dart containing phencyclidine, the drug produced an alarming degree of excitement and distress which persisted for hours. But in monkeys and apes, the big cats and some other carnivores it was superb. We never saw any signs of the long-lasting sexual stimulant effects or burning sensations of the fingertips and toes which humans treated with the drug had reported, although big cats under phencyclidine anaesthesia do regularly extend and contract their claws.

For Mary's operation phencyclidine was the best drug I had at the time. Checking that evening through my library I found one or two reports of its previous use on elephants, but details were scanty. What was suitable as an experimental dose in the African bush where elephants were plentiful was not necessarily right for Mary, a valuable and much loved animal in a city zoo in the industrial north of England. I had to get the dose right. Another problem is estimating the weight of an animal such as Mary. My usual practice is to walk the animal or take it in a lorry to a public weighbridge, but the toothache had made Mary crotchety and unco-operative and I could not risk taking her out of the elephant house. If an animal cannot actually be weighed I take the average of three estimates made by myself and two other people accustomed to working with animals, which is what I had to do in Mary's case. With the small amount of information which I had accumulated I was able to calculate a dose for the following morning. Certain nagging problems remained: how long would the anaesthetic last and what would be the cumulative effect of any further doses once she was down? What awkward physiological changes would several hours' unconsciousness produce in the ponderous creature? How was I to ensure that she went down with her bad tooth uppermost? It is not easy to turn a four and a half ton elephant when she is collapsed unconscious like a great pile of coal.

The next morning I was up early. My first call was to the local ironmongers. Dental instruments for human or ordinary veterinary use are far too puny for the granite-hard teeth of an elephant and the thick, resilient bone in which they are embedded. What I needed was a set of high-quality, all-metal masonry chisels. The ironmonger produced exactly what I wanted, a set of tough tungsten-edged tools specially intended for punching holes in hard stone. When I explained what they were for, the shopkeeper said he would sell them to me at trademan's price.

'After all,' he said, 'you're using them for your trade, I suppose. Never thought I'd find myself selling surgical instruments!'

At the zoo I found Mary suffering considerably from the diseased tooth. The pain-killing drug had worn off and she

23

was in a black mood. As I entered her quarters she glowered down at me and shuffled agitatedly around, whisking and flailing her trunk. It was going to be difficult keeping her still enough even for the normally simple under-skin injection of phencyclidine. I decided to leave all the instruments outside until she was anaesthetised. How she would go down and whether, during the few seconds that the anaesthetic first affected her brain cells, she would feel dizzy and become alarmed, I did not know. But I remembered having cases of horses run amok during the first stages of barbiturate dosage, with disastrous effects on the surrounding and carefully sterilised equipment, and I was not taking any chances.

Matt Kelly solved the problem of keeping Mary still for a second or two while I gave her the dope. Mary had one great weakness – an unbridled appetite for custard pies, the open, nutmeg-sprinkled, Lancashire variety. Even though the tooth-ache had quenched her desire for more conventional foods, Matt guessed that she would still be quite unable to resist these delicacies and he sent up to the zoo restaurant for some. Sure enough, when a keeper appeared with a box full of the newly baked golden pastries, the demeanour of the miserable animal immediately changed. Her black mood became, well, charcoal-grey, she stopped roaming irritably about and proceeded with obvious enjoyment to roll the custards one after another into her mouth, carefully avoiding the offending left side of her jaw. While she was thus engaged I slapped three times on her rump with the flat of my hand and then, when she was accustomed to the contact, slapped her again with equal force but this time with a three-inch needle held between my fingers. She did not feel a thing as I connected the syringe full of anaesthetic to the needle and pressed the plunger. It was in. I had begun the general anaesthesia of my first elephant.

Mary continued to consume the last of the custard pies, still standing calmly as we silently watched her. The elephant's soft munching was the only sound to be heard. Now I was going to be faced with the answers to the questions with which

24

my mind was racing. What was the effect of the drug going to be? Was my dose adequate or perhaps even too large? Had my needle squirted it deep into a layer of fat where its absorption would be greatly delayed and the effect minimised? A minute passed. Mary cleared the last flakes of pie pastry from her lips and looked at Matt for more. No signs of grogginess. At what time should I consider giving another dose, I wondered, clenching my fists. How would a second injection act in relation to the first? What would the cumulative effects be? Suppose the first effects on Mary were indeed to make her feel dizzy and alarmed. What if she ran amok while still sufficiently conscious to stay on her feet? For a moment I almost wished myself back in the everyday vet's world of anaesthetising dogs with fractured legs and ponies for castration.

Two minutes passed, then five. Suddenly, as if chilled by a gust of icy air, Mary began to tremble. Her knees buckled and she sagged down on legs of jelly. With a drowsy sigh and a boom as her leathery side hit the thick carpet of straw on the floor, she crashed over. She was flat out with the operation site and the bad tooth fortuitously uppermost. Matt and Mr Legge, the zoo director, positioned her legs and trunk as comfortably as they could and I checked her breathing and the working of the massive heart with my stethoscope. The operation was under way.

The peeling back of a large flap of gum over the root area took only a few minutes and the bleeding was very quickly controlled with forceps. Then began the slow business of chipping away the bone. It was fantastically hard. I struck the sharp chisels with a heavy metal mallet, working to a guideline painted on the bone in purple antiseptic dye. I was working naked from the waist up, as I prefer to do during prolonged large animal operations, particularly in warm animal houses. The effort was making my arms ache and the sweat streamed down my face and chest. Hordes of little red mites from the straw saw it as their duty to climb aboard and stroll about my body, making me itch annoyingly. Bit by bit, but far slower

25

than anticipated, I chipped my pathway along the jawbone. It was so hard that the jarring as the mallet and chisel rebounded from the dense tissue began to numb my hands. Mary remained perfectly unconscious. From time to time I stopped my chiselling to examine her pulse and breathing – so far all was well.

After two hours I had at last broken through the jawbone right along the line I had marked. Then, using a strong stainless steel bone 'pin' rather like a small crowbar, I levered the plate of bone off. There below it was the whole of the troublesome molar's complex root system. Like an iceberg, there was far more of the tooth below the surface than protruded above the gum, and the roots were still hideously intertwined with a lace-work of bony bridges. On and on I chipped, gradually freeing the broad, curved root branches. With my crowbar I tested my progress now and again by attempting to lever the great tooth outwards. Still it remained firmly implanted. After four hours I could at last see the inflamed area on the root that was the cause of all our problems. It was not much to look at: just a pinkish-yellow blob about the size of a pea. Another hour passed and then, as I tried levering outwards yet again, there was a loud cracking noise and the largest tooth I have ever extracted heeled over and fell out of the jaw with a thud.

From now on it was plain sailing: replace the plate of bone, fill the gaping hole in the gum (it was as big as a house brick) with a four-pound ball of sterilized dental wax, and stitch up. As I began the last lap, replacing the gum flap, I noticed that the colour of the gum was not as bright pink in colour as it had been. The colour was now distinctly tinged with lilac. I hurriedly completed the last knots in the catgut and sat back exhausted on my haunches. The colour change in the gum had diluted some of the elation in finishing the job. Now to attend to the animal's general condition and protect it from post-operative complications. Mary still lay dreaming on her side. Her reflexes were becoming a bit stronger. First I checked the heart and lungs again. Her heart was thumping strongly but faster now. As I listened to her lungs, with the stethoscope placed on the uppermost part of her chest, all sounded normal.

Then, faintly, from far away, I heard the deep rumble of a new sound, a dull bubbling noise far below the healthy swoosh of air in and out of the lung nearest to me. I went round to the other side of the animal and knelt down, pushing my stethoscope hard into the tight space between the underneath side of the chest and the floor. I could not get very far in but the bubbling noise was distinct, rather like a cauldron of jam gently boiling. I knew what was beginning to happen. The immense weight of the animal pressing down on the lung nearest to the floor was interfering severely with the flow of air and blood through the vital tissues, and fluid was collecting in the underneath lung. It is something to be watched for in all animals lying on their sides under anaesthetic and it can usually be prevented by turning the animal frequently from side to side.

'Let's get her over as quickly as possible,' I said. 'I don't like the sound of the right lung.'

Matt and his keepers hurried to attach ropes to Mary's feet and to push planks as levers beneath the bulging belly. Everyone pushed or pulled. Keepers braced themselves with their feet against walls and their backs wedged beneath Mary's legs.

Gradually we raised her until she was lying on her backbone with all four feet in the air. Then we let her down gently on the other side. I gave injections of heart and lung stimulants and drugs against shock and infection. The bubbling noise was now less noticeable in the right lung but, to my horror, I detected the first sounds of it in the other lung. Mary had been down under anaesthetic for too long. Although she was beginning to rouse, she had a long way to go and I had no way of speeding up the process. The lungs were becoming fatigued. We were in trouble. Mary was beginning to drown.

Her breathing became steadily more laboured and abnormal. She was more restless and moved her legs and trunk erratically. She even tried to raise her head a few inches from the ground. The unpleasant sounds in both lungs increased and, more ominously, some areas of the lung tissue became silent: they had filled completely with liquid and there was no longer any movement of air through them. An oxygen cylinder was set up and the gas was fed by tube under a sheet placed over Mary's head. For a moment I saw again, as if in a nightmare, Chota's tarpaulin-covered body as I had seen it on my first visit to this very zoo. Although now the tube which led under the sheet carried not deadly carbon monoxide but life-giving oxygen, it was beginning to look as though the end result would be the same, for Mary's breathing was steadily weakening. If only I could have reversed the effects of the injected anaesthetic! A full return to consciousness and the ability to stand and move would soon have restored good circulation in the chest.

Mary's colour was changing for the worse. The gums were now grey-blue with only a hint of pink. The respiration was weaker and seemed more laboured. The interval between breaths became agonisingly longer.

'Stand next to me and we'll try artificial respiration,' I said to Matt, who was standing glum and tight-lipped. 'Both together we'll get on and off the chest to see if our weight can compress the ribs.'

Simultaneously we both jumped onto the rounded grey chest of the recumbent giant. The rib cage sank a little. We immediately jumped off again. There was a slight expansion of the chest, but it was impossible to tell how much air had been sucked in. We repeated the process. On, off, on, off: at five-second intervals we jumped with all our weight onto Mary's chest. We tried jumping up and down on the chest itself. Our exertions produced some wheezing as small amounts of air were forced in and out but it was not enough. I stopped and listened again with the stethoscope. The lungs

28

were in dire trouble, with fluid building up, and the heart was beginning to fail fast. I gave more injections, more circulation stimulant and a chemical to give a kick in the pants to the centre in the brain that controls breathing. It was no good. Five minutes later Mary stopped breathing altogether and the heart-beats faded away fainter and fainter until I could hear them no longer. Mary, the most famous of Manchester Zoo's elephants and voted by schoolchildren their favourite animal in the park, was dead.

The autopsy on Mary confirmed that the long operation under phencyclidine had produced serious fluid build-up in the lungs with a resulting fatal lack of oxygen and heart failure. The zoo director and I had a meeting with the Board to report on Mary's loss. It was miserable explaining how my technique, up to date as it was, just had not been safe enough for a long operation on an elephant. I told the Board that if another elephant developed the same problem as Mary on the following day I would have to do the same again, using the same anaesthetic. It would be so until someone developed a new way of tackling anaesthesia in the elephant.

Four

Phencyclidine was the first breakthrough in the anaesthesia of most exotic species, and the invention of the dart-gun solved almost completely the problem of getting the anaesthetic to the patient while the vet stayed well out of range of its claws, teeth, hooves or horns. Gradually, pharmaceutical firms began to develop new experimental chemicals. They did the laboratory work; it was up to me to test the drugs in real live wild animals in the field. The bottles of prototype drugs with labels bearing only code numbers arrived regularly on my desk, accompanied by all available data concerning their effects on cats, rabbits, dogs or pigs. I could not risk losing or injuring any animals, but the new drugs were badly needed and very cautiously I began to try them out on my zoo patients. Bit by bit, feeling my way with the dosage levels, varying the strengths of the injected solutions, ringing the changes on 'cocktails' made up of mixtures of drugs, and working with emergency cases in a widening circle of species, I began to find means of sedating almost all zoo animals safely and quickly to any desired level. The process continued until eventually there were only two species which I found particularly difficult to anaesthetise without worry, the sealion and the giraffe.

In other ways, too, there have been dramatic advances in zoo medicine over the past twenty-five years. I doubt, for example, whether I shall ever again see an elephant destroyed because of osteo-arthritis. Powerful X-ray machines can easily pene-trate the tree-trunks that are an elephant's legs and pick out the first signs of disease. With ingenious fine fibre-optic tubes carrying lights and lenses I can actually look inside the joint cavities and inspect the diseased surfaces. Although I still use poultices of freshly-brewed infusions of comfrey leaves, the herbal 'knitbone' therapy so popular among the older Lancashire people of the Pennines where I was born, on the legs of elephants, now I can reinforce such time-honoured methods with injection into the joint of modern cortico-steroids, the feeding of tasteless new anti-arthritic drugs in the food, and courses of healing and pain-relieving ultrasonics.

Chota and Mary, the Manchester elephants, both died because the drugs, equipment and techniques available could not cope with the special problems posed by their massive bulk. Because of its sheer size the elephant is the species which illustrates most clearly and dramatically the developments in zoo medicine, and it was through his elephants that I first met Billy Smart junior, when he brought his troupe to Manchester for the Christmas circus. The animals were quartered in stables behind the King's Hall in Belle Vue. One of the elephants had begun to show signs of arthritis identical to those displayed by the ill-fated Chota. The pain had affected her normally placid temperament and on the evening before my visit she had attacked and beaten a circus elephant keeper so badly that he had had to be taken to hospital for emergency removal of a ruptured spleen. The keeper had made things much worse for himself by going into the elephant lines late at night after returning somewhat the worse for an evening's drinking. Elephants, like many other animals, are very sensitive to changes in the manner and mood of those who attend them. Reeking of beer, with perhaps a louder voice and rougher style of speech than normal, and probably moving on his feet less deliberately and calmly than usual, the keeper was not recognised as its friend by the aching elephant which had settled down in its usual place for the night. The man was on his own and could easily have been killed.

It is always risky as a stranger to move among elephants unaccompanied. Elephants look after one another. They have special friends and mates among their companions from whom, in sickness or health, they are usually inseparable. As I move between two elephants to prod or feel at something they will tend to press together, making me a filling inside a great living elephant sandwich. It can be difficult to sqeeze out, and I usually find myself dropping down and wriggling out between the forest of massive legs. If I inject one elephant its protective neighbour will often reach out and clout me sternly with its trunk or, worse, if it has tusks, lunge out with the ivory points at my body. One has to keep talking gently but firmly, to move steadily and decisively and to bear gifts: Polo mints are very well received.

The Smarts' elephant was indeed in the early stages of arthritis, but after a fortnight's treatment with the new arsenal of anti-arthritic drugs that were just becoming available, the animal was back to normal. When the troupe left Manchester at the end of the Christmas season she was walking normally and showed no sign of joint damage. Billy Smart seemed pleased with the result and said that he would contact me when next he had problems with the elephants, his special love. A few months later I was in Cyprus on holiday with my family when we saw a large photograph on a Cypriot magazine cover displayed in a bookshop in Nicosia. It showed Billy Smart standing in a car-wash with an elephant which was being shampooed in this modern and rather novel way. Prominently visible on the thigh of the animal was a lump the size of a cricket ball. An abscess or a tumour, I remarked to Shelagh, my wife. We had no way of knowing when the photograph had been taken. Perhaps it was something which had been dealt with long ago. I soon forgot about it.

When I returned to England I found myself busy with elephants again, this time a group of baby African elephants which had been brought to Flamingo Park in Yorkshire. They were a wild and riotous bunch, fourteen in number and all about four feet high. They had come straight from the African bush and although youngsters were fearless and aggressive. They had to be examined carefully: some had weak and bent ankle joints, others I suspected of being ruptured at the navels. But as soon as I approached closely to inspect them, they flared their ear flaps and charged at me, squealing angrily. One young male took such a dislike to my attentions that he chased me across the elephant house and beat me against the concrete wall with a blow of his broad bony forehead. I literally saw stars. It was obviously going to be necessary to use anaesthetic on these young tearaways if I was to have any chance of giving them a thorough check-up.

First supplies of a new anaesthetic drug called M99 were just coming in. Good reports about it were being published by vets working with wildlife in Africa and I had already found it first-class for knocking out deer and wildebeest, but this would be my first attempt to anaesthetise an elephant since the sad affair of Mary. M99 is a drug of the morphine family but thousands of times stronger. It is effective in minute doses, particularly in elephants, and most important of all it can be instantly neutralised by an antidote drug. So efficient is the antidote that animals return from anaesthesia to complete normality within seconds and without any grogginess or hangover. For the young African elephants at Flamingo Park I decided to use M99 even though at that time it was costing approximately £480,000 per pound. Very little, just a few milligrammes, would be required for each animal, I was assured.

Each young elephant was injected by a flying dart fired from a special gas-powered rifle. One to two minutes after the dart had struck an elephant's plump buttocks, the animal would sink quietly without any sign of alarm or dizziness to the ground. The medical inspection over, I slipped a small dose of antidote into the ear vein and within two minutes the animal was on its feet, eating food and glaring suspiciously at me once more. It looked as if M99 was going to be the answer to the terrible problem of doping elephants.

Two months later the telephone rang. It was Billy Smart junior. Gilda, one of his elephant troupe, was having trouble with a strange lump on her hind leg. Apparently the lump, the size of a large apple, had been there for about a year, but over the past three weeks it had begun to grow very rapidly and was now as big as a melon. I drove down to Leicester where Smart's Circus was playing and went into the elephant lines. Sure enough, Gilda was the elephant I had seen in the photograph in Cyprus. The swelling in her leg was hard but apparently painless. Its base was deep below the skin in the great thigh muscles.

'What do you think it is?' asked Billy. He had had years of experience with elephants and with the abscesses, cysts and skin diseases which are commonly seen in the species, but he had never seen a lump behaving like this one.

'It doesn't look like an abscess or cyst to me,' I replied, exploring the consistency and shape of the thing with my fingers. 'I think it's a tumour.'

Billy had trained the elephants himself and thanks to his remarkable rapport with them I was able to push a special biopsy needle deep into the lump in order to sample the tissue without the animal reacting or making a fuss. Billy just stood at Gilda's head talking firmly and kindly to her and stroking her trunk while she gazed devotedly down at him. The speck of flesh on the end of the biopsy needle was sent to the laboratory for microscopic examination. A few days later the result came back that it was a tumour, with areas of cancerous change. A major operation to remove it was imperative.

This time the anaesthetic would be M99. My experiences with it in the African elephants and other animals had impressed me, but I travelled down to Leicester again with a slight feeling of apprehension. Everything had been beautifully arranged in the elephant tent for the operation. Deep straw had been piled on the ground and covered with new canvas sheeting. The other elephants had been moved far away to the other end of the tent, where they stood with necks bent and eyes popping inquisitively as they watched with an air of disapproval what we were preparing to do to their companion. Gilda had not been given any solid food for twelve hours prior to the operation and was grumbling a bit about this as she was led onto the canvas sheets. She tried to grab bits of straw from the bedding as an illicit snack and became irritable when Billy Smart stopped her.

'I think I'll bring Burma over to stand by her,' said Billy. 'It will give her more confidence.'

Burma is the gorgeous old matriarch of Smart's Circus elephants. The first elephant that the famous Billy Smart himself bought, very big, looking always uniquely old and wise, she is the most intelligent, gentle and patient elephant I have ever met. She is just the sort of companion you want next to you in time of trouble, reliable, a rock. The Smart family worship her and see that at Christmas, weddings and other festivals, or if she looks a little peeky, she receives a bottle or two of her favourite tipple, neat Bisquit de Bouche cognac. The presence of Burma near a nervous, distraught or ailing elephant always seems to bring calm and confidence to the sufferer. I have often been glad of her help when treating sick or injured animals in the Smarts' winter quarters at Winkfield.

Burma came and stood impassively and quietly next to Gilda, who seemed immediately reassured. It was not necessary even to drop the anaesthetised elephant onto the floor. Billy simply gave Gilda the command to lie down (this is just one of the advantages of working with circus as opposed to zoo elephants) and the elephant obediently lay down with the tumorous leg uppermost. I could almost hear Burma murmur in approval. It was easy to inject just two c.c.'s of the M99 solution painlessly into Gilda's ear vein, and within half a minute and without any problems she passed from conscious rest into a deep and satisfactory sleep. It took me about an hour and a half to cut out the great growth. Although elephant skin is tough, it is nothing like as thick and awkward to work with as, say, rhinoceros skin, and ordinary scalpels cut through it with the greatest of ease. The time-consuming part was the tying-off of all the blood vessels that supplied the hidden depths of the tumour.

When at last the mass had been totally dissected out (I had been at great pains not to leave behind even one particle that might multiply into another tumour) there was left a gaping hole in the thigh which had to be closed. The skin was virtually impossible to slide across the hole, the gap was so large and I had been forced to remove such a great expanse of skin. For a moment I was frightened. The hole had to be closed, but how? Using double lengths of the thickest stitch material I had, a sort of plaited nylon fishing line with a breaking strain of 250 lb, I inserted 'relaxation sutures', which go through the skin far behind the wound edges and take the main strain. I put dozens of them in place and gradually tightened them. Slowly the wound began to close. As the first relaxation sutures went slack I tightened them and reinforced with more. At last it was finished. The hole was sealed, although the operation site looked like a spider's web of interweaving green nylon. I prayed it would be strong enough to withstand the pressures when Gilda moved about. After tidying up the wound I filled my syringe with the anaesthetic antidote, injected it into the ear vein and looked at my watch. Thirty seconds later Gilda sighed deeply, switched her trunk and rolled her eyes. Then she heaved herself over onto her brisket and with a little grunt rose to her feet. No wobbling, no dizziness. Gilda looked round, touched trunks briefly with Burma and then grabbed a tuft of straw protruding from beneath the canvas. She stuffed it hungrily into her mouth. The stitches held.

There was no further trouble with Gilda and her growth. The last sign of it was the faint white scar which could just be detected the following Christmas when I sat with Shelagh and watched Billy Smart's Circus on television. The audience in the big top and the millions of television viewers undoubtedly enjoyed the scintillating and colourful display as the elephants carried clowns and glamorous girls about the ring. But the glimpse of that thin and fading line on the prancing grey hams of an elephant made me the proudest person on earth that Boxing Day afternoon.

Five

The only bit of advice on treating exotic animals that students were given when I was at University was that wallabies go dotty over Fox's glacier mints! My Professor of Surgery, Sir William Weipers, told us how he had discovered this fact when called in to a case of frostbite on the tails of wallabies kept on the lawns of some Scottish country house. Wallabies, a highly-strung species liable to drop dead from shock if harassed or handled roughly, are like most other zoo animals in that they must be approached gently, patiently and bearing gifts of sweetmeats. It is amazing what can be done at the back end of a correctly approached and undoped animal as long as it is being fed something it fancies at the front end. At Belle Vue Zoo a special brown bread used to be baked daily for the animals. Almost all of them, whether herbivore, carnivore or something in between, adored it, and while a keeper supplied one chunk of loaf after another to the drooling camel or bison or brown bear, I would be taking temperatures or injecting at the rear.

Before the days of reliable and compact sedatives for zoo animals Matt Kelly, head keeper at Manchester, had showed me some of the knack of coming to grips with his animals. From him I learned how to catch a lion's or a leopard's tail as it sauntered by the bars of the cage and then to drop down so that the tail was bent over the edge of the cage floor. With the indignant lion roaring and pulling horizontally, and me using my weight vertically on the bit I was holding, the edge of the floor took most of the pressure and I could hold a fully grown big cat with his bottom up against the bars in a perfect position for injecting. From Matt I learned how to hypnotise a crocodile by turning it onto its back and stroking its belly, and how to baffle a bloody-minded parrot, bent on a mouthful of human finger, by a neat piece of kung-fu that leaves the astonished bird flat on its back and safely immobilised in less time than it takes to tell.

The learned journals are full of papers on the pathology and physiology of aardvarks and axolotls but the vital scraps of information that make life easy for the zoo vet, and save wear and tear on fingers and horn-holes in various parts of the anatomy, have to be gathered from experienced men like Matt Kelly. From Matt I learned how to root out an absconding porcupine that has installed itself under a fairground carousel and is gleefully gnawing away at the works, and how to negotiate with a monkey that has stolen a packet of razor blades and, like some Indian fakir, is packing the lethal leaves of steel into its cheek pouches. A gazelle or antelope, released suddenly from its carrying crate, may dash headlong into the walls or netting surrounding its paddock and injure its head and limbs terribly, even breaking its neck and dying instantly: I had seen it happen with zebra. Matt showed me how to use double-doored crates so that animals could be made to emerge rear ends first. This stops the frantic dash and allows them to get their bearings as they turn. I may never know whether some of the things Matt told me will work in practice. What to do when an enraged and highly dangerous male chimpanzee charges at you? Matt swore that he had once been in this position and that quick as a flash he had dropped his trousers and stuck his bottom in the air to impersonate a chimp in the submission posture. It worked. The chimpanzee reacted predictably to this signal which says 'OK, I give in. You're the greatest' and checked his attack. I hope that if I am ever in a similar predicament my zipper does not stick!

Some of the things I saw at zoos and circuses were not for learning, like the chimpanzees' tea party whose animals were not just as good as gold, they were almost automata. The audience marvelled at the obedience of the little apes and smiled as the trainer fondled their hairy heads. It was all in the fondling. The man showed me his thumbnail which had been allowed to grow long and then filed into a vicious point. It was strong and horny and he used it with cruel skill to gouge and twist the sensitive flaps of the chimpanzee's ears. It was really a display of brutal sleight of hand carried on in full view of the public. I was to find that this method of controlling chimps by their delicate ears was commonplace in the world of chimpanzee training: even mature specimens were subdued by the agony of a quickly applied hold.

Although many circus animals are trained without cruelty, there are still terrible black spots. You will find them in the smaller, tatty circuses and menageries if you can penetrate the closed, suspicious, obstructive world behind the scenes. It is a world skilled in repelling outsiders and deceiving RSPCA inspectors and, most important, able to move on if trouble is brewing. At first hand I have seen bears encouraged to move from travelling box to circus ring by lighted newspapers thrust underneath them, and I have heard the regular, sickening thuds as a chained African elephant was beaten systematically with bamboo rods by two keepers to break it by literally torturing it until it collapsed. The most repellent feature of the process was the calm clinical way in which the keepers administered the beating. It was a job, just like grooming, which called for a repetitive movement for long periods of time. No anger, no emotion, just a boring job of beating. Of course when the police arrived the men were indeed grooming the elephant. Bamboo rods applied with all a man's might across the rib-cage of an elephant leave no marks.

One hard-bitten old lion trainer showed me his method for giving pills to lions. 'Watch this, young fella,' he said, running the big male lion into the barred tunnel between ring and travelling cage. 'Quicker and better than all your dart-guns and powders on the meat.'

When the lion was halfway down the tunnel the trainer slipped a board between the bars in front of it and a similar

40

one behind to make a simple treatment cage. He picked up a crowbar and a bottle of aspirins, shoved the crowbar through the bars and cracked it hard down on the animal's head. The lion was at his mercy, unable to back away or turn around. It roared thunderously, opening its jaws and raising its head. The lion trainer dropped in a couple of aspirins. Down they went and the lion closed its mouth. The trainer hit the lion's skull again. The sound was sharp and revolting, the clang of metal on bone. The lion roared again in frantic impotence. Two more aspirins went in.

'See? How's that, eh?' said the trainer proudly. 'No problem, eh?'

'Bloody horrible,' I replied. He would never understand, never.

Sadly there will always be some showman who is prepared to use inhumane methods to create a new crowd puller. At one marineland in the United States the high spot of the show was a water-skiing elephant. I was there on the day that the elephant was persuaded by much use of the feathered spike to mount a pair of specially constructed giant skis. The rolling anxious eyes and the shrill trumpeting showed clearly that the elephant was an unwilling amphibian – so unwilling that once in position it was chained to the skis and the chains were secured, not by padlocks as is usual when tethering elephants, but by heavy nuts and bolts. To the applause of the crowd and the smooth spiel of the loudspeakers the motor boat towing the skiing elephant pulled away onto the smooth water of the lake. The animal waved its trunk and seemed to hang back on its chains. The skis tipped up at the front as the boat accelerated.

'Look at Herbie go, folks!' enthused the loudspeakers. 'My, he's sure enjoying himself?'

The skis were supported beneath by large buoyancy chambers so Herbie did not have to do much in the way of balancing. The boat accelerated into a turn. Herbie's ears flapped in the wind and he waved his trunk more furiously. It must have been too tight a turn. With a squeal of despair, a mighty crash and an

41

eruption of white water, Herbie lurched over and capsized into the lake. Only the upturned bottoms of the ski floats were to be seen. Somewhere under the surface, still chained to the skis, was Herbie. I struggled through the horrified crowds with the vet attached to the marineland, but by the time we had got round to the point on the lakeside closest to the scene of the accident it was too late. Boats had gone out and found Herbie drowned. Without the chains he would have stood a good chance.

There are other ways of training animals: the results come from the rapport between man and animal and from understanding of animal behaviour rather than from fear and pain. My friends who train dolphins and whales and sealions, Bobby Roberts with his camels, Billy Smart with his elephants, Katja Schumann and her horses, Eddie Wiesinger and his big cats, and hundreds of other trainers of parrots, dogs and kangaroos, get superb results by kindness and communication. Of course there are cruel and abominable methods of training animals just as there are cruel and abominable animal trainers. They are the more despicable because they know that there are better and humane methods that can be and are used. In fact I have found the exponents of fear and torture in animal control to be markedly less successful than those who do it all through a combination of patience, observation, knowledge of animal behaviour and psychology, real affection coupled with respect for the creature, precise oral and visual commands, a consistent attitude, quick and sensitive response to an animal's movements and moods and, most important of all, long training themselves at the hands of good and experienced teachers.

Working in a good circus or marineland where humane methods are practised is immensely enjoyable. In the disreputable few I hope always to be an influence for better standards. Even in a scruffy hell-hole of a travelling menagerie, someone must look after the health of the animals. Moving on from town to town, they receive at best scant attention from a succession of different vets, almost all inexperienced in exotic animal medicine, who rarely have the opportunity to follow through the progress of a case and may well be left with an unpaid bill and a truculent attitude to the next travelling show that passes through. But the bears and monkeys and pumas in these caravans need attention. To spurn them would be to condemn them to even worse miseries, so I try to stimulate improvement of such set-ups from within rather than criticise impotently from without.

From the crucial central point of view, that of the animal, most performing animal acts are in no way detrimental. Some species such as dolphins, sealions, dogs and horses positively revel in their routines, play up to audience applause, benefit from the exercise and go distinctly mopy and morose if laid off for a long time. Of course the elephant awkwardly waltzing on its stand or the chimpanzee that lifts the skirt of its companion and saucily pulls down its knickers are undignified, embarassing and, in some senses, exploited. Elephants are seen at their best charging across the savannahs of Africa, and to watch chimpanzees organizing their lives in the forests is gloriously fascinating. But the embarrassment and shame that we feel is one of guilt in knowing what we are like, what we enjoy, what we have asked them to do. We feel uncomfortable about being part of a human audience that laughs at such outrageous anthropomorphism. The animals are not ashamed and do not have our hang-ups. From their point of view, and that is what matters to me, life is not bad. In a well-run circus nobody hurts them, the bananas are plentiful and at hand, the quarters are snug and warm and they are groomed and cleaned and stroked and fussed over. Many of these animals have been born into the zoo or circus and hand-reared into the business. They are as artificial, as domesticated, as toy poodles or budgerigars or Siamese cats and are far removed from the truly wild members of their species. They have no conception of what life on the outside might be like, they thrive and grow fat and breed and enjoy more freedom in most cases

43

than many lap dogs, pub parrots or flat-bound pussy cats.

Some tricks can only be achieved through cruel methods, to be sure, but they are only a tiny minority and do not figure in the repertoire of a reputable trainer. Provided an animal trusts its trainer and suffers no pain or discomfort, the most complicated 'artificial' behaviour can be achieved. Food, and the greed for it, is the commonest method of persuasion. It is interesting that there seem to be few, if any, occupational diseases of circus animals. I have never heard of a case of waltzing elephant's foot-rot, punch-drunk boxing kangaroos or liberty horse lumbago. Contrast that with the occupational diseases of broiler calves, racing greyhounds, battery hens, sweat-box pigs and hunting horses.

Typically skilled and humane animal trainers are the Naumann family from Germany. They travel all over the world with their big cats and I have spent many hours watching their methods with lions, tigers and pumas. They raise their cats from cubs and work patiently long hours each day, teaching the animals to perform by reward – reward in the form of finger-sized pieces of tender meat, in stroking, patting and praise from familiar voices. No coercion, no pain, no fear. Firmness of course, but that is necessary to train a police horse in its duties or even your own pet dog to fetch the newspaper from the letter box. Do it so, do it right, and see, here is a nice juicy morsel.

By these methods the Naumanns created a unique high-diving tiger act, in which a fully grown Bengal tiger dived into a circular swimming pool from a platform twenty feet above the water. Several years ago the Naumanns arrived with all their gear and their cats for a summer season in the grounds at Belle Vue, Manchester. Work went ahead to assemble the pool, ladder and platform. Everything was set up, but not exactly to order. Somehow the platform was not positioned directly over the centre of the pool as it should have been. This mistake was not apparent to anyone looking from below. Nor, it seems, did the tiger realise anything was wrong when it climbed up the

44

ladder for its first Manchester performance and, after suitable fanfares and drumrolls, launched itself into the air. The flying tiger plunged down into the water but in doing so rapped its back sharply against the metal edge of the pool. In great pain and partially paralysed, the poor animal struggled out of the water and dragged itself to its trainer. The Naumanns were distraught at the pain caused to one of their beloved cats by the carelessness of a member of their team. Within minutes I arrived at the scene to examine the patient.

The collision had produced bleeding and severe tissue damage in the canal carrying the spinal cord down the lower back. The pressure of the blood and swollen soft tissues was pinching the nerve within its bony passageway and as every minute passed the tiger was suffering more pain in the spine and losing the use of its hind legs. The front end of the animal was distinctly aggrieved and in a foul temper. Whatever might be the case with the two hind feet, the front pair and the jaws were in fine fettle. We would have to handle the tiger in its small travelling cage. This was where the kindness and patience of Herr Naumann in training his animals personally since they were tiny cubs paid off.

'Don't worry,' he said to me, opening the little door into the cage. 'You will be able to do whatever you need. I will look after that.'

He squeezed through the opening into the cage and beckoned me to follow. I went in and Herr Naumann's wife closed the door and locked it behind us. There was not much room for the two of us and the tiger. It lay growling and groaning in pain, its tail lying limply, too numb to be switched irritably. Naumann went to the front of the animal and knelt down. Affectionately he took the tiger's head in his hands and brought it onto his lap. He stroked it and talked soothingly in German. The tiger stopped growling and lay impassively.

'Go ahead,' said the trainer, 'He'll be OK now.'

Inwardly I marvelled at his confidence. If there were any fractures waiting for my probing fingers, disturbance of the

45

tortured tissues might well make the animal feel anything but OK. Very gingerly I placed my hands on the muscular back of the big cat, pressing gradually deeper into the tissues, feeling for the spine, tracing the outlines of the vertebrae and running down the sides of the pelvis. The tiger tensed whenever I came across damaged areas and sometimes growled. Naumann tightened his embrace on its head.

The next stage was more delicate. I wanted to feel the inside contours of the pelvis as far as possible, which meant putting two fingers deep inside the anus. I slipped on a finger stall, lubricated my hand and slowly introduced my fingers into the rectum – the first and I suppose the only time that I will ever do that to a conscious adult tiger. The tiger growled and wriggled the front end a bit. He was not amused by this approach, but I was able to satisfy myself that there were no palpable pelvic fractures. It looked as if the lower spine had been badly bruised and jarred. With any luck the soft tissue swelling could be dispelled and the spinal cord would in time return to its normal function. I prepared injections of pain-killers, inflammation-shrinkers and enzymes to speed the removal of damaged cells and blood clots. Naumann continued to mur-mur away reassuringly while I selected new sharp disposable needles. If there was going to be a sudden nasty reaction it would surely be now as I pricked deep into the muscles. I glanced at Naumann's face, only an inch away from the cat's curved fang teeth. One short-distance blow from the left forefoot would open up his chest like a fork impaling boiled ham. Gritting my teeth, I indicated to Naumann that I was about to strike.

'Go ahead,' he said again. 'He understands we're not here to tease him.'

I stabbed the needle as quickly as I could through the tough skin and deep into the muscle. To my relief the tiger was apparently unaware of the injection and did not stir. Eventu-ally all the drugs were safely inside it. We left the cage and discussed the setting up of an infra-red lamp above the patient's back and the preparation of my favourite invalid food for sick big cats, a sort of steak tartare made of minced steak, raw egg, dried milk powder and sterilised bone flour.

Next day the tiger was much easier but still largely paralysed at the rear, which was causing secondary constipation. It would be necessary to give an enema. I made up a small pail of warm water and soap flakes and primed an ordinary human enema pump. Once again Naumann cradled the head of the tiger in his arms while I filled it up with the soapy solution. Soon I was gratified to be covered in an explosive eruption of froth and tiger excrement, to the apparent relief of the tiger.

Each day the tiger made more and more progress towards recovery. Little by little the power of its hind legs returned although the sluggish bowel action remained for almost two weeks. As the animal became more mobile we had more difficulty in giving the enema. It would rise to its feet with me and my pump still attached to its rectum and, leaving Naumann behind, would spin round in the small cage in an effort to reach the person doing the embarrassing things to its stern. Until Naumann could catch up with the head again and return it firmly to his lap, I had to keep myself, pumping merrily away with one hand and dragging my slopping pail with the other, as close to the animal's bottom as possible. As long as I spun round in the constricted space and did not let the anus get away from me, the cat could not quite reach me with tooth or claw. If the cage had been any larger, constipation might well have triumphed. At last the enemas were over, and a heap of laxative breakfast cereal sliced into the patient's meat for a few days was all that was needed. The tiger made a complete recovery and when I was satisfied that he was a hundred per cent up to scratch I let him go back to the diving board.

Tigers frequently need a little chiropody. Like all cats they try to keep their claws in trim by scratching the earth and, best of all, by dislodging the overgrown outer shell of their nails by raking tree bark. Unfortunately it does not always work and a claw will continue to grow out and round until it digs into the

47

pad of the foot. Then things become unpleasant. The point of the nail produces a painful sore that rapidly becomes infected, and until the nail is cut and the offending portion pulled out of the pad there is no possibility of its healing. It is my job to stop things reaching this stage by regularly looking over the big cats in my care and doing pedicures where necessary. Rather than giving a general anaesthetic for a minor job like this, I try to do it with the animal conscious, by using specially designed restraint cages. At many zoos and safari parks special trapping cages for tigers, lions, leopards and cheetahs have been built with a variety of ingenious devices to immobilise the animals speedily, humanely and conveniently for the veterinary surgeon. Some of these cages have walls that travel in towards one another, controlled by cables and winches from outside. Others have silent descending ceilings like the evil four-posters of Edgar Allan Poe.

One of the most complex systems was built at Manchester by Mr Legge, the former zoo director. A passageway through which the animals pass unconcernedly each day to and from their paddocks conceals a false floor and a roof which can be brought down after the creature has been captured by doors closed in front of and behind it. The roof is a strong mesh of soft rope, stretched within a metal frame, which presses down firmly over the contours of the animal and permits not a flicker of movement. The false floor is removed, revealing a grille of bars on which the underside of the cat is forced to rest. Underneath all this is an inspection pit where I crouch with, of course, an inspection lamp and look up at the belly and feet of my patient. By reaching up I can bring one foot at a time down through the bars, shear off excessive nail and dress any wounds. If necessary I can take a blood sample, give an injection or lance an abscess.

Naturally I found snags in the procedure when I went down to service my first feline. Like the common or garden moggy which finds itself suddenly grabbed and incarcerated out of the blue, the big cat vents its feelings of amazement and apprehension by doing the only things possible in the circumstances, opening its bladder. But between the moggy and the big cat there is one difference in this respect, a difference of enormous degree. Whereas the bladder of your average ginger tom can accommodate a smallish, if noisome, quantity of liquid, the same organ in an adult tiger or lion often holds a pint or two, and somehow the cunning beast contrives always to have it brimming when the chiropodist calls. I was not aware of this prescient control of the feline waterworks when I began working in the newly built cat house in Manchester. I was yet to meet the lion who would wander amiably up to the netting separating him from a small crowd of admiring visitors, turn with his buttocks towards them and expertly spray the front row of the audience with urine. As the dismayed and dampened victims fell about in confusion to the laughter and ridicule of those standing behind, the lion waited patiently in the same position while the dry and unsuspecting guffawers moved forwards into the now vacant stalls. Little did they know that he had, as it were, one barrel still loaded, that all his powder was not spent. When the crowd, now swelled by others who had come running to see what all the fuss was about, was correctly positioned, the cat would look winningly over his shoulder at the clicking cameras and then empty the second half of his bladderful into the throng.

The first time I went down into the cat house inspection pit was for a visit by a photographer from *The Observer* who wanted pictures of a zoo vet for the colour supplement. I would do the chiropody in style, I decided, clad in a surgeon's gown of neat green cotton. The cat was trapped and I slipped down into the narrow sump. Taking up a suitable pose for the photographer who peered down over the edge, I trimmed off a nail or two and held up the bits for the camera. Then it happened. The tiger above opened his water valve to the limit and a cascade of warm yellow liquid poured down onto me and soaked through my gown and underclothes. There was no escaping it. I tried backing off towards the head end. No use. Turning my back

49

simply hastened the soaking of my trousers. Cats have a way of doing these things, as if they have an adjustable nozzle like a rose-spray, and the whole of the air space of the pit was filled with a sort of aerosol effect. I lunged for the metal steps in the wall of the pit and clambered out. Every since then I have made a point of carrying out cat chiropody in oilskins and sou'wester, even though folk in Lancashire used to say that external application of urine was good for the complexion. What would they know about the tiger variety?

Six

Since the principles of good management of performing animals are frequently ignored in the richer, so-called advanced countries, perhaps one should not be surprised that in countries where poverty forces a lower value on human life itself the treatment of exotic animals in captivity would send an appalled shudder through a vet or any animal lover. To dolphins the Far East recently has been like Devil's Island to French convicts: once arrived there they rarely return alive. There has been a lucrative business, largely organised by German theatrical agents, sending pairs of European dolphins out on tours of Thailand, the Philippines, Indonesia, Singapore and Taiwan. Asians adore circuses, travelling shows and novelty exhibitions, particularly where animals are involved. The 'intelligent giant fish', which I believe a majority of the audiences confuse with the feared shark, is immensely popular. The Flipper series of TV shows has been broadcast widely in the Far East and has heightened the interest: every travelling dolphin show naturally has as one of its performers 'the original Flipper direct from Florida, USA'.

The German agents procure the animals in Europe and America and hire them out to Chinese sponsors, who in turn sub-let the shows and sell pieces of the action to syndicates of more Chinese. This is the root of the problem and the key to the numerous disasters that have befallen these hapless creatures. Interested only in the cash return on their investments, totally ignorant of what dolphins are and what they require for good health and condition, often speaking no European language, and ruthless in their commercial dealings, the syndicates have time and again murdered dolphins by incompetence, obduracy and wilful neglect.

Because of the complex network of sub-contracting, the person actually responsible for providing good pool and water conditions and first-class food for the animals is frequently difficult to pin down. Anyway the poor guy with the problem when the animals fall sick or run out of water or find themselves swimming in three feet of thick sewage is the European dolphin trainer. He cannot communicate with the Chinese sponsors direct. His boss has an agreement with the German agent, but both of them are half the world away and in any case the German agent has no more chance of controlling the intricate machinations of an ever-changing group of Chinese businessmen than he has of destroying the Mafia.

So gay little Atlantic bottle-nosed dolphins find themselves in the backyards of Buddhist temples in Singapore's China-town, up in the sweating hills of Borneo, or slipped into the bill of a wrestling championship held in a football stadium in downtown Manila. Transport costs are pared down to a minimum: instead of taking a direct jet from Europe to Hong Kong, the animals and trainers find themselves droning along in ancient Dakotas that stop perhaps ten times or more along the route. It is bad enough for the human attendants, who arrive haggard and exhausted after three to four days in the air. But what must the dolphins be experiencing, out of water, unfed and subjected to the din of the engines for half a week?

That is how Andrew and I often come to be flying at a moment's notice to Jakarta or Taipei to try to pick up the pieces of yet another animal tragedy. It may be purely a disease problem or there may be complicating political and economic factors. I have had to wrangle with Chinese entrepreneurs who were trying to save electricity by turning off the big fans that cooled the air in a Singapore stadium. I was not concerned for the audiences, who had to endure the stifling humidity for only three quarters of an hour, but I was anxious about the water temperature of the dolphin pool. It was rising steadily towards the danger point above which the creatures might have difficulty in dispersing their excess body heat. The negotiations were difficult and carried out through an interpreter. It was important not to lose my temper or cause them to lose face. After hours of almost surrealistic exchanges over a matter which to any animal man is painfully, ridiculously obvious, they conceded the point. The fans would be started again.

'What impressed them about you, Dr Taylor,' said the interpreter afterwards, 'was that you are rich and must therefore be someone to be respected as knowing his business.'

'Rich!' I exclaimed. 'Why on earth should they get that idea?' I was hardly well dressed and was sporting no gold teeth or expensive jewellery.

'Your tummy,' replied the interpreter, tapping the results of too much car driving and sitting in aircraft seats. 'You are getting a belly, they said, the sign of the prosperous one.'

The following year I was in Sumatra, dealing with skin disease caused by filthy water when the sponsors had refused to mend a filter pump. A few months later I was called to Bandung in the hill country of Java: a dolphin was seriously ill and there were big problems. I flew out to Jakarta and was met by a representative of the German agents. He had not received the telegram giving my arrival time but had sat on the airport for three days and met every passenger disembarking with 'Dr Taylor, yes?' He whipped me through customs and immigration and took me to a car.

'Only four hours drive to Bandung,' he said.

I was very tired by my long but relatively comfortable jet flight, and wondered what it must have been like for the poor dolphins. After being unloaded from the aircraft they too must have set off by road, but in a wagon taking far longer than four hours over the bumpy roads into the high country.

I am not sure what my companion was thinking nor to which branch of the show-biz fraternity I belonged when he said: 'Before we go any further, Doctor, I should warn you that all artistes who have come to Java up to this time, without exception, have caught VD.'

'Oh, thank you very much,' I murmured.

We passed over a wooden bridge spanning a shallow wooded valley. Below in the stream a young woman with long gleaming black hair and a green and red batik sarong paddled naked from the waist upwards. It was a warm, scented evening with a sky of fluorescent salmon pink. We bounced along, climbing steadily through hills neatly stepped with paddy fields and crusted with dense green tea plantations. We slipped over the range and dropped down into Bandung, a bustling, friendly city, full of colour and the babble of voices, of old Dutch colonial villas, neat little houses covered with lush tropical vegetation, higgledy-piggledy conglomerations of shanties, temples, and colourful bird markets, swarms of rickshaws and charming, beautiful people. I went straight to the dolphin pool, in one of the poorer quarters. A simple pair of portable plastic swimming pools stood in the middle of an arena made from wooden laths and partly roofed with palm leaves. The water was brown and contained a high concentration of particles: it looked for all the world like oxtail soup but smelled like rotten fish. Juan the dolphin trainer, an old friend from England, was in a terrible state over his animals. One was very ill and losing weight by the hour, and to cap it all the Chinese sponsors had cut up rough. Sick dolphin, they had said, meant no show. No show meant no people. No people meant they were not going to pay money for electricity or water or salt or food. Two people had been killed the day before in the crush trying to get into the arena to see Flipper. Now the police were on guard outside.

In my usual tropical kit, my underpants, I jumped into the pool to examine the sick dolphin, Rocky. He was in a bad way, with thin, diseased skin and half-closed, lethargic eyes. I went over him carefully and found an enlarged liver lobe bulging back beyond the last rib which suggested liver disease. When working in the East I rarely have problems getting blood samples processed, since there is usually a mission hospital or similar institution with a lab only too willing to help out in an emergency. Sure enough, within half an hour I had located an American Pentecostal hospital who readily agreed to analyse a blood sample from Rocky. A couple of hours later the results came back. It was hepatitis. The dolphin was in danger of complete liver collapse and death within a very short space of time. I went back to the pool and opened the bag of tricks that I always carry with me. I had little doubt that the infection had come from the foul water, though the fish that were being fed to the dolphins looked none too wholesome either. It would take a few days to identify exactly the bacterium responsible, and by then Rocky might be dead. I decided to assume that the germ causing the liver infection was one of a group which often affects dolphins: a frequenter of water and bad fish, it is totally resistant to penicillin and most antibiotics. I would have to use a drug rarely employed as yet in treating animals in Britain, the highly efficient gentamycin. Years before at Flamingo Park in Yorkshire I had experimented and found that because dolphin kidneys are more efficient at throwing the stuff out, three times the dose for an equivalent weight of human being was needed to achieve a curative level of gentamycin in the dolphin blood-stream. At this rate it would cost around sixty pounds a day for Rocky's antibiotic alone, without the drugs to aid the weakening liver cells and replace chemicals that the organ was too weak to manufacture. Also, it is no good giving gentamycin by mouth as it just is not absorbed from the bowel. Rocky would need to be injected four times a day.

So began an intensive course of treatment to clear the dolphin's system of the poisons building up because of the liver failure. He was unable to take part in any performances and Flipper his mate was unwilling to do any tricks without him. The management were up in arms about it; it was most uncooperative and inconsiderate of the animal to fall ill. What about the paying customers, who would give their right arms to get in? And why, now that the dolphin doctor from England had given the animal the once-over and an injection of golden liquid, wasn't the wretched Rocky hard at it again? Hadn't he heard? The show must go on!

A compromise of sorts had to be reached. I was adamant that Rocky would rest like the serious hospital case he was; they wanted rupiahs from the punters. So it came about that the public were admitted four times a day to watch an extraordinary kind of dolphin show. When all the customers were packed into the rows of seats around the pool, the compère would do his usual warm-up introduction to the amazing 'lumba-lumbas' as the dolphins are called in Indonesian. He would explain that Rocky was a bit off colour so Flipper would not do his stuff very well, but, he would add, he had a special treat for the crowd. At great expense, all the way from England, the management had brought that unique, that amazing, that incredible per-forming dolphin doctor! Applause from the audience. For the first time ever in Asia, complete with hypodermic needle, stethoscope but no baggy trousers, Dr David Taylor will examine and inject the sick Rocky! At this point ninety-five per cent of the audience stand on their seats for a better view. And now to introduce the man who knows all the secrets of a lumba-lumba's sex life! The tape-recording of 'A Life on the Ocean Wave' is turned up to maximum volume. Your friend and mine, Dr Taylor from Lancashire, England!

Out from the fish-kitchen I walk. The audience grin, cheer and applaud enthusiastically. With a great show of net-twirling Juan and his assistants catch the torpid dolphin. I bow to the crowd, wave my stethoscope in the air, then get down to the serious business of giving Rocky his essential treatment. When it comes to the filling of the syringe with the gentamycin I hold up the bottles so that the audience can see every detail of the process. The empty vials are eagerly sought after by small boys in the front row. There is a great a-a-a-ah from the crowd as I insert the needle and more clapping as I withdraw it and rub the site with an antiseptic swab.

Four times a day, *pace* Equity and the Royal College of Veterinary Surgeons, I trod the boards, and by the end of the week Rocky was coming back strongly and the sponsors had coined a small fortune. The trouble was that the fortune was not big enough, nowhere near what they had hoped for. A few days after I began my act I had bigger trouble than ever. The leader of the syndicate came to the arena one evening and personally removed all the fuses, venting his anger with the German agent on the innocent dolphins. Now they were totally unfiltered. Without an amp of electricity in the place there were no lights for my night injections and the fish in the refrigerator were rapidly going bad. I was livid. The sponsor had gone into a deep huff and refused to see Juan or the representative of the German agent. Flipper and Rocky cruised around in even thicker oxtail soup. I put a ban on feeding the putrefying fish and went to see the Chinese sponsor. Whether he liked it or not, I would sit on his doorstep until I had words with him. Eventually I was let in and invited to talk with him.

'I bear you personally no ill will,' he said, 'but these animals that cannot work are causing me much anguish. It is not just money, it is a political problem. You see, we Chinese in countries like Indonesia have to be very careful. There are racial tensions here although you may not sense it at the moment. Last year a Chinese sponsor promoted a show here in Bandung and something went wrong, he didn't give the people what he'd promised, and it sparked off an explosion of resentment among the native Indonesian majority. They took it out on all the Chinese community, not just the sponsor. Cars of Chinese had their windscreens broken and tyres slashed. Some houses were set on fire. It could easily happen again. Chinese businessmen in the Far East are widely resented by other races in the community. I really believe we Chinese sit on a tinder box. So if the dolphin show that I promote this year is regarded as a wash-out and doesn't come up to the Indonesians' expectations, I could have big trouble. And so could all

57

the other Chinese in Bandung. That is why we don't use banks for our savings but hoard little gold ingots. You can never tell what will happen tomorrow.'

So it was yet another political affair involving dolphins.

'But you must see my point of view also,' I replied. 'I am here solely to look after the health of the dolphins. The sooner Rocky is OK, the sooner the show can be a big hit.'

The Chinaman nodded impassively but returned to his theme of racial tension. 'Three days ago two people were killed, you know, trying to get into the show. How many next time? And suppose they blame it on me? I'd be crucified.'

On and on we wrangled but I made no headway. He was not going to spend money on keeping the dolphins unless they worked. In desperation I tried a different tack.

'Right then,' I said, standing up to go, 'as you can do nothing for the animals, I myself personally must pay for the replacement of the fuses and the water and electricity bills. The animals are not my property. I have no interest in the show. I am not an employee of the German agent nor a shareholder in your syndicate. But we British are at least humane and civilised enough to protect the weak and innocent' (I hoped he had not heard of our fine English stag- and otter-hunters and the hare-coursing fraternity) 'and, though I cannot afford it, I cannot see the dolphins die. Good evening.'

I walked smartly towards the door. Can't the bastard lose some of this notorious Oriental face, I thought. Perhaps it doesn't exist. As I reached the door, to my astounded delight he called me back.

'Dr Taylor,' he said, 'I have no quarrel with you. I will make enquiries to see who removed the fuses. The electricity will be on within the hour.'

Good Lord, I thought, it really has worked. I've shamed him, and to avoid losing face he's suggesting that someone else turned off the power. Still, I had no wish to embarrass him and did not let on that I knew who had pulled the fuses.

'How very good of you!' I said, shaking his hand heartily. 'I'll do my best to have Rocky in A1 shape as soon as possible.' To improve things further I offered to mediate between him and the German agents and to thrash out a more reasonable arrangement for the rest of the tour.

Rocky recovered splendidly and eventually he and Flipper came back to Europe for a well-earned rest. But they brought something else back with them. From some batch of contaminated fish or pool of unwholesome water in Asia they had picked up a virus. This evil little germ lay dormant in their bodies for many weeks but in time it became active and began to multiply rapidly within the cells of the dolphins. Intensive efforts were made to destroy the germ, which like all viruses was resistant to antibiotics, but after a long period of illness both Rocky and Flipper died.

No-one ever really escaped from Devil's Island.

Seven

When the whale trainer walked into the dolphinarium at Flamingo Park early one morning he could not believe his eyes. The deep, hour-glass-shaped pool in which the killer whale, Cuddles, had lived for three years was no longer brimming with clear blue artificial sea water. Instead the entire pool was filled with murky scarlet liquid. He felt a sickening contraction of his stomach. Something terrible had happened to the whale. Surely the sixteen-foot-long animal must be lying disembowelled on the bottom of the pool. But no – with the usual blast of steaming breath, Cuddles' shining black head suddenly emerged from the red soup. He was alive. The trainer dashed down to the basement and peered through the underwater windows. It was like looking into a crimson fog, a pea-souper with less than six inches visibility.

It was only a few days after my return from Java and my theatrical debut with Rocky and Flipper, but when I received the frantic telephone call I set off for the zoo immediately. Obviously, I thought, someone is exaggerating rather in the heat of the moment. Whales bleed like any other animal when injured, but to turn 250,000 gallons completely red? Impossible! OK, whales are big creatures and Cuddles weighed over two and a half tons, but how much blood did they think such an animal could carry in his circulation system? Horror erased such thoughts the instant I saw the pool. It was actually true. The water looked like somewhat anaemic blood. We all know that blood stains easily and that a little goes a long way: every veterinary surgeon has been called to see a dog with a cut foot where the scene of the accident or the house in which it is being attended looks as if a dozen pigs had been slaughtered there. But this was something unbelievable.

Cuddles floated quietly in the middle of the pool. His deep black body colour had taken on more of a dark grey shade. When I called him over to the side he responded slowly. This was not the perky, mischievous creature that I knew so well, who would call to me with his high-pitched piggy squeal whenever I passed through the crowd of spectators. He was torpid and depressed. His gums and the membrane round his eye, normally a deep pink colour, were now a death-like white. I enquired about his appetite. Zero. For the first time since he had arrived in Yorkshire, Cuddles' enormous appetite for herring and mackerel had vanished. He would not face even a single fish.

I was highly alarmed. Of all the animals with which I have worked I have been closer to none than to Cuddles. Despite the species' fearsome-sounding name, and although in the wild state they are voracious and deadly hunters, killer whales in captivity are generally amenable and gentle to the humans who look after them. I had been with Cuddles when he arrived one frosty winter night, a plump and genial baby with teeth just cutting through his gums. Through the summers we had played daily together in the water. He loved to hug you with his flippers while he floated vertically and you tickled his smooth round belly with your toes. Tug-of-war with an old car tyre, carrying a rider round on his back either in front of his dorsal fin or behind, on what I called the rumble seat where the ride was bumpy and exhilarating; he had played eagerly all day. As a patient he had been impeccable. Martin Padley, his trainer, and I had designed a special examination sling that ran out over Cuddles' pool on telescopic girders. Not only was he easy to get into it for routine blood sampling or vaccination but he was positively reluctant to leave this aquatic examination couch! Martin always had to entice him out rather than in. There had been the awful time when he swallowed a child's plastic trumpet and submitted placidly to stomach pumping, and he had been highly co-operative as a donor in a unique attempt at long-distance artificial insemination of another whale in Cleethorpes. I had learnt most of my techniques of whale handling and medication on this fellow. Now it seemed that I was about to lose him through some systerious calamity.

The first priority was to find out where the blood was coming from. There was no sign of a wound on his upper surface as he bobbed in the water. I put on a wet-suit and jumped into the pool. The crimson water smelt dank and unpleasant. I paddled across to my friend and hugged his head. Cuddles gazed at me with his round dark eyes but made no move to cuddle up to me as he usually did. Ominously, the healthy syrupy tears no longer flowed from his eyelids. Cuddles was dehydrating somehow, bleeding to death.

I went all over his back and tail flukes: so sign of any injury. Then, using his paddle-like left flipper as a lever, I laboriously rolled him over in the water. His gleaming white abdomen broke the water surface. Not a trace of a wound could I see. There were now only two possibilities: the blood was coming out either with his urine or in his stools. Suddenly, as he floated like a great capsized plastic boat, a massive welter of what seemed to be almost pure blood gushed out of his anus. That was it. Cuddles was bleeding massively somewhere in his intestines.

Climbing out of the pool, I gave instructions for it to be emptied immediately. Whatever the problem was, it had struck rapidly out of the blue. Cuddles had been normal up to the previous evening when all the dolphinarium staff went home. It seemed to be affecting the lower bowel: if the bleeding source was in the stomach or high in the bowel the blood would have been partly digested and changed to a much darker brown or black colour on its way through the intestinal tract. I suspected bacterial or virus infection producing rapid ulceration of the bowel lining. If it was a bacterium, perhaps the culprit was the evil salmonella, a food poisoning germ which causes diarrhoea and the passing of blood in other animals.

Whatever the cause, my first priority now was to get Cuddles down onto the dry bottom of the pool, examine him thoroughly and take blood samples to see how bad the damage was. Next I had to stop the bleeding and replace some of the liquid that his circulation had lost. When the volume of circulating blood becomes too small to carry enough oxygen and other vital supplies to key organs, shock and death speedily set in. How to expand Cuddles' blood volume? I decided that in any event I had to make preparations for some sort of transfusion. Ideally I wanted many pints of killer whale blood, not quite the sort of stuff that is usually available at the local blood bank! We knew that there were certainly three major blood groups in bottle-nosed dolphins, but no-one knew anything about the blood groups of whales. The nearest captive killers were in America. Perhaps some of my colleagues out there had some suitable blood stored.

I telephoned all the major marinelands in the United States and explained my predicament. No-one had any killer whale blood stored and no-one had come across a similar problem. My friend Dr White at Miami Seaquarium had had a case of severe bleeding in a whale that had crashed through an underwater viewing window. It had needed lots of surgery and supportive medical therapy but no blood transfusions had been given. Would anyone fancy volunteering one of their whales as a donor of a dozen or two pints? I could easily get the stuff shipped over express on the next Pan-Am or TWA flight. The answer was always the same. Highly valuable animals. The difficulty of having to drain pools in the middle of the show season in order to take blood. Anyway, how were we to be sure without wasting days testing samples whether any particular whale's blood would be compatible with Cuddles'? Whole blood transfusion was out.

The fire brigade arrived. Whenever we needed to speed up the emptying of the pools they were called in. Half an hour later, an unusually dark grey and very white whale was lying passively on the concrete bottom of the pool while hoses and buckets were used to keep his skin moist. I went down and took blood from the big blood vessel in his tail. Even to the naked eye the sample appeared watery and thin. The crucial analyses were quickly done in the laboratory at the pool side. As I had feared, Cuddles had lost a great deal of blood into the intestines. Normally he carried a regular seventeen grammes of haemoglobin, the red oxygen-carrying constituent, in every hundred c.c.'s of his blood. Now it was down to only ten grammes. The total number of red blood cells had also dropped precipitously. Other tests showed no sign of active bacterial infection or liver or kidney damage.

A trainer came into the laboratory carrying what looked like a fragment of wet white paper. 'He's just passed another load of blood,' he reported, 'and there was this in it.'

The specimen was sticky and fragile. I dropped it into a beaker of cold water and teased it out with a needle. It unfolded into a delicate white film as big as a postage stamp. The film was not completely intact for at three or four points there were round holes ringed distinctly by reddish-brown material. It was a piece of intestinal lining membrane and the holes were ulcers surrounded by blood pigment, a valuable find but a depressing one. Cuddles had actively bleeding multiple ulcers in his bowels. If there were so many on this small fragment, how many thousands more might there be if the entire hundred feet of his intestines were similarly involved?

The bit of bowel lining and some swabs went to the bacteriology laboratory for urgent examination and I then returned to the problem of replacing Cuddles' lost blood volume. I had to take second best. Although it had no oxygen-carrying power, transfusions of artificial plasma would combat many of the shock-producing factors and would stop the blood vessels from literally collapsing. It was going to mean putting Cuddles on an intravenous drip, and I estimated that at least forty pints would be required. An urgent call for help was sent out to Leeds General Hospital. They readily agreed to supply us with a hundred bottles of the life-saving liquid and it was despatched by fast car under police escort. Meanwhile I filled Cuddles with other important drugs to tackle the sadly abused bowels. Through the giant one-foot-long needle I injected things like vitamins, anti-inflammatory drugs and antibiotics. Although it would take ten to fourteen days for it to be assembled into the essential haemoglobin, I gave big shots of iron liquid. He would need the iron reserves if he recovered.

When the cases of artificial plasma arrived I started work on the transfusion. I used a special needle-like tube of the sort we had employed when doing electrocardiographic investigations on Cuddles some weeks before. The tube had to be inserted accurately into a tail vein. In both dolphins and killer whales, veins and arteries near the surface are closely intermingled for heat-exchange purposes, and if any of the liquid from an intravenous injection goes into an artery there can be nasty repercussions including profound sloughing and death of a large area of tail skin. Kneeling with Cuddles' great tail held above my head I inserted the tube and checked and double-checked that the blood oozing from it was coming only from a vein. When I was satisfied that all was well I connected the plastic tubes to the plasma bottle and adjusted the dosage regulator. A keeper stood on a chair holding the bottle high in the air so that the flow of liquid was not counteracted by Cuddles' massive heart pressure.

Slowly the golden fluid seeped into the whale's system. After ten minutes I switched to the second bottle. Although whale blood does not clot easily, I had anticipated trouble with the tube in the vein and had used a chemical to inhibit clotting and consequent blockage, but I felt sure that frequent changes of the tube would be necessary. In fact, as the hours passed slowly by, the keepers holding the bottles and the bottles themselves were the only things to be changed. The tube remained unblocked throughout the whole ten hours of the transfusion. Cuddles was as good as gold. Not once did he protest or wriggle.

The man holding the tail up during all this time refused to be relieved. He, too, was deeply involved with the animal and wanted to do everything in his power to help. It was cold and damp in the pool bottom so I sent for a bottle of rum to ward off inner chills. From time to time I insisted on the tail holder taking a good pull from the rum bottle. So solicitous was I for the man's health that I did not realise how many tots he had taken during the long hours of waiting. When it was all finished we discovered the good man to be totally drunk and incapable and had to hoist him out of the pool in a dolphin sling.

We refilled the pool. To my delight, when it was up to the six-foot mark Cuddles accepted a few fish. It was terrible to see the chalk-white back of his throat when he opened his jaws to take them but at least the boy was eating again! I stopped the refilling at eight feet. It was good to see clear blue water again but what if he continued to bleed?

Next morning I held my breath as I went into the dolphinarium. My heart sank like an express lift when I saw the glum expressions on the faces of the trainers. The pool water was deep scarlet again. We drained immediately and once more I took a blood sample. The haemoglobin and red cell counts were lower than before, below the point at which, in humans, a blood transfusion becomes imperative. I transfused the plasma again, gave more injections and passed a stomach tube. Cuddles took it all philosophically. Through the stomach tube I pumped in a peculiar pink mixture which I had concocted in a large unused plastic dustbin. It contained water and honey, mineral salts to replace those lost in the bleeding, glucose, rose-hip syrup, invalid food, kaolin to soothe the inflamed bowel, and Guinness. As it by-passed his taste buds I do not suppose Cuddles relished it or otherwise. The next day things looked much brighter – Cuddles had not bled overnight and showed an improved appetite. The following day dawn broke for the third time on a scene of gory water, but analysis showed the blood loss to have been much reduced and the haemoglobin level, though still below the critical minimum, was levelling out. Still seriously worried, but no longer in complete despair, I repeated my injections and the dustbin mixture.

By now the laboratory results were all back. No bacteria were involved. The cause of the ulcers remained a mystery, as it does to this day, although I strongly believe a virus to have been the culprit. Cuddles continued to eat quite well and even agreed to play gently. He did not haemorrhage on the day after the third bleeding, nor on the next day or the one after that. I became increasingly hopeful. The whale was still very pale but steadily growing stronger and I fortified his fish by packing them with chunks of cooked Lancashire black puddings, rare delicacies made from blood and fat.

Cuddles never bled again. His recovery was fast and free from further incident. Two weeks after the first attack his blood analysis was halfway back to normal and in a further three weeks it was completely satisfactory. By this time he was greedily gulping down whole undisguised black puddings by the dozen and opening his now salmon-pink mouth with alacrity to have foaming quarts of Guinness poured straight into his gullet.

Many things about Cuddles' bleeding disease I do not understand, and which if any of my lines of treatment helped to save the day will never be known. Certainly the transfusions only averted death from shock and tackled some of the circulatory complications. Perhaps it was the kaolin or the anti-inflammatory drugs or the black puddings that turned the tide against the ulcers. Perhaps if a virus was involved Cuddles developed a rapid immunity which effectively combated the attack. A Devonshire woman working at Flamingo Park as personal secretary to the director had a different view on the affair. When it was all over we were talking and she told me what she had done to help the dying killer whale.

'When he bled the third time I went and phoned a wise woman in my home village in the West Country,' she told me. 'She's a person who uses white magic on warts and styes and rheumatism. Marvellous reputation. Never known to fail.'

'What did you say to her?' I asked.

'I told her briefly what was wrong at the dolphinarium and she just said that everything would be all right, and that the bleeding would stop when I put the receiver down.'

It sounded like the most ridiculous humbug to me, but I respected the director's secretary as an astute and intelligent woman.

'Well,' I said, 'can you remember the time when you finished speaking to your wise woman acquaintance?'

'Of course I can,' she replied with an odd smile. 'It was eight-thirty in the morning.'

I walked down to the dolphinarium and looked in the record book. Every minute item concerning the whale and dolphins in health and sickness is logged there day by day, year in and year out. On the morning of the third and final episode of Cuddles' bleeding a trainer had recorded the last occasion on which the whale was seen to pass blood. The time was entered as 8.31 a.m.

Eight

Although the fascination of tending exotic animals is endless, it is not every day that a vet is faced with a life and death emergency like the drama of Cuddles' bleeding. All the same, what may start as a comparatively simple task (if such a thing may be said to exist in a zoo vet's work) can develop into a situation calling for rapid action if a valuable animal is to be saved. For example, a new hippopotamus, Hercules, arrived one afternoon at the zoo in Manchester. He had been sent from Whipsnade in a massive crate made out of thick wooden beams reinforced with steel bands. The hippo is not a creature to be trifled with. He can hurl himself forwards or spin round on his hind feet with remarkable agility, he is as unstoppable as a tank and he delivers a fearsome chomping, crushing bite. To be on the safe side, Whipsnade had given Hercules a dose of phencyclidine before sending him off and had strongly recommended that he should receive a further shot just before he was uncrated in Manchester. They feared that otherwise, once the door of the crate was opened, a highly irascible hippo might emerge and make his way like an express train, walls and so on notwithstanding, towards the city centre.

Hercules' crate was open-topped and by climbing up the side I could look down on the steaming armour-plating of the big hippopotamus. He was standing calmly enough without any sign of agitation and showing little sign of the effects of the sedative. I had not unloaded a hippo before. My inclination would have been to forgo the second phencyclidine injection but Whipsnade, with much more experience of these matters at the time, had made the point strongly. They had even sent a measured dose of the drug. I filled a syringe, bent down over the side of the crate and slapped my stoutest needle through the hippo's rump. Hercules reacted by slamming my wrist hard against the wooden side of the crate. I was trapped securely. Hercules maintained the pressure against my wrist with all his might. He wiggled his hips a bit and ground my hand excruciatingly into the wood. Biting my tongue, I slapped vainly at the hippo's bottom with my other hand. It was some minutes before he conceded to pull away and I could retrieve my extremity, now numb, black and horribly scuffed. Twenty years later I still have no feeling in that part of my wrist.

After a quarter of an hour Hercules was still standing but his ears were drooping slightly and there was a string of saliva hanging from his jaw. I decided to let him out. The bolts were removed from the reinforced door and the door was opened wide. We were using the rear door to make him back out so that he would be less likely to charge. Hercules did not budge. No matter what we did, tapping his nose with a stick, tempting him with food or slapping his back, he was not inclined to go into reverse gear. So we cautiously opened the front door, revealing fully the bucolic features of Hercules for the first time. He stared blandly at the inside of the tropical river house where he was now to live, sniffed disdainfully and blinked his drowsy eyelids. Then he saw the shining pool of warm water for him, its surface wreathed in misty vapour. Very sedately Hercules began to move forwards. He emerged from the crate, paused briefly, then walked slowly towards the pool. He went down the ramp at the side of the pool as if on tiptoe, sniffed at the water, found it to his liking and very gracefully slipped in. Through the clear water, not yet sullied by hippo droppings, we could see him settle peacefully on the bottom of the pool and then, gradually it seemed, fall asleep. The second dose of phencyclidine, together with the soothing warm bath, was having an understandable but potentially lethal effect. A conscious hippo can hold its breath underwater for many minutes but will eventually come to the surface to take in a fresh gulp of air. A doped hippo might very well be a different matter. Suppose Hercules inhaled blissfully while dreaming on the bottom of his pool? A cluster of icicles formed in the pit of my stomach.

'It looks as if he's going to sleep,' I told the keepers around me. 'Get some ropes – fast. We could be in big trouble!'

Some of the men dashed off. The zoo director and I stood at the water's edge looking anxiously down at the recumbent form of the hippo three feet below the surface. When the ropes arrived there was only one thing for it. Stripping off to our underpants, Matt Kelly and I jumped into the water and dived for the submerged hulk. It is no easy task to feel one's way over a hippo's anatomy without the benefit of a pair of goggles and towing a length of thick rope. Spluttering we both surfaced for a quick discussion on a plan of action.

'You try to get a rope on the back legs, Matt,' I said. 'I'll see if I can get one round the neck.'

Matt dived again and I followed. Hercules slumbered on, unaware of the visitors struggling clumsily about his submarine bedroom. I would not dare to take such liberties with a hippo in full possession of its senses. After much effort and repeated returns to the surface with bursting lungs we managed to place the ropes more or less as we wanted them. The keepers hauled on the ropes and to my relief Hercules, most un-Venus-like, rose to the surface. The great nostrils opened as his head cleared the water and he exhaled gently. His eyes were half closed and there was a pleasant softening of the hippo's usual grim smile.

It was impossible to drag the heavy creature onto land. There were not enough of us, hippos have no convenient handles, and I was afraid that the excessive use of ropes on Hercules' limbs and neck might injure him. In water he weighed much less, so we would have to support him in the pool by passing ropes under his belly until he was no longer under the influence. We kept the crucial head up by wrapping towels round it and slinging it to a beam. Hercules looked for all the world as if he was suffering an attack of toothache and had taken to the whisky bottle to alleviate the pain.

After some hours Hercules began to wriggle on the supporting ropes. His eyes opened fully and he surveyed the strange scene sombrely. When he realised that his towel bandage inhibited chomping he became restless and we decided that he had come round enough to look after himself. After being untangled he retired to the bottom of the pool from which secure position he looked up at us lugubriously. Several minutes later I watched him come to the surface to breathe deeply. Hercules was going to be all right.

Hercules was indeed all right. He immediately fell in love with his pool set in an imitation tropical jungle with waterfalls, islands and luscious vegetation. His arrival, however, spelt disaster for some other denizens of the Manchester jungle. Sharing his habitat were tapirs, capybaras and an assortment of exotic birds. These Hercules proceeded to stalk and, if possible, eat. He would play the crocodile, lurking beneath the surface of the water now dark with his droppings, and using his protuberant eyes as mini-periscopes. When a tapir came down to drink or a bird perched on a rock at the water's edge, Hercules would glide stealthily in like a killer submarine. With a sudden charge when he was within inches of his prey he would seize it in his jaws and kill it instantly with one powerful crunch. Then Hercules the hippo would feast until not a scrap remained. So much for vegetarianism: Hercules fancied meat and he still does. Sometimes when he is off colour I stand on the rocks by his pool and toss him loaves packed with pick-me-ups or stimulants. I have to watch carefully for the pair of gleaming eyes that just about break the water surface and come slowly but steadily towards my feet. At such moments I skip smartly backwards.

Hercules would seem to relish a taste of vet's meat to break the monotony of his orthodox diet, and perhaps it is for the same reason that zoo animals so often swallow unusual objects. Sometimes these things are ingested accidentally but at other times there may be special reasons for them being taken in voluntarily, as in the case of the sealion, which in the wild can often be found carrying a few stones quite harmlessly in its stomach. These stones act as ballast to help the animal dive, rather like the weighted belt of a skin diver: thus deeper diving species of sealion tend to carry more ballast than the shallower diving species. In captivity this natural, fairly limited taking on of stones can go wrong. Where sealions are kept in fresh water with no access to salt, particularly if the pool is a simple one scooped out of the earth, the animal may attempt to satisfy its craving for salt in its diet by eating soil and stones. To avoid this I try to see that all the sealions and seals in my care that are not in saltwater pools have table salt added daily to their fish diet.

Unfortunately, I still see the results of stone-swallowing by sealions over a long period, as when a sealion at a safari park in England died suddenly after a lengthy spell of erratic eating. For months it had been keen to feed but quickly lost its appetite after being given one or two fish. Then, as if it had just had a Chinese meal, it would be hungry and calling for fish within half an hour. The owners had not worried unduly because the sealion seemed to be actually gaining weight. Indeed it was! When I looked at the body it had a plump rounded belly that must surely be full of fat. I began the autopsy and within seconds of slicing through the abdominal wall was faced with an amazing sight. The sealion was, in fact, skinny and free of healthy fat stores. The stomach, which is normally about the same size and shape as a human's and lies tucked neatly away under the rib cage, was horribly distended. It filled the abdomen, squeezing the liver and kidneys and intestines. It bulged everywhere, particularly back towards the tail. I could not see the end of it; it continued on into the pelvic cavity where only the bladder and associated organs should be found. Inside the stomach were stones, hundreds and hundreds of them packing every bit of available space and stretching the stomach wall until it was as thin as tissue paper. When they were all removed they filled three gallon buckets and weighed almost forty pounds. It was the worst foreign body load I had ever seen.

There were other sealions in the safari park of the same age as the poor dead individual. What about them? They were fit-looking animals who delighted in performing their skilful feats of balance before the visitors. All looked well, but I was of a mind to X-ray the lot of them to make certain that no more were carrying around stomachs like gravel pits. I asked the trainer whether there were any abnormal symptoms to report. He thought for a moment and began to shake his head.

'No, I don't think so except . . .' He frowned and then carried on. 'Except for Mimi. She's a little bit like Otto, the dead one, always hungry but very easily filled.'

I walked over to where Mimi stood elegantly on her show stand. She sniffed diffidently at me and clapped her front flippers hopefully. I could see no sign of trouble brewing. Then the trainer called Mimi off the stand and she slipped down onto the ground and hauled herself towards the fish bucket. As she passed I heard a soft and unusual sound, like the lapping of water on a shingle beach, the rush of pebbles one upon another. There was too much incidental noise from the other animals and the visitors to hear it clearly so I had Mimi taken to the quiet of the hospital. There I listened again. When she moved it was possible to hear the crunching, grinding noise of gravel. I stroked her and made friends and then carefully pressed her stomach. Scr-r-runch. It was exactly like digging into a bag of marbles. Mimi was full of rocks.

Although, along with the giraffe, the sealion is one of the more difficult animals to anaesthetise (its ability to hold its breath as if diving can cause problems with anaesthetic gas machines), I decided to operate. Opening the stomach of a dog to remove swallowed objects is a common and not very diffcult operation but the sealion is somewhat trickier. A particular risk is post-operative infection from the skin, which literally teems with all sorts of nasty bacteria. For the surgeon, too, contact with sealion skin and other tissues can be risky if there are any cuts in his rubber gloves and abrasions on his hands. A germ often found living harmlessly on sealion skin can attack pigs, dolphins and other animals dramatically, and in humans may set up the unpleasant infection known as 'blubber finger' or 'seal hand' to generations of seal skinners and whaling men.

From Mimi's stomach one by one I retrieved 124 stones weighing almost sixteen pounds altogether. No wonder she had been hungry, with nowhere to accommodate a decent meal. When she was stitched up Mimi was a much more streamlined creature. I looked forward to seeing her eat a hearty meal of three or four pounds of herring in a few days after the stomach sutures had done their work and she could come off the post-operative diet of liquidised fish and water.

Other animals have eaten odd things as well. The elephant at Belle Vue Zoo that took an umbrella did not seem to suffer the slightest twinge of the collywobbles, although an enormous old elephant seal at Cleethorpes found a woolly cardigan too much for it and tragically choked to death. It is not always necessary to approach the stomach by operation through the abdomen, since increasingly nowadays, particularly in dolphins, the arch-swallowers of bric-à-brac, we employ an ingenious piece of equipment normally used for exploring the higher reaches of the human bowel. This is the Olympus fibre-optic gastroscope, a very expensive device which can do wonders when slipped simply and without anaesthetic down the animal's throat. It is thin and flexible and carries a powerful light source, a mobile viewing tip, a water spray, an air tube for inflating organs to be inspected, and a host of special attachments. Looking through the eyepiece we can see magnified and in full colour every nook and cranny in the stomach and even further down into the intestine or up the bile duct. The tip can be made to go round corners and to look backwards towards the viewer. By passing minute instruments down within the tube we can cauterise bleeding points, take biopsy samples of diseased tissue and grab or lasso objects. The stomach and bowels expanded by air from the gastroscope become fascinating caverns and grottoes through which by remote control we can wander in search of the bizarre and the diseased.

It was by using this machine that we took the first colour photographs ever made of the inside of a living dolphin. Since then we have begun to build up a reference library of slides of the various bacterial, fungal and other ailments that can attack the crucial three stomachs of our cetacean friends. One of the first patients on which we used the fibre-optic gastroscope was Brandy, a talented star of the dolphin show at Marineland in Palma Nova, Majorca. One day, for no apparent reason, Brandy swallowed one of the soft plastic rings, six inches across, which he played with during his performances. Down into his stomach it went and down it stayed. Nothing untoward happened at first, and Brandy continued to eat and work normally. But the powerful acids in his stomach were slowly vulcanising the plastic and turning the soft ring into something much more hard and irritant. David Mudge, the director of Marineland and an old friend in the dolphin business, became worried when the ring was not regurgitated as he had hoped. What was more, after some days Brandy began to look unwell. He became irritable, his work became erratic and his appetite disappeared. David was certain that Brandy was experiencing stomach pain.

We had talked together over the telephone when the ring was first swallowed and had decided to observe the animal and to treat him conservatively at first. Now it became obvious that we would have to intervene with strong positive measures. Andrew, my partner, flew out to Majorca with the fibre-optic gastroscope and accompanied by David Wild, the most skilled 'driver', as he calls himself, of the complex instrument in the country. Brandy certainly looked ill. He was pale, seemed tense and in pain, and his usual cheeky, vivacious temperament had changed to one of irritable misery. No longer was he cock of the male dolphins in Palma Nova, forever paying court to his harem of admiring females. Blood analysis showed strong evidence of bleeding ulcers in his stomach. Without further ado Brandy was caught, hauled out of the pool and placed on a soft rubber mattress.

Dolphins out of water produce a lot of body heat and unless they are kept wet may overheat and show dangerous cracking and peeling of the skin. A man stood by with a bucket wetting the animal down while Andrew completed his preparations. First, wet towels were wrapped round Brandy's upper and lower jaws and used to pull the mouth open and hold it open. Gently, Andrew passed the lubricated gastroscope over the back of the dolphin's tongue, to one side of the larynx and then down the gullet into the first stomach. Kneeling behind him David Wild watched through the eyepiece as the tip of the instrument moved onwards, spraying the lens with water when stomach juices threatened to cloud the vision and pushing the walls of the stomach away from the tube with air so that he could have space to look around. Through a side attachment to the eye-piece Andrew was able to monitor progress as well. Before long they both saw the first of a series of ugly bleeding ulcers in the stomach lining. Everywhere there was black blood from the ulcers, partly digested. Brandy's digestion was in a terrible state. David swung the tip of the gastroscope round, and there was the ring! They could see a segment of the red plastic lying in a black pool of blood. The natural contractions of the stomach muscles against the hardening ring were grinding one ulcer after another through the delicate velvety lining of the organ.

Now to get the ring out. A special attachment to the gastroscope allowed the introduction of a wire loop which was guided round the ring and back to the gastroscope again. When the ring was firmly snared it was pulled to the tip of the instrument and then both ring and gastroscope were withdrawn together. Brandy gave an enormous gulp as the ring travelled back up his gullet. Luckily dolphins have remarkably elastic gullets for swallowing large fish whole, otherwise there would have been a risk of rupturing the organ. With the ring gone Brandy looked much relieved, but Andrew reintroduced the gastroscope to inspect the ulcer damage. Some of the worst bleeding points were electrically cauterised and photographs were taken. Then Brandy was returned, to his great relief, to the pool and his wives, and his complete recovery was ensured by a course of tablets normally given to dyspeptic middle-aged business executives. To celebrate his sense of well-being after the poolside operation, Brandy was seen to mate long and amorously with one of the female dolphins, and eleven and a half months later, on the following Boxing Day, a little baby dolphin was born in the pool at Palma Nova.

Nine

Even stranger jobs than saving a drowning hippo or emptying a sealion of gravel have come my way. Arnold was a bloody-minded and malevolent African grey parrot with a powerful liking for the flesh of human fingers, a black hatred of dogs, particularly of Bimbo, the amiable and pacific retriever that lived in the same household, and a remarkable talent for vocal mimicry. Arnold had a pornographer's vocabulary but he did not limit himself to impersonating only human speech. He was also superb as a vacuum cleaner and as the clatter of the cover on the letter box. His *pièce de résistance*, however, was the characteristic click and squeak of the refrigerator door being opened. Arnold used his talent with what I can only describe as grim malice aforethought. When he had had a particularly liverish day, when perhaps the doting mother of the family had neglected to produce his customary after-lunch teaspoon-ful of Advocaat or the window cleaner had pulled faces at him, Arnold would take it out on Bimbo – indirectly, of course. Bimbo may have been rather dumb but he valued his hide too dearly to go within a yard of the parrot cage and its choleric occupant with the red-rimmed eyes and assiduously shar-pened bill.

In the past Bimbo had occasionally been guilty of flicking open the refrigerator door in search of goodies, but he had been duly chastised and was now fully rehabilitated into society, a reformed character. When Arnold and Bimbo were alone in the living room and the parrot could see that the kitchen where the ice-box stood was also empty, that malign bird would loudly imitate the opening of the refrigerator door.

Immediately he would scream loudly 'Bimbo's at the chops, mother!' or 'The bloody dog's got the weekend joint, for Christ's sake!' The response, sadly, to this display of dastardly misrepresentation was predictable, unvarying. A member of the family ensconced in the parlour watching telly would emerge and boot Bimbo roughly out of the back door, invariably without checking whether the psittacine accusation was true or not. It did Arnold's black heart good to witness the affair, particularly if it was raining and he could watch the luckless dog standing dejectedly in the yard.

But the meek shall inherit the earth. Time ran out for Arnold. He was caught several times in the act of perjury by the family, who resented being hauled away from 'Coronation Street', and his bad language became positively disgusting. Mother had loved Arnold dearly since an old sailor boy friend had brought him as a present thirty years before, but it was decided that he would have to stop the ventriloquism. They came to me with Arnold and asked me to make him dumb.

Arnold took an instant dislike to me and I cannot say that he exactly turned me on, but I refused the request. To render animals voiceless by surgical techniques which take chunks out of their vocal chords is mutilation that can rarely be justified. There may be a point in silencing mules used for transporting military supplies in jungle terrain, as was done by the army in the Far East during the last war, but I have never agreed with the idea of removing the screeches or hoots or Arnoldian language from creatures, particularly exotic ones, just for the convenience of an owner who acquired them without first considering all the aspects of keeping such animals in captivity. Many owners of birds of prey or peafowl enjoy the appearance and activity of the birds but object to the natural noises that go with them: the eerie wail of a peacock at dead of night may put the wind up the more imaginative of your neighbours but if you and they cannot come to terms about having such gorgeous birds on your property, don't ask me to insert red hot cautery needles into the peacocks' voice boxes to destroy the source of the noise. People have even asked me to obliterate the honking of sealions by surgery. To them as to Arnold's owners I gave my stock reply: 'If you don't like the voice you shouldn't be keeping the animal.'

There have been much more bizarre requests. Tigers in the wild are fairly solitary beasts. Unlike lions they do not consort with their prides. After the success of the first safari parks, where lions adapted well, the constant entrepreneurial search for something new turned towards the idea of a tiger or leopard reserve, but there were fears that a group of tigers kept in a relatively small area might slaughter one another mercilessly in battles over artificial territory. With tigers worth ten times as much as lions such prospects deterred many park owners for some years. One English businessman was anxious to be the first to exhibit a big group of tigers living peacefully together and he asked me to meet him to discuss his idea of how it might be done. It was quite simple, he said as we sat in his walnut-panelled office sipping gin and tonics. All we had to do was to remove aggressive impulses from the minds of the tigers – make 'em placid and disinclined to squabble. It was, after all, being done all the time in mental hospitals and institutions for the criminally insane. He had read about it in *Reveille* and seen something on television. So why not do it in tigers? It was all quite simple: just perform a lobotomy on every tiger before introducing it into the reserve!

Imagine. The idea was to drill a hole in each tiger's skull and then to insert special neurosurgical saws to cut off the frontal lobe of the brain, to separate the 'personality' of the animal from the other functions of the brain which were essential for basic living. I marvelled at the man's sheer, stupid audacity in even conceiving such a plan. Apart from the need for highly delicate surgery of a kind never before undertaken in creatures of such a size, its precise effects would be unpredictable and irreversible. It had been performed experimentally on domestic cats in the laboratory but they were at least contributing to the serious scientific study of mental disorders in man.

81

What was being proposed to me was the creation of a pack of tiger zombies, orange and black striped organisms that would feed and breathe, defecate and sneeze, walk and stretch out in the sunshine for the benefit of carloads of paying punters, but would be no more tigers than the colourful paper models of Chinese New Year. It was a frightening proposition.

Even if it were legal, which I doubt, the last thing I would want to deal with is a Frankensteinesque tiger which has been tamed artificially by surgery. I have tiger friends who are gentle and fond of certain human beings because they have been brought up that way and there are others whom I greatly respect and who give me lots of trouble when I am called to examine or treat them. At least I understand their reluctance to be poked and pricked by people like me, and their indignation when restrained in a crush cage, for they are real, complete, magnificent animals. If I should become careless and drop my guard when examining an unanaesthetised wild animal, then I am quite rightly rewarded by a claw hooking my Achilles tendon through the bars or a horn smacked painfully into my backside. I do not want vegetable animals.

My meeting with the businessman lasted about three minutes, just long enough for him to describe his idea and for me to tell him what abominable nonsense it was.

Another businessman, wanting to cash in on the publicity for the Loch Ness monster, approached me with a different kind of request. Instead of faking up a 'monster' from plastic or canvas or upturned boats or oil drums he wanted to have a real live monster swimming in the loch and available for capture before the lenses of the world's breathless media men.

'I want to make a monster out of a big sealion or elephant seal,' he confided. 'If I get hold of a really big sealion will you stitch a plastic dragon's wing along the length of its back?'

He actually wanted me to suture a tall, spiky contraption painted in fearsome black and red to the delicate skin and thick blubber of a living creature. The wing had been made before he even mentioned his scheme to me. When I gave my reply, again brief and to the point, he became angry and spiteful.

'You vets may be all right with all this medical stuff but you'll never make any money. No commercial sense. All book learning and science. No idea of business.'

The meeting ended abruptly.

The possibility of the existence of a real Loch Ness monster has always fascinated me. The circumstantial evidence seems remarkably strong in favour of some type of large, possibly plesiosaur-like animal inhabiting the black depths of this immense stretch of water. Over the years I have been in touch with both scientists and lay people interested in various aspects of the monster problem. Folk who have been within six yards of the beast both in the water and on land and who have claimed to have infallible means of capturing, killing, biopsying, photographing or otherwise identifying the monster have asked me to join their expeditions.

There was the Dutchman who was certain he could kill the monster by setting a net studded with hand-grenades right across the loch and driving the creature to its doom by noise-making machines. There was the American who wanted me to help design an underwater dart fired from a spear-gun which would take a blood sample for later analysis so that we could identify the animal at our leisure from its blood protein characteristics. It seemed to be asking a lot to expect a dart to be fired underwater accurately into a blood vessel of an animal about whose anatomy no-one knows much.

'Ah, but it's bound to have a jugular vein!' enthused the American.

He had never seen the murky gloom that faces anyone swimming underwater in the loch, like being submerged in a vat of flat brown ale. Anyway I would not rely on being able to dart the jugular vein of, say, a crocodile or a hippopotamus on land in the most favourable conditions. Then there was the Englishman who wanted me to drive the monsters to the surface of the loch by a method used in Japan to catch dolphins. A long pole with a flat plate on the bottom end is pushed down into the water. The end of the pole above water is then hammered by the fisherman to produce irritating metallic noises underwater, a terrible din which causes the dolphins to rise, presumably with their ears ringing. It might work if the monsters have got sensitive ears but the Englishman could only afford to sponsor an expedition lasting one day!

'But we'll have one by lunchtime,' he said, pressing me to join his group.

More seriously, I have studied carefully all the written records of monster sightings at Loch Ness and in some other waters and have spoken to several people of integrity, teachers, clergymen and professional men, who claim actually to have seen the beast. The theoretical biological and ecological implications of the monster's existence interest me particularly. Being specially concerned with marine mammals I have studied the evidence to see whether the monster might have similarities to a freshwater seal or dolphin, possibly of the type that still exists in the Tung Ting Hu Lake in China and elsewhere. Like most scientists who have looked objectively at the problem I have come to the conclusion that a more likely candidate is a reptile, or possibly a warm-blooded dinosaur, with many similarities to the apparently extinct plesiosaur.

Certainly it must be carnivore, eating fish and particularly the eels which abound in the loch. There just is not enough vegetable matter in the lake's rather forbidding waters and the evidence suggests that land visits are infrequent and probably out of character. Martin Padley, the Flamingo Park whale trainer, and I had for some time been toying with the idea of making a bait suitable for a carnivorous reptile. It would have a strong, attractive underwater smell and would be fortified with hormones which are active in high dilution and which have a sexually stimulating effect on reptiles. The opportunity to try out our bait came when Independent Television, in conjunction with the Loch Ness Investigation Bureau, the Royal Navy (noise-making machines), the Plessey Company (underwater detection apparatus and two mini-subs), Birmingham University (sonar scanning) and many other experts from Britain and the United States, mounted a two-week expedition to sort out the elusive 'Nessie' once and for all. Martin and I were asked to join the expedition, both to conduct baiting experiments and to take along the dart-gun and a selection of knock-out drugs. This was a Loch Ness expedition I was prepared to join.

Before setting out for the north of Scotland we prepared our bait. It was, as Vincent Mulchrone of the *Daily Mail* was later to describe it, 'a foul-smelling black pudding'. We bought hundreds of pounds of dried blood, anchovy paste and gelatine. Sawdust was used as a filler. The ingredients, including small quantities of the reptile hormone, were mixed into a dark red jelly moulded in plastic buckets. When they had set, the contents of the buckets were put in plastic bags and loaded into the boot of my car.

By the time we had driven up to Inverness through boiling hot weather the giant raspberry-coloured 'lollipops' in the boot were beginning to smell ripely even through the plastic. If the strong fishy-bloody smell was as powerful underwater as it was on land and evoked a positive response in the monster population, they should come rushing from miles around! We unloaded the bait at the ITV base on the shores of the loch near Drumnadrochit. The place was teeming with newspapermen, television engineers, scientists of one discipline or another, skin divers, submariners and crowds of sightseers. In the first few minutes after our arrival excitement reached fever pitch. Two men had come into the camp with what looked like some great pre-historic monster's thigh bone which they claimed to have found nearby. The television people went wild about it. It was massive, obviously fossilized bone, and you could see the head of the femur, the bony projections and the holes for blood vessels. They had struck oil on the first day of the expedition!

Film was rushed to Inverness for 'News at Ten' and vast sums of cash were paid to the two bone finders for portions to be scientifically analysed. There was only one problem. Surprisingly, among all the experts of one sort or another at the lochside headquarters there was not one single person with biological training until I arrived. The TV producer and the journalists besieged me in a frenzy once they knew they had found someone familiar with animal anatomy. Would I please examine the monster thigh bone as a matter of urgency and pronounce upon it in front of the camera? I went to look at the find. It was about four feet high, weighing perhaps 150 pounds, definitely bone but greatly weathered rather than fossilized. I recognized it at once. Bones like it were often made into gate arches in places like Whitby and the Orkneys. It was part of a whale's lower jawbone.

Certainly there was a knobbly articulating surface at the thick end, but it fits into the upper jaw, not the pelvis. There were not tooth holes as giveaways since the bone came from a toothless species of baleen whale, the mighty blue. The television team, already in a state of high excitement, became ecstatic when I pronounced the find to be bone rather than fossilized wood. A well-known TV science correspondent stood it on end and pointed out the monster blood vessel apertures ('Surely the femoral artery emerged here!') and the bit where the thigh would join and support a pelvis that must have belonged to an animal weighing fifteen tons or more and adapted to wading in water. When I managed to get another word in edgeways I revealed what the bone really was. Sudden gloom descended and the television team, grown silent and wan, moved off as one man to the Drumnadrochit Hotel for restoratives. Later it was found that the 'monster bone' was identical to one which was missing from the garden of a museum in York.

When we got back to our dried-blood bait, the warm weather was continuing to produce an understandable effect. Nobody would come within fifty yards of us and we were attracting the attention of half the fly population of the north of Scotland. We loaded the bait, ten pounds at a time, into muslin bags.

These were to be suspended from buoys in areas of the loch where monster sightings had been most frequent. We were also going to groundbait an area of the loch with the stuff at a point where batteries of both fixed and shipboard sonar equipment would be scanning. In addition, the monsters would be driven into this area by boats carrying noise machines and moving up from either end of the loch. Only the sonar-covered, baited area would remain free of noise. With any luck this is where the monsters would arrive as the noise-makers approached one another. I, together with my dart-gun and dozens of photographers and TV cameras, would wait silently on a launch moored in the centre of the target area and surrounded by water redolent with the special bait.

There had been some problems in deciding my duties as anaesthetist/marksman. A strong Scottish conservationist element was breathing terrible threats of what would happen should the monster be inadvertently killed. How was I to calculate my dose for the flying syringe when I had no idea of species or weight? A biopsy would enable us to identify the creature and I had experimented using the syringe needles as biopsy samplers, recovering the darts by means of very strong but fine nylon line attached to the missile before firing. I was not impressed: the technique was clumsy and unreliable. In the end I decided to dart any monster that made an appearance with valium, a tranquilliser which is effective in a very wide range of wild animals but which would not produce anaesthesia and possible death if the monster dived below the surface. Perhaps a tranquillised Nessie would be more forthcoming and lose some of her obsessive shyness.

On the day of the big sweep the noise-makers came slowly towards us, while I stood on the prow of the launch looking down at the black water and Martin bobbed about in a dinghy scattering dried-blood bait onto the waves as an extra enticement. Everyone was in position. Anything moving underwater at any depth in the silent target zone would be picked up and recorded on the sonar tapes. Somewhere in the black water beneath our launch lurked out two one-man submarines carrying powerful searchlights and cameras. They should be the first to catch a glimpse of the monsters. Then, so the planning ran, the animals would break the surface just over there, a few yards from where I stood, and within a few minutes the dozens of cameras mounted on the launch and the other boats would prove once and for all the nature of Scotland's most famous inhabitant. It was foolproof and precise, according to the Director of Operations. Any monster was bound to surface in camera for the benefit of the TV people. Nessie, for the first time in a millennia of her existence, was about to be produced.

With our hearts in our mouths we saw the noise-making boats reach their final positions just outside the target area and stop. There was not a sound as we stared intently at the small area of choppy water where the monster must now be lying. Cameramen focused on the water surface where Nessie must surely now emerge. I aimed my rifle at the spot. There was a loaded syringe up the spout and the safety catch was off. Then, breaking the silence, the radio telephone laconically announced that the sonar scanners could find nothing in the area. The monsters had failed to co-operate. We would try again, but next time at night.

The expedition persevered but Nessie either snoozed in her underwater caverns or cared not a fig for the puny noise-maker brought along by the Navy. Just before we left Loch Ness at the end of the venture we used the remainder of our bait in bags attached to free-floating oil drums. The drifting drums would be kept under observation by the members of the Investigation Bureau who manned strategic points on the banks of the loch throughout the summer and autumn. Some days later when we were back in England we received a report that the crew of a fishing boat, the *Snowdrop*, passing through the loch on their way to the Caledonian Canal, had been frightened out of their wits by two monsters apparently fighting over a yellow oil drum. It would be nice to think that the beasts were squabbling over the free meal which we had cooked up for them.

Undoubtedly the most exciting aspect of zoo animal medicine is that concerning birth. Most exotic creatures have little trouble in giving birth to their young and although there are fertility problems in many species, obstetric complications are rare. It is always a privilege to be able to witness the birth of a young chimpanzee or antelope or dolphin, but to be called on to give assistance in a difficult labour has a magic of its own. The mothers almost always seem to understand that you are there to give a hand and rarely, even with the wildest species, react badly when you get down to brass tacks at their rear ends. I have never been kicked by a giraffe or wildebeest as I have followed it around with my arm deep inside the womb straightening out the knotted legs and badly positioned head of a wriggling calf that has jammed on the way out. For giraffes there is usually a man carrying an orange-box for me to stand on. The straining mother moves slowly about her pen. When she stops the box is placed for me and, with an arm coated in lubricant antiseptic jelly, I feel inside to determine the problem. If I pull the calf's limb or head the mother will normally push and bear down with her powerful abdominal muscles, but if she moves on I quickly jump off the box and chase after her with my assistant. Getting someone to feed the mother pieces of brown bread on such occasions is a considerable help.

All the baby dolphins I have been called to see so far have arrived speedily and unaided. My only difficult dolphin birth was one where my patient and I were 1400 miles apart: an animal in Malta was having great difficulty giving birth and I conducted the calving over the telephone. A nurse and the local government vet worked on the dolphin while an assistant standing at the telephone at the side of the pool relayed my instructions. After exchanging information and advice to and fro continuously for about three quarters of an hour, I was relieved to hear above the crackle and hum on the wires the sudden cries of delight from the midwives as the pointed head of the baby dolphin at last came free.

Occasionally I have to give the mother an anaesthetic in order to tackle a more complicated delivery snarl-up, as in the case of a powerfully built zebra belonging to Flamingo Park Zoo in Yorkshire. The keepers had seen afterbirth hanging from her for some hours and assumed that she had foaled and that the foal was somewhere in the zebra reserve, but a careful search revealed nothing. I was called in and examined the nervous animal at a distance through binoculars. She still had the afterbirth dangling. The fact that her tummy was rounded and bulging did not necessarily mean that a foal was still in there, as zebras' shapes can be very deceptive. Then I saw her stand and lift the floor of her abdomen in a long, powerful contraction. A small white object appeared outside the birth canal and then popped back in again as she stopped straining. It was the delicate little hoof of the baby zebra emerging under pressure. I decided to leave well alone for two hours and then re-assess the position. Two hours later I returned to the zebra reserve. Peering through the binoculars I saw no sign of straining, although the baby had still not been born. No part of the foal was visible and the mother seemed to be duller and more tired. All was not going well, and I decided to intervene.

Because the animal could not be closely approached I would use the long-range dart-gun. I had found that it was possible to get closer to groups of deer, antelope and zebra by taking vehicles into their large paddocks rather than by going in on foot, so I decided to take my car in and shoot from that. At the time I had a Citroën saloon whose adjustable suspension made riding at speed over rough ground and firing a rifle at the same time, as if from a Western stagecoach, fairly easy. A keeper drove my car towards the mother-to-be and when in range I pulled the trigger. The syringe thwacked into her buttocks and she moved a few paces, flicking at it with her tail. The missile hits so fast that it produces no more pain than a smack of a hand so the target rarely runs off in alarm. Five minutes later the zebra was asleep on the ground and I began my internal examination. The foal was terribly tangled up with itself and I could detect no sign of life in it. Although I could unravel the awkwardly bent legs, struggle as I might I could not position correctly the foal's head, which was bent backwards deep into the womb and also twisted round on itself. The mother's natural lubricating liquids were drying up. I had no choice but to try a Caesarean operation.

Caesareans in the horse family, of which the zebra is a member, are still not common. Horses were at one time far greater risks for this type of operation than cattle or sheep, since they get peritonitis after abdominal surgery at the drop of a hat and until the development of modern anaesthetics and antibiotics did not have much of a chance: even today there are unsolved problems in major abdominal surgery of the horse. Cattle, on the other hand, have a tough constitution and an abdominal cavity whose design resists the onset of peritonitis, while Caesarean operations on domestic animals are of course very common. In fact, the first successful operation on the bitch was carried out as long ago as 1824, by a vet in my home town of Rochdale. In zoo animals Caesareans are quite often performed on the big cats and on primates, but on zebras and other exotic horses nothing had been done before this case. But I had no option. I had to open her up.

A tractor pulled the sleeping zebra into the stable on a sledge improvised from an old door. For a large animal like this there is rarely a spotless, aseptic operating theatre at hand so we have to operate literally in the field. After reinforcing the anaesthesia by numbing the belly with local anaesthetic I cut quickly through the skin and muscle and peritoneal tissues, bringing the bulging uterus into the light of day. As usual with wild animals there was none of the messy fat tissue which clogs up the operation site in so many obese and pampered pets. I opened the womb and the striped leg of the foal popped out. Perhaps there was still a flicker of life. I pulled, and the slim

91

and perfect form of the baby zebra slid out onto the side of its unconscious dam. Ignoring the mother for the moment I quickly opened her foal's mouth and hooked the mucus out of its throat with my fingers. Then I took it by its hind fetlocks and whirled it round and round my body as fast as possible, trying to clear its breathing tubes by centrifugal force. I stopped and listened. If its heart was beating I could not detect it. I gave an injection of stimulant and dropped some liquid on the back of the tiny tongue to kick the breathing centres into action. Still nothing. Finally I tried mouth to mouth respiration, packing the slippery little muzzle into my mouth and blowing as hard as I could. It was no use. The foal could not respond. It was dead.

The mother still had to be saved for her next son. I scrubbed up again and went back to work stitching up the layers in the operation wound. Before closing the abdomen I left behind in the peritoneal cavity a handful of antibiotic tablets and sprayed the bowels with a chemical to stop peritonitis sticking them together. Finally I sutured the tough skin, tearing my fingers as I gripped the large curved needles with their cutting edges. Finished. The zebra was breathing strongly. Surprisingly little blood had been lost during the operation, hardly more than a tablespoonful. I gave her a precautionary dose of antibiotics injected into her neck, then the anaesthetic antidote. Two minutes later she snorted, righted herself, rose and walked sedately out to the reserve. I was happy to see her go, for the reserve was a cleaner place for post-operative recovery than a dusty stable.

The zebra never looked back. She recovered superbly from the operation without the slightest hint of complications. The following year she was proudly to produce unaided and unobserved the most charming little zebra filly one could wish to see.

Ten

'Can you go out straightaway to Pakistan?' the question came over the telephone. 'There's a chap near the border with Afghanistan who claims he's got pigmy sperm whales.'

I was accustomed to all manner of unusual requests from Pentland Hick, the owner of Flamingo Park in Yorkshire and of the zebra on which I had just performed the first Caesarean operation in the species. An expert entomologist and a pioneer of the boom in displays of performing dolphins in Europe, he was an entrepreneur of imagination and audacity. He was always looking for new ideas in animal exhibition, and was responsible for Cuddles, the first killer whale to be brought to England. He was also responsible for my initiation into the fascinating world of marine mammal medicine: realising that medical care and water management were the keys to the successful management of porpoises, dolphins and whales, he sent me all over the world, but most importantly to the United States on several occasions, to learn at first hand about the catching, handling and water requirements of these amazing creatures. It was through his enthusiastic support that I spent time with the undersea warfare division of the US Navy, and went clambering about the ice floes of Greenland in search of the strange unicorn of the sea, the narwhal. Now here was Pentland Hick off on yet another tack.

Kogia breviceps, the pigmy sperm whale, is a charming miniaturisation of the cachalot or sperm whale. Never growing much above seven feet in length, as compared to the sperm whale's length of fifty to sixty feet, it appears to be widely distributed throughout the oceans of the world although it is

93

very rarely seen by man. It tends to swim alone or in small groups and feeds on squid and probably crabs. Virtually nothing is known about its habits or reproduction, but the facts that it was small, weighed only 600 to 700 pounds, and would therefore be easy to transport, and that it had teeth and preferred food which is readily available in Britain, made it a suitable and exciting prospect for Hick's expanding collection of cetacean species. Two other small whales on which we were working at the time, the beluga and the narwhal, needed refrigeration equipment to keep the temperature of their pool down to Arctic levels. Kogia seemed to be a frequenter of much more temperate waters and therefore easier to keep.

The man who had written to Pentland Hick with the offer of pigmy sperm whales was unknown to us. He was apparently a Scottish naturalist living in Quetta, the provincial capital of Baluchistan, and dealing in birds and animals of that part of the world which he claimed to supply to zoos in various countries. His name, let us say, was McPherson. Apart from friends at the Steinhart Aquarium in San Francisco who said that they had met a man of that name while collecting freshwater dolphins in Pakistan some weeks earlier, I could find no-one in the zoo or animal business who had heard of him. Still, his letter stated plainly and without ambiguity that he had got *Kogia breviceps* for sale and at a reasonable price.

'I want you to go out as soon as possible and see what McPherson has got to offer,' said Hick. 'We can't afford to run the risk of anyone else in Europe beating us to it.'

As soon as possible was the next day. I booked my flight to Karachi by radio telephone while driving back from Flamingo Park to Rochdale. One thing that puzzled me when I got back and consulted the atlas was that Quetta is situated hundreds of miles from the sea in the rugged hills of the north-west frontier – an unusual base for whale-catching. I could not recall any reference to such goings-on in those stirring films that featured Errol Flynn and his lancers.

I flew out to Karachi via Moscow on PIA, a thoroughly

miserable flight; within thirty minutes of leaving Heathrow almost all the passengers had been air-sick. After a brief rest in Karachi I took off again, this time in a small and rather ancient aeroplane, for Quetta. The passenger sitting next to me was a pleasant but loquacious character with a brother in England whom, he felt sure, I must have met. He was carrying a block of what looked like fudge wrapped in silver paper and weighing about three pounds. It was high-quality cannabis resin and mine to take home as a souvenir for a mere twenty pounds, my companion suggested. After all, he posted it regularly to his brother in Birmingham. I tried to disengage from the conversation by concentrating on the view through the aircraft window as we flew north over red desert country but my neighbour had not finished with me yet. After downing the best part of a pint of whisky from a bottle he produced from his bag, he was apologetically sick all over my trousers. The Pakistan adventure was not beginning well.

The red desert suddenly gave way to a mountainous grey lunar landscape. Valleys and peaks looked uniformly sterile and forbidding, unrelieved by any streams or trees or signs of habitation. As we came in to land at the airfield which serves Quetta, the resemblance to the moon surface was even more striking. We glided down onto a grim grey plateau, the centre of a vast crater in the middle of the mountains. Apart from a small building that served as the air terminal nothing but pallid dust could be seen in any direction. Having collected my bags and discovered that the hotel in Quetta to which PIA in Manchester had cabled to reserve a room for me had been pulled down five years earlier, I found myself standing alone in the dusk outside the terminal wondering where to go and how. Apparently there was no way of getting into the town, some miles away. Apart from the man in the tiny control tower, who did not seem interested in opening his door or window to discover what it was I kept shouting at him, there was no-one about. The aircraft had taken off for its next destination, Peshawar, and the light was beginning to fade.

95

Just then a decrepit old station wagon came rattling down the road. It was tightly packed with fierce-looking Pathans and an assortment of skinny goats and sheep. Desperate to get moving, I ran out into the road and flagged the vehicle down. It stopped and I scrambled thankfully into the tight press of smelly animals. The men said not a word to me and hardly cast a glance in my direction. It was as if they had not noticed the addition to their load. We rumbled off in clouds of dust and eventually arrived at the town. When the wagon stopped in a narrow street of dilapidated wooden shacks and stinking open sewers, I got out and thanked the driver, who drove on without acknowledging my farewells in any way. By this time I was very dishevelled and reeked of an outlandish mixture of human vomit and goat.

It was a long time before I found someone who spoke English and who could direct me to the only hotel in Quetta, a decaying wooden relic of the British Empire called, of all things, the Regina Coeli. An unprepossessing character, unshaven and with a wall eye, who spoke a little English, informed me that I would be their sole guest and showed me to the filthest suite of rooms I have ever seen. Darkness had fallen and it had grown bitterly cold. My host brought a home-made metal stove and set it up in my room. He explained its intricacies and temperamental ways and sold me a quantity of oil for it at an astronomical price. By the light of its noisy, fluctuating flame I was able, once I was alone, to explore the four rooms I had been given, including a lavatory built directly over an evil cesspit. There were doors everywhere, behind which I could hear people shuffling about and murmuring. Whoever they were they seemed to be constantly on the threshold of the other side of the doors. It was eerie and disturbing. With much difficulty, for apart from a low wooden bed and the stove there was not a scrap of furniture in the rooms, I secured all the entrances with bits of wood or stone wedged under the doors. I closed the shutters and wired them so that they could not be opened from outside and went to bed.

As I lay on the low bed I noticed an irregular pattern of red dots decorating the crumbling white plaster of the walls. It was difficult to tell what they were by the light of the stove so I struck a match for closer inspection. They were the bloody patches where countless fingers had squashed bed bugs into oblivion. I could see the thumbprints and the fragments of corpses ground into the plaster. Thoroughly dismayed I got up and took the cowl off the stove. The flames soared up to the ceiling and coated it with oily soot. Now I could see better. I had never actually met *Cimex lectularius*, the bed bug, in person but I had studied him and his kind when doing my Fellowship and knew where he was likely to be found. Sure enough, from the cracks in the dry rot of the skirting board and from wide cracks in the wall plaster, like climbers from a rock chimney, the flat and unmistakable insects were beginning to emerge. I stripped the bed, found and eradicated more of them. Finally, with oil from the stove I made shallow pools on the stone floor round the bed legs and painted a strip of oil round all four walls to prevent my unwelcome companions from climbing up to the ceiling and launching parachute attacks. Exhausted and miserable, cold and damp, still smelling of goat and other things, I eventually fell asleep fully clothed on the top of the bed.

A peep into the kitchen the following morning and I decided to fast for as long as I was in the hotel. The cook thought it most strange that I would take nothing but tea and that without milk. Hunger was now added to my miseries, but I was reluctant to share their repast with the two enormous brown rats that I had just seen sitting in a cooling pan of vegetables and eating unhurriedly from the warm pottage in which they reclined.

My job was to find McPherson and his pigmy sperm whales and then to get out of Quetta with all speed. Finding him proved to be almost impossible. The hotel owner knew of no Englishman or Scot with such a name in the town. He could not think of any Europeans in the place at all, except for the strange young people who passed through from time to time on their way from Afghanistan to India: Quetta is a watering place on the twentieth-century pilgrims' way. I went into the town past the derelict barracks and rusting cannon still bearing the names of famous British regiments, down streets lined by windowless wooden dwellings as small as police boxes and with sacks for doors, and across weedy fields where white mosques gleamed against the grey backdrop of the mountains. Quetta looks like what it in fact is, a frontier town. It was devastated by an earthquake in 1935 and has never recovered. I found the police station, the office of the agriculture ministry and the municipal headquarters. No-one had heard of McPherson nor of any naturalists working in the area. As for whales, even the English-speaking people that I met did not understand the meaning of the word. When I drew a picture of a whale to make matters clearer their eyes opened wide and they looked at me curiously. 'But the sea is far away, sir,' said one puzzled policeman.

All day I wandered through the town looking for clues to the whereabouts of McPherson. Knots of tall, striking-looking Baluch tribesmen standing on the corners found me an object of great curiosity and some amusement as I tried to orientate myself with the aid of a street map of 1940 vintage. McPherson's letter naturally bore an address. Not only could I not find the street on my map, but no-one I spoke to admitted any knowledge of such a place. The day ended with me no nearer finding the elusive naturalist but my hunger was growing and the weather was becoming colder, threatening rain. I spent another unhappy night at the hotel fortified only by tea and lay awake most of the night as a great storm swept down from the mountains and the wind threatened to blow the building away.

Off I went round the town again the next morning. I was becoming convinced that McPherson was some sort of confidence trickster trying to extract money by false pretences from Pentland Hick. Perhaps he had been hoping to obtain a deposit in advance. But in that case why pick on Quetta as a supposed base for his marine operations? And if the address was false, as seemed likely, how could money sent by mail possibly reach him? I decided to try the post office again. The day before I had drawn a blank but surely if the man or his address had ever existed in Quetta he must have received post. I went into the post office building and stood looking at the rows of numbered post boxes. Someone tapped me on my shoulder. I looked round to find a large, smartly dressed policeman with a swagger stick confronting me.

'Dr Taylor, sir?' he enquired politely. 'I wonder if you would be kind enough to come with me. My Superintendent would like to meet you.'

He led me out to his jeep. A fat man with bloodshot eyes and a nude blonde painted on his tie sat silently in the back seat. We bounced through the rough, rubble-strewn streets and stopped outside a tall building covered with peeling pink paint. The policeman led me inside and the fat man followed behind. We entered an office where another policeman sat at a desk and a civilian wearing gumboots on a settee against one wall. The man behind the desk smiled, introduced himself as the Superintendent and asked me to sit down. This must be something to do with the guy on the plane, I thought, my sick friend with the cannabis.

'Dr Taylor, I have asked you to come in to see us,' the Superintendent began, 'because we believe you are having difficulties finding an acquaintance of yours.'

Very civil, I thought, perhaps they have located him for me. 'Yes,' I said, 'Mr McPherson, the naturalist.'

The man with bloodshot eyes grunted loudly. There was silence for a few moments.

'McPherson, the naturalist.' The Superintendent repeated my words slowly as if reflecting on them. 'Are you here to see him on business or on pleasure?'

'Business. I'm up here to see him about whales. I'm a veterinary surgeon.'

Now the fat bloodshot individual grunted again and spoke

for the first time. 'Dr Taylor, a veterinary surgeon, eh? An animal doctor from England, eh? To see McPherson the naturalist, eh?'

'Yes indeed,' I replied, beginning to feel a little uneasy. 'Why? Is there something odd about that?'

The Superintendent spoke again. 'This is Major Darwish,' he said, indicating the fat man, 'Major Darwish of Military Security.'

For the next hour I sat while Major Darwish explained the reason for this interview. There was political trouble in Baluchistan, moves for regional autonomy, even secession. It was a sensitive area, border problems, big power interest and so on. The Pakistan Government had detected American CIA activity in the border area based on Quetta. Some Americans had been asked to leave the country and McPherson was thought to be implicated in the whole business.

'We've got our eye on your Mr McPherson,' said Major Darwish, 'and we've got our eye on anyone who comes up here trying to fish in troubled waters. The tribal problems are delicate enough for Karachi without foreigners making matters worse.' He leaned forward towards me and spoke in a mock confidential tone. 'Do you know Quetta has been crawling with CIA men?'

The penny dropped. I had been hauled in as a possible agent of a foreign power!

'You don't think I'm a CIA man, do you?' I laughed, perhaps a shade too heartily.

There was silence, then the Superintendent said, 'But we are told, Dr Taylor, that you are an animal doctor looking for a man who has whales, that you have been enquiring around town as to where he lives and saying to people that you are here to inspect sea animals. We do not have whales or sea animals in Quetta. The sea is far away. And we are wishing to assure ourselves that what you tell us is right.'

'It is right,' I said with some annoyance. 'That's why I'm here.'

100

'We would like to be sure that you are indeed an animal doctor,' cut in Darwish. 'What university did you attend?'

I gave them a terse curriculum vitae and finished by saying that if they would produce a horse or a goat for a demonstration of my trade I would prove I was telling the truth by castrating it neatly on the spot.

'Well,' said Darwish, 'that won't be necessary. This gentleman is Dr Mohammed, a veterinary graduate of Lahore who works in the government service here.' He pointed to the man sitting silently in his gumboots. 'I think Dr Mohammed might ask you a couple of questions to validate your claim to be a veterinary surgeon. I'm sure you will understand.'

I was stunned. Here was I, suspected of being a spy in the fastnesses of the north-west frontier, about to be given a viva voce by another vet about whom I knew nothing. What if he had firm but erroneous opinions on some matter on which he questioned me? And was there not a good chance that he would ask me about some local malady about which I knew little or nothing? Dr Mohammed stood up importantly and cleared his throat.

'Now, sir,' he began with an air of great solemnity, 'would you kindly answer the following three questions. Firstly, what is the volume of the gall bladder in the mule? Secondly, for what do I use butter of antimony? And thirdly, what is Bang's disease?'

He sat down with a satisfied smile. Everyone looked at me. The first question was a trick one.

'Well, Dr Mohammed,' I said, 'the answer to the one about the gall bladder of the mule is that its volume is exactly the same as that of the dolphin's gall bladder.'

Dr Mohammed jumped to his feet with gleaming eyes. 'Aha,' he exclaimed, somewhat theatrically, 'you really will have to be more explicit than that. I asked you the volume. Approximately how many c.c.'s?'

'Like I said, the same as a dolphin or in other words, zero.' Horses and mules and whales and dolphins do not possess gall

101

bladders although they do produce bile and have bile ducts.

Mohammed sat down again looking a trifle crestfallen.

'The second question about butter of antimony is a bit old-fashioned,' I continued. 'I've not seen it used for years but it was applied to foot infections in cattle. Bang's disease is contagious brucella abortion.'

There was another long silence and then Darwish began a lengthy questioning of Dr Mohammed in Urdu. Eventually he turned to me.

'Dr Taylor, you may go, we are satisfied. We wish you well in your search for Mr McPherson.'

'But I assume you know where he is,' I said. 'You say you're keeping an eye on him. How do I find him?'

'I'm sorry,' replied the Superintendent. 'He was here but we don't know where he is now.'

Everyone looked a bit sheepish and I realised that my interview was over and that I was not going to get any more out of them. Thanking them I left the building and took a bicycle rickshaw back to the hotel. I would leave next morning for Karachi. McPherson had been the cause of a wild goose chase. Pigmy sperm whales indeed!

The hotel keeper said that there would be no flights out on the following day. The storms were still blowing in the mountains and the small aircraft could not make it over the high peaks encircling the town. In low spirits I sat in my room drinking tea and hungrier than ever. Somehow I felt that it might be worth one more try at finding McPherson, especially as I would have to spend at least another day in this dreary place anyway.

The next morning dawned grey and showery. Walking down into the town I puzzled over where to make more enquiries. As I stood looking round, a sign on a small bungalow across the road caught my eye. 'Ministry of Forests' it read. Perhaps they knew of naturalists going on expeditions in areas under their supervision. I went in and asked the first person I saw for the director. He got my meaning and took me through dim corridors cluttered with ragged figures squatting in corners and against walls. The Director of Forestry was a pleasant little man who spoke some English. To my delight, when I brought up the question of McPherson, the naturalist, I did not receive the expected blank look and shake of the head.

'I think I know who you mean,' he said. 'I'm not certain of the name but there is an Englishman.' He rang a bell and an assistant appeared. 'I'll get Hussein here to take you.'

I was elated. It looked as if I had done it at last. Hussein hailed a bicycle rickshaw and we climbed in. Through the middle of the town we went and into an area which I had not explored on foot. The streets became narrower and the tarmac gave way to dirt tracks between tightly packed wooden hovels. We rattled through a maze of muddy lanes where beggars crouched over open sewers and thin dogs covered with sores barked and howled. We were in the worst of the slums, surely on the wrong track. Abruptly we came upon the only proper building in the middle of that odorous shanty town, a dirty white bungalow that had known far better days and was surrounded by a high wall of dried mud. We stopped and paid off the rickshaw driver and knocked on the gate. After much barking of dogs it opened and a young man in baggy trousers whom I took to be a house-boy let us in. I explained why we were there and he took us into the house.

Inside it was dim and smoky. We were led into a large room that looked like a curio shop. Stuffed animals were piled around the walls, trinkets and weapons and articles of falconry equipment hung in clusters from the ceiling. Three hawks sat on blocks in the middle of the stone floor. In the light of the log fire, lying on a sofa drawn up close to the hearth, lay a European of about forty with tangled hair and a reddish beard. He was sleeping fully dressed in grubby clothes. His face was covered in big drops of sweat and his hands and arms were a mass of nasty sores. The house-boy gently roused the sleeping figure, who opened his eyes but made no attempt to rise.

'Good morning,' I said, as he blinked at me and wiped his eyes feebly. 'I'm Dr Taylor from Flamingo Park, England. Are you Mr McPherson by any chance?'

In a polished public-school accent he replied, 'I am, but I'm afraid I'm not well at present. You shouldn't have come out here until I asked you to come.'

His voice was weak and tired. The sores on his arms were going septic and the lymphatic channels stood out in dull red lines. I asked him what was wrong. Apparently he had been severely bitten by some falcons and was obviously at least on the brink of septicaemia. I always carry a selection of broad-spectrum antibiotics when visiting the East, so I gave him all the terramycin tablets I had. He accepted them gratefully. Apparently antibiotics were hard to come by and expensive, and it was clear that he was very short of cash. I told him I would give the antibiotics time to take effect and start reducing his fever, then I would return later in the day and talk with him.

After spending the day in the foothills outside the town I returned alone to McPherson's house with the aid of a scrap of paper on which his house-boy had written the directions for the rickshaw driver. McPherson was looking a bit better, sitting up and dressing his wounds. I got straight down to brass tacks – I had come to see his pigmy sperm whales. He had problems there, it appeared. The whales were six hundred miles away by the coast. Could I go down to see them? No, because he hadn't known I was arriving and would be unable to accompany me. Alone then? Well, no, that would be difficult.

I began to realise that my whole trip had been in vain. As we talked I found him anxious to discuss the financial aspects of the matter and keen to describe how he had trapped the animals, but gradually I pressed him to tell me precisely how many whales he actually had and exactly where. Of course he had none, nor did his catching facilities and holding pools seem to have much substance. He showed me photographs of sea-scapes and muddy estuaries but on none were there any traces of sea mammals. They could have been taken anywhere. He was adamant that he could not accompany me to the coast.

'I shall go alone and look around for myself,' I said.

'If only you had waited until I told you to come,' McPherson replied, 'I could have shown you pigmy sperms.'

He could not explain why his letter had so enthusiastically assured customers that the whales were ready and waiting for inspection. I asked him about Major Darwish and the CIA. He agreed that some of his friends had been expelled and showed me the Land Rover they had had to leave behind but he was reluctant to talk further about the matter or to tell me how and why he existed in such an odd place. Apart from the dogs and hawks there were no animals to be seen or heard.

Before I left to pack my bags McPherson said there was something else I might be interested in. What would Pentland Hick offer for a pair of giant pandas? It is impossible to put a price on this most popular and rare of exotic animals but I said that I was sure he would give a million pounds. McPherson had a scheme, on which he was shortly to embark, for smuggling pandas out of China. Would I like to join the expedition? The plan was breathtaking. A team of men, including me as vet to tranquillise the animals and watch their health, would leave Bangladesh (East Pakistan as it then was) and travel by mule and on foot across Assam, skirt the foothills of the Nyenchen-tanglha Mountains of Tibet and reach the panda country of Szechwan in China. The distance was about 850 miles over high uninhabited regions for the second half of the journey. The pandas would be brought back into Pakistan, dyed brown and shipped out as low-value brown bears! McPherson showed me the maps and other documents he had collected in preparation for the expedition.

'Will you join us?' he asked. 'It'll be worth £25,000 to you.'

'I'll wait until we've got some pigmy sperm whales first,' I said. 'Then I might consider it.'

Two days later the weather improved and I took a flight back to Karachi. I decided to visit the fishing villages on the coastline near the city to see what the fishermen knew about sea mammals in the area. My first call was to the offices of the Port Authorities where I asked about whale and dolphin catching by the fishing fleets.

'The fishermen take great pains not to catch or injure dolphins or whales,' the director explained. 'You would not find it possible to persuade them to help you.'

The fishing folk apparently consider cetaceans to be half human and therefore sacred. They base their belief on their knowledge that the sea mammals, unlike fish, produce milk to suckle their young and also make sounds similar to the human voice under certain conditions. What the director had said turned out to be true. I visited a number of primitive fishing communities on the salt flats north-west and south of the city, accompanied by a helpful employee of the Dutch airline KLM, who have a reputation for superb animal transporting facilities. I took with me a book of coloured illustrations of various species of sea mammal. The fact that the labelling and text was all in Japanese did not matter, as the man from KLM asked the fishermen just to point to pictures of any animals that they had ever encountered. I would stand in the middle of a cluster of dried mud dwellings while the people gathered round to stare at the pictures. Men at every village nodded when I pointed to the spinner dolphin. Some knew the pilot whale and the killer. At only one village could I find a man who had apparently seen a pigmy sperm whale and that only in deep water and very infrequently. They smiled and nodded at pictures of the dugong, probable origin of the mermaid myth. Yes, they were well acquainted with her and was she not a cross between man and dolphin? In one village the dugong picture brought much shuffling of feet and embarrassed lowering of heads. The KLM man said that they knew of fishermen who had taken dugong as lovers, but that they did not like to talk about it with strangers. Dugong were trouble. Their wives would scold them for days if they knew that they had even discussed them.

So pigmy sperm whales were not to be. Before leaving

Karachi for home I cabled McPherson to say that there was nothing doing at the coast. Just before I left my hotel to go to the airport he telephoned me from Quetta saying that he had some more of the elusive creatures in a set of ponds about twenty miles east of Karachi. If only I would wait a few days I would see. I was sceptical, but he protested vehemently that he could prove he was telling the truth. To my astonishment McPherson revealed that his house-boy, the young fellow who had let us into his house and stood quietly in the shadows during our conversations, was a qualified vet; McPherson had sent him down to the ponds near Karachi to look after the animals. If I looked over the side of a certain bridge near a Parsee fire temple I would see the animals and the house-boy in two large pools cut out of the rock. If he had had time he would have come down to Karachi to show me himself, he said, and pleaded with me to go to the pools before going home. I told him I would try, and bade him farewell.

Consulting my timetable, I worked out that I had just about enough time to make a forty-mile round trip by taxi before checking in for the flight to England, so off I set in a noisy Chevrolet with wheel wobble. The driver was a diminutive man who came originally from Goa and before letting out the clutch he informed me that he was, undoubtedly like myself, a Christian in an Islamic state. Also he had thirteen children, so would I ensure that his tip at the end of the journey was suitably lavish. I believe he was hinting that in doing so I would be actively supporting the conversion of Pakistan.

We reached the Parsee temple and the bridge. I got out and walked to the side. Below the bridge was a wide dried-out river bed. A number of holes had been scooped out of the rocky bank. Women washed clothes in murky green water from a drain that emptied onto the rocks above them, the liquid finding its way in a dozen trickling streams down to the pools, the solid matter being left behind on the stone to bake in the sunshine. Other women were spreading laundry on the rocks to dry. Two of the pools were much larger than the others and were not being used. In the foul green water of one of them something floated half submerged.

I went down the rocks to the pool and looked at the dark shape hanging motionless in the water. It was a dead baby whale. Its umbilical cord could just be seen running down from the belly into the cloudy depths. There was a rusty old car spring on the ground not far away. I used it to pull in the corpse and flip it out onto the rocks. A new-born pigmy sperm whale! Unable to believe my eyes, I looked around. There was no sign of any other whales nor of McPherson's house-boy/vet nor of anything to suggest that this was the centre for a whale-catching operation. I examined the little body. It was a female and only the second member of the species that I had ever seen in the flesh. How had it got to this place? No-one seemed to take any notice as I began to do a makeshift autopsy on the spot with a penknife produced by the taxi driver. Two things I found that were of importance. One, the animal had not been born dead: it had breathed, for the lungs were fully expanded. Two, there was severe bruising, haemorrhage, splitting of flesh and scorching in the rectal area. The burnt-out case of a firework, the sort English boys call 'bangers', was jammed deep inside the anus.

My head spinning with rage and shock, numb with incomprehension, I was driven to the airport. The whole affair was bitter and bizarre. I never learned any more about that poor little soul, nor how it came to so cruel an end nor at whose hands. I have not heard any more from McPherson, nor to my knowledge has anyone else. I sent a final caustic cable to him in Quetta before leaving Karachi Airport but had no reply. About pigmy sperm whales in Pakistan we are no wiser, although some three months after I returned from this strange visit there arrived at Flamingo Park an unsigned cable that read 'PLEASE SEND FORTY YARDS STRONG TAPE FOR CONSTRUCTING CARRYING SLINGS PIGMY SPERMS URGENT'. The telegraph office of origin was Quetta.

Eleven

So little research has been done in exotic animal medicine compared to the other branches of veterinary science that a zoo vet must seize on any scraps of information which might help him in his work. Thus it was that I took my first lessons in the care of the camel from the manual of the Royal Army Veterinary Corps. Not much has been published about the health problems of camels, but somewhere I had found an ancient copy of this work and among the masses of information on unlikely things such as how to dispose of dead horses at sea and how many miles a pack mule can be expected to go on so many pounds of groundsel, I found what the Army knew about camels and their problems in days when military men considered such knowledge essential.

A camel in the Manchester Zoo which had been in England for almost three years was becoming thin and debilitated for no apparent reason. Try as I might I could not find any firm cause, and tonics, pick-me-ups and vitamins were not having much effect. After some weeks of illness swellings began to appear on the camel's sides and legs. The tissues in these regions were soggy: if you pushed your finger in you left a dent that stayed for hours as if in putty. The camel was developing dropsy. I checked and re-checked the heart, took urine samples for more tests of kidney function, and sent blood to the laboratory for analysis of liver function. But no, the dropsy was coming from none of the expected sources. There did not seem to be much wrong with heart, liver or kidneys.

The case puzzled me. I read what little I could find in the

pathology books I had available without getting much further. One day I remembered that the Army manual had talked about certain important diseases and I vaguely recalled something about surra, a kind of sleeping sickness similar to the well-known tropical disease of humans and caused by a trypanosome parasite which is carried by biting flies. It attacks camels in Africa and Asia and other animals including the horse, buffalo, elephant and tapir. Surra does not occur naturally in Europe. I searched for the manual but could not find it, indeed I never have found it again, but I had remembered enough to set out on a new trail. Surra produced lumps or bumps of some kind. I went to the Medical School library in Manchester to consult the books on protozoology. There it was. Surra: trypanosomiasis of camels. Caused by a rather elegant protozoan parasite in the blood. Common in Egypt, Africa, etc.

Could this be a case of tropical trypanosomiasis in darkest Manchester? I examined the camel once more and took more blood, this time to make smears which I could examine myself for the presence of the parasite. Not a thing. No parasite. More blood, more smears. Still nothing. I sat at the microscope with my eyes aching and my hopes of a clinching diagnosis receding. I decided to take more blood from the animal but at a different time of day, since some of these parasites are creatures of habit and only seem to go promenading in the blood at certain times of day. I took blood at night. Still nothing. Then I tried a sample first thing in the morning. The camel, miserable as it was, was becoming thoroughly fed up at the repeated jabs from my needle. I was having trouble washing the smell of camel puke from my hair. The latest sample was stained in the usual way with dyes to bring out contrasting colours in the blood corpuscles and anything else that might be there. I scanned field after field through the lenses until little red discs filled my eyes. Suddenly there it was! A beautiful object to look at, coloured by the stains at the moment of its death and preserved for ever, a sinuous twist of

110

lilac and purple veil. A trypanosome. You only need one to clinch it. I had a case of surra.

When I rang up ICI and asked for what I needed the man at the other end of the telephone thought I was pulling his leg.

'You're D. C. Taylor of Rochdale and you've got a case of camel trypanosomiasis?' He paused. 'Rochdale in Lancashire, you mean?'

'Yes,' I said, 'and I believe you make a drug to cure it.'

The ICI man said he would have to have a word with somebody and I could faintly hear the comments as he left the telephone and recounted the gist of my request to the office at large. There was some guffawing and something about somebody having somebody else on. The man returned to the phone.

'Well, how many doses will you need? We only sell it for export normally. It's in packs of a hundred doses.'

'I only need enough to treat one camel,' I replied. 'Can you split the pack?' Rochdale doesn't see many camels. I imagined having difficulty getting rid of the other ninety-nine doses.

ICI turned out to be most co-operative. They sent me a specially packed single course of treatment for my surra case. The animal had obviously been infected with the parasite when it first came to Britain nearly three years previously. All that time the bug had been slowly nibbling away inside it. At least things turned out well: the anti-surra compound worked as efficiently in Manchester as it is said to do in Africa, the dropsy subsided and in due course the camel regained a plump, healthy weight.

Camels are fascinating animals, tough, uncomplaining about work and beautifully and functionally built, but the contents of their stomachs seem to have an affinity for suede leather. Once together the two cannot be parted. This I discovered when, clad in an expensive and much prized suede jacket but unprotected by an overall, I examined my first camel. I knew as we all do that camels spit but I did not realise what little it takes to make them spit. Camels will spit for the slightest provocation, real or imagined, they will spit pre-emptively to start trouble or defensively even if only looked at in the wrong way. What is more, the word 'spit' conjures up a picture of relatively limited quantities of frothy saliva, the sort schoolboys eject, whereas camel spit is in fact a bottomless well of smelly, green, partly digested stomach contents that are sprayed as a broadside or aimed in a single noxious blob of flying soup. This makes examining camels something of a specialised art. Putting an old jacket over the camel's head is said to help but I have known a wily beast spit accurately down the sleeves of the garment.

Camels can also kick in any direction with any or all of their legs, if necessary at the same time, and they try to heighten the effect of spitting by making awful gurgling noises and extruding a heaving pink sausage, part of the lining of the mouth, from between yellow teeth. They can bite very severely and with purpose and Moses, a magnificent but stroppy male Bactrian camel at Manchester, is one of the most dangerous zoo animals I know. I saw what he did to a kindly old man who, without permission, went into the camel pen to stroke him. Camels can build up a pressure cooker of resentment towards human beings, then the lid suddenly blows off and they go berserk. In Asia when a camel gets to this high pitch of bottled-up tension the camel driver senses the brooding trouble and takes off his coat and gives it to the animal. Then, rather like the Japanese workers who are provided with special rooms where they can work off their frustrations and resentments by beating up models of their executives, the camel gives the garment hell. He jumps on it, rips it, bites it, tears it to pieces. When it is all over and the camel feels that it has blown its top enough, man and animal can live together in harmony again.

Andrew and I had ample opportunity to study the contrariness of the species at close quarters when we went twice in the same day from Manchester to Prague to pick up a consignment of Bactrian camels. The camels were from Asian Russia, semi-wild and grumpy. Some had vicious rope halters running

112

tightly round their heads and through holes bored in their ears. They had been branded on the cheeks with hot irons months or years before and had been fitted with the halters when quite small. As the camels had grown the halters had cut deep into the flesh and in some places had disappeared completely beneath the skin. Before loading in Prague our first job was to cut off these evil devices but, even so, for one poor creature it was too late. The dirty rope sawing away interminably at its head had introduced tetanus germs into the body and it was showing the first symptoms of lockjaw, a terrible disease to witness. At least when we got it back to Manchester we were able to give it treatment and relieve the agonising muscular spasms, but the unfortunate animal died.

Everything went well with the loading at Prague. A communist soldier stood guard outside the aircraft's lavatory door to ensure that no-one stowed away in there, while the poor veterinary surgeon from Prague Zoo who handed the animals over to us was not even allowed to set foot inside the cargo hold or cabin at all. He would dearly have liked to see his charges settled down in the plane but the authorities were not taking any chances that he might somehow disappear amongst the grunting, shuffling crowd of Bactrians. Instead we gave him a bottle of whisky and some bottles of a superb new zoo animal anaesthetic and he gave us in exchange some Czech aerosols for treating skin diseases.

The camels behaved themselves perfectly. Once aboard the aircraft almost all of them sat quietly down and we did not need to use a single dose of sedative. The flight back to Manchester was uneventful, with not so much as a peep out of the animals. We landed at Ringway Airport where transport and lots of keepers from the zoo were waiting to help us unload. By this time all the camels were sitting down and relaxing. They were superb air travellers. Now we had to get them onto their feet to walk them down the ramp into the special fly-screened quarantine van that would take them to the zoo. Camels and their relatives, the llamas, alpacas and vicunas, are easily offended. They sit down for a variety of reasons such as annoyance, disgust, boredom, fright or just to be unco-operative. Sometimes, of course, they sit down for the pleasure of it. When sitting down they may insist on rising for the same reasons. The general rule is that they will do the exact opposite of what the humans round them want them to do. This was a typical case: the complete cargo of camels in the aircraft decided, as one camel, not to get to their feet. Presumably they felt that they had done us enough favours that day in allowing themselves to be loaded so easily and then transported across Europe and that it was time for them to give us a bit of stick.

We tried shouting, slapping, lifting tails, blowing down ears and prodding with a stick. Nothing worked. Camel spittle began to fly around. Not one solitary camel was prepared to budge. They sat quietly resting on their briskets as if bolted to the floor. In the end they won. Each one had to be lifted by hand and carried bodily down to the van. It breaks the backs of five or six men to pick up a mature camel in this way and we had fifteen on board and another fifteen in the second consignment waiting in Prague. At last it was done. We flew back to Czechoslovakia and collected the rest. Again they travelled perfectly but, once they had landed at Manchester, became completely unco-operative and had to be carried out like the first bunch. It made the sweating keepers curse when some strapping great bull, who had just insisted on being borne out like a pitiful stretcher case, stood up voluntarily when deposited in the quarantine van and projected a gurgling stream of stomach contents at his erstwhile bearers.

Once in quarantine in Manchester the camels had to be observed carefully for any sign of disease. As usual we found on the skin of several of them dry scaly areas where the hair had fallen out. They had mange, a very common complaint caused by a minute mite which burrows into the skin. That meant giving the camels special shampoos, spraying every square inch of their body surfaces with a stirrup pump. It is not easy to be sure that the animal is totally wetted by the shampoo

114

but if it is not, a few mites may escape destruction and survive to spread rapidly over the body during the next few weeks. Ideally the camels should be made to swim through a deep dipping tank and their heads dunked under the surface briefly to ensure complete application of the anti-mange chemicals, but very few zoos have that facility.

Another problem Andrew and I found in the camels was the appearance in the droppings of a bacterium related to the tuberculosis germ. We arranged with Cambridge University to perform a delicate and accurate test on the droppings which would spot these germs, the cause of an illness named Johne's disease even when present in only minute numbers. Johne's disease, or paratuberculosis as it is sometimes called, can attack cattle, sheep and goats. Little is known about the effect of the germ on exotic ruminants, so when we began to find large numbers of the bacteria in some of the camels we became rather worried. The camels were not showing the typical symptom of chronic diarrhoea. Were they just carrying the germ harmlessly? Then after some weeks one of the animals began to lose weight and condition steadily. Despite intensive investigation and treatment it became a walking skeleton, but the only thing we could find were clusters of the Johne's bacterium in its droppings. Virtually nothing had been written about Johne's disease in species other than farm animals but we did stumble across a Russian scientific paper which said that the disease had been recorded in a substantial proportion of Bactrian camels and that it could cause death. Our camel in Manchester became in the end so weak and emaciated that it could no longer rise to its feet and the keepers had to bottle-feed it with gruel. One morning it was found dead. An autopsy found the wall of the intestine to be extensively damaged, and the microscope showed lying in the wall the little red rods that are Johne's bacteria.

So Johne's disease was able to treat camels with as little respect as it does domestic cattle. What was worse was that I soon spotted what looked like another case of the disease, this time in a rare sitatunga, a beautiful but very nervous antelope from the secluded swampy forests of Africa. Again there was no persistent diarrhoea as might have been expected but the other symptoms were highly suggestive and we found the germ lurking in the droppings. By now we were very alarmed. Through how many species could this tiny red rod that looks so insignificant under the microscope spread its havoc? No-one had ever seen a case of Johne's disease in sitatunga before. What other new ground were we doomed to break?

One major snag was that there was no certain cure for Johne's disease and vaccination was still being developed. We decided to try an experiment. The germ looks like and indeed is a close relative of the human tuberculosis bacterium. What if we did something not normally feasible for economic reasons in domestic cattle or sheep affected by Johne's disease and treated the sitatunga with a long course of drugs designed to combat TB in humans? We had no choice. Tragically, one of the sitatunga, a younster bred in the zoo, had died and we had found his bowels riddled with the complaint. The others must all go onto the treatment immediately.

Sitatunga panic violently for the slightest reason so handling them provides many headaches. Open the door into their paddock or startle them by some unusual noise after lights-out and they may dash frantically about, colliding with walls or fences and damaging themselves severely. The pop of the dartgun and the slap of the flying syringe are asking for trouble so to examine the sitatunga closely, except in urgent emergencies, I use crushed tranquilliser tablets mixed with their food. Like all antelopes and similar creatures, sitatunga require a far larger dose than a human being of twice the weight or more. To treat the sitatunga with daily doses of streptomycin or even twice-weekly shots of viomycin as used for TB was simply not practical. We would have to rely on rather more old-fashioned anti-tuberculosis chemicals mixed daily in the food.

The treatment seemed promising at first. Symptoms of the

disease faded, but although the numbers of bacteria in the droppings diminished it was impossible to eradicate them altogether and even after months of treatment the animals were not fully cured. The entrenched germs meant that recurrences were likely to occur – sadly, they did.

The finding of this disease in two zoo species prompted us to screen other likely candidates for possible unsuspected infection. More tests at Cambridge found it in a few other ruminants in the zoo. The management at Manchester, who always supported enthusiastically any health programme for the good of their stock, were keen to find out the extent of this hidden problem. In order to compare the position in Manchester with that elsewhere we obtained samples from animals in other British zoos. In a remarkable number of samples from a range of antelope, deer, gazelles and exotic cattle we found the germ.

Although all the zoos had been most willing to co-operate in supplying the samples, the reaction of a few zoos when we found evidence of Johne's disease was surprising. Ostrich-like, they stuck their heads in the sand. They were actually piqued that we had provided evidence that their stock had a potentially dangerous infection in its midst. There was nothing wrong with their stock, they protested. The whole things was absolute nonsense. It must have been some other harmless bug picked up from the grass and simply passed out through the intestines into the droppings! This latter possibility had been provided for in the test developed at Cambridge and we were certain that we were not dealing with cases of bacterial mistaken identity. Despite this, and although we had seen the bug chewing away at the bowel tissues of camels and sitatunga, some very respectable zoological collections dropped the whole matter like a hot potato. They could not contemplate the possibility that all was not well with the animals in their care. There is quite a grapevine in the zoo world and from time to time I hear of animals dying in some of the parks where we found positive samples. The post-mortem findings, so it is whispered, strongly suggest Johne's disease.

Twelve

What happens when a unicorn falls ill? You might suppose that along with mermaids, phoenixes, rocs and griffins these creatures are immune to earthly ills in their faery realms and come more within the province of the sorcerer or elf than the veterinary surgeon. Not so, for in the deserts of Arabia I have attended one of the rarest and most beautiful species on earth and the probable source of the fabulous unicorn.

The Arabian oryx is the most stunning in appearance of all the antelopes. A dazzling creamy colour, with crisp brown face and leg markings, tall and elegant, its head topped with a pair of long, tapering, backward pointing horns, it is superb. So symmetrically are the horns set on its head that viewed from the side it appears to have only one (unicorn) horn. Its colouring is perfectly suited to blend into a background of bleached and blazing sand. Similarly, its anatomy and physiology beneath the handsome exterior have evolved over the millennia into an amazing organism capable of living and reproducing in one of the world's most terrible deserts, the Empty Quarter of Arabia. With ingenious internal tricks to cope with the shortage of natural water and to stop its blood rising to boiling point in the searing heat, with finely tuned senses that can detect danger at great distances in shimmering air or locate springs of water under the sand, and with the ability to outrun all but the fastest carnivore, the Arabian oryx once prospered. Then came the hunters. It was a strong and brave collector of skin and horn who could penetrate the fastnesses of the oryx and at first, because of the risk and effort involved, the number of animals killed was not excessive. But when Arab sheiks with big air-conditioned Chevrolets and sub-machine guns took to updating the hunting, the death warrant for this wild, beautiful animal was sealed. They were slaughtered as trophies until it was believed that not one remained in the wild free state. At least the species did not become extinct, for one Arab sheik, Sheik Qassim of Qatar, captured a number of the oryx and set up a precious breeding herd on his desert farm. Another small herd was established at Phoenix Zoo, Arizona, and a programme started to reintroduce zoo-bred stock into the wild in Oman.

One grey, drizzly breakfast-time in November the telephone rang. It was the Director of Medical Services in Qatar, Dr Gotting. Sheik Qassim's oryx were dying like flies. Could I go at once to see what was up? A first-class ticket on the next flight to the Arabian Gulf would be waiting for me at London Airport.

My bag is always packed. As well as clothing, maps, notebooks and credit cards there are emergency drugs, a basic surgical kit, syringes and needles in sizes suitable for humming birds or hippopotamuses, bottles and plastic bags for samples and a complete range of anaesthetics. To save time on arrival the bag and its contents are just compact enough to be carried as hand baggage. While Shelagh checked that it was all in order I telephoned the Foreign Office: I would need to take the dart-gun which meant getting assistance in oiling the official wheels so that it could be carried out of the country with me. This weapon, designed to carry sleep and healing instead of death, fires an ingenious metal hypodermic syringe by means of carbon dioxide gas pressure. It is loaded with canisters containing carbon dioxide and can throw a syringe fast and accurately up to thirty yards or more. When the syringe hits the target it automatically injects the contents into the animal by means of a small explosive charge that powers the rubber plunger inside. I carry all types of needle in my bag, some suitable for the armour-plating of rhinoceros, some fine and slightly barbed for monkeys, and others with collars on them to ensure the right degree of penetration where under-skin vaccination is required. I never use the crossbow, a powerful weapon which caused the death of a number of deer when I was a student. It throws the syringe with such force that there is a possibility of the whole thing, syringe, needle and flight, going in one side of an animal and out the other.

The dart-gun is a so-called prohibited weapon classed along with machine guns and the like, an odd arrangement for it is slow to load and no more lethal than the drug it is filled with, which may be penicillin or a vitamin solution. Nevertheless the authorities make a great fuss about it and insist on special Home Office licences as well as the usual firearms certificate. Taking the dart-gun overseas can mean days of form-filling and delay.

On this occasion, however, the Foreign Office Qatar Desk turned out to be most enthusiastic. There were political overtones to my visit, it seemed. The Qatar Government had their reasons for not wanting American assistance on the oryx problem and had asked the British for help. It was important that I handled the affair properly. After all, Sheik Qassim was the brother of the ruler of the tiny oil-rich state that juts out of Saudi Arabia into the waters of the Gulf. There would be no trouble over taking the gun and the embassy in Doha, the capital of Qatar, would smooth things for me at the other end. I was informed that the French were taking a lot of interest in Qatar and trying to extend their influence there. They had shown willing to involve themselves in the oryx problem too. The FO thought that it would be first-class if I could beat them to it, get to Doha first, sort the trouble out and generally fly the flag for British veterinary science!

Later that day I flew out to Doha and as night fell I had my first glimpses of Arabia, the bright flares at the oil well-heads flickering thousands of feet below in the darkness. When we landed at Doha in the early hours of the morning the scene on the tarmac was like something out of *The Seven Pillars of Wisdom*. Arabs in black robes and white turbans, carrying rifles and automatic machine guns and with bandoliers of gleaming bullets criss-crossing their chests, clustered round the bottom of the steps. At first I thought they were there for me, but then I saw that they were exchanging greetings with a small Arab gentleman in traditional dress who had preceded me down the gangway. Later I found out that he was the very man whose oryx I had come to examine, Sheik Qassim, and that the armed men were his personal bodyguard.

Dr Gotting, Dr Qayyum, whose was the Chief Veterinary Officer, and the Chief of Police made up my welcoming party, the latter having come specially to examine my dart-gun. With the minimum of formalities I was whisked through customs and immigration and taken to a hotel. I was impressed by the speed and efficiency; they certainly were not wasting any time. Over a cup of camomile tea I asked Dr Qayyum about the outbreak of disease in the oryx. I was anxious to begin work as soon as dawn broke and any history learned now would save valuable time.

'When was the last death, how many have died and do you have any fresh post-mortem material for me?' I asked.

Dr Qayyum looked a little embarrassed. 'Twelve animals died,' he replied, 'but I'm afraid we have no post-mortem material.'

'But when was the last death? Are any others likely to die in the next day or two?'

'The last death, Dr Taylor, was in April but on exactly which date in April I cannot recall.'

I was flabbergasted. It was now the middle of November and the last deaths in this apparent emergency had occurred in April, over six months before.

'But I believe you are having serious problems with the oryx,' I said after I had regained my composure. 'Are any ill at all at present?'

Qayyum shrugged his shoulders and made a despairing grimace. 'I am not sure,' he said, 'but His Excellency the Sheik is very worried about them. That is why he has returned today from London where he has been himself for treatment.

He is very, very fond of the animals. He says no more must die.'

'So you have no post-mortem reports or specimens from the last deaths?'

'Well, no. But we opened one or two.'

'What did you find in those, Dr Qayyum?'

'Nothing much; perhaps the lungs were redder than normal.'

'And you have no preserved specimens?'

He shook his head sadly.

'Well, how many oryx are left now?' I asked.

Dr Qayyum shrugged again. 'I do not know exactly, but tomorrow if you wish you can go to see them with my assistant, Dr Iftikhar. Then you can see exactly how many there are.'

At daybreak the following morning I set out from the hotel with Dr Iftikhar, a smartly dressed young Pakistani who had recently arrived in Qatar. Doha is a small town of dusty buildings set on the water's edge and backed by desert which rolls away into the vast Rub'al Khali, the Empty Quarter. Graceful dhows lie in the harbour side by side with modern steamships carrying fertiliser and chicken feed for the embryo livestock industry. There are opulent palaces surrounded by trees and elegant pierced walls, and a modern, cool, emerald-green mosque. Women in black veils, their faces hidden behind beaked black-gold masks, ride by in Lincoln Continentals and knots of men squat at street corners inspecting trussed hunting hawks. There are dim, bustling souks filled with the tinsmith's wares, vegetables, sherbet, spices and Kraft margarine. The dust swirls in the street as diggers and excavators work to build this new city out of the rocky desert. Nowhere can one escape the sound of Radio Cairo carried by the ubiquitous transistor radio.

We drove out into the desert, a flat khaki plain covered by rocks and rubble for as far as the eye could see. Small grey-green tufts of wiry shrubbery somehow survive in places and on these the nomadic shepherds graze their flocks of sheep and goats. On and on we travelled across the depressing flat land until a small oasis of trees came into view. As we got nearer I could see that a cluster of farm buildings and paddocks was set beneath the trees and nearby was a small unpretentious palace. This was Al Zubarrah, Sheik Qassim's weekend retreat, from where he keeps in touch with events in the capital by radio telephone. A tall radio antenna was fixed to the roof of the little mosque within the palace garden. A man sleeping on the ground in the shade of a windowless one-room hut by the gate of a large paddock awoke as we rumbled up and came forward to greet us. Dr Iftikhar introduced him as the man who looked after the oryx.

The paddocks were built on the desert sand with high walls of grey breeze blocks and wide wooden doors. It was impossible to see what was inside them. Dense clouds of pigeons wheeled over the farm and the entire area was littered with rubbish and crusted with birds' droppings. Even so, I was excited. Within a few moments I would see for the first time the largest existing herd of an animal rarer than the giant panda or the komodo dragon. Few European zoologists had been to see Sheik Qassim's farm in the desert. The oryx keeper took us over to the paddock gate, struggled with a rusty lock and pushed open the heavy doors. We walked through into a sunlit compound which had a line of green trees planted all along one side.

Standing glowing in the morning sun at the far end of the paddock, all heads turned in our direction, were the oryx, about three dozen beautiful creatures of all sizes from calf to old bull, all motionless and alert with ears pricked and nostrils distended. This was *Oryx leucoryx*, the famed Arabian oryx. Quietly we walked towards them across the sand. There were troughs of sparkling fresh water, barley and some sort of rough salt supplement set out under the trees. Piles of lush, freshly cut lucerne lay on the ground nearby. The oryx certainly seemed to be fed and watered carefully. As we came within fifty yards of the herd they moved off, circling round us

123

close to the grey walls. What gorgeous creatures they were. Beige-coloured calves not yet grown into perfect proportion pressed between cantering adults with flanks of dazzling whiteness and horns as straight and even and shiny as rapiers. I had worked with other species of oryx such as the beisa and the scimitar-horned oryx, and my first short scientific paper published in my early days with zoo animals had concerned a fatal case of tapeworm cysts in a beisa oryx, but, handsome as these other species undoubtedly are, the Arabian oryx surely wins first prize in the oryx beauty contest.

There were thirty-three animals and all of them looked in tip-top condition, plump and well-rounded. Only one elderly female had a hygroma, a sac of fluid the size of a grapefruit (a sort of chronic housemaid's knee) on one knee joint.

'They look very well, Dr Iftikhar,' I said. 'Do they breed well?'

'We get six or eight calves each year,' he replied. 'The herd size increases quite rapidly, but then the disease seems to strike and we're down to around thirty again.'

Questioning him in detail about the last deaths in April produced little of importance. There was not much to go on, just the vaguest of histories. Whatever it was that was killing the oryx, it struck suddenly as a rapidly fatal epidemic and then apparently disappeared when the numbers of oryx had been trimmed back. This pattern suggested that overcrowding and population density might be important factors. But suppose one day the disease just went on spreading through the herd until it wiped out the lot or at least a minimum breeding group? It was a frightening thought. One minute the animals had appeared to be ill, dull and off their food and the next they were found dead: that would be consistent with anthrax, the deadly illness that crams the blood vessels with fast-multiplying, lethal bacteria. There must be millions of anthrax spores in the rubbish and offal lying around the farm.

While I stood and watched the oryx and they circled warily round us, there was a commotion in the air above us as a flock of pigeons numbering about two thousand swept over the wall of the oryx paddock and descended on the troughs of barley. The oryx keeper chased them away and they rose in a noisy, dusty blue-black cloud.

'I've never seen so many pigeons in my life,' I remarked. 'Why does the Sheik keep so many?'

'To feed and train his falcons,' was the reply. 'After the oryx, Sheik Qassim's great love is to hunt the houbara.'

The houbara is a fast-flying species of bustard living in the desert. Rich Arab falconers will take fleets of air-conditioned cars, dozens of trained hawks and falcons and a retinue of staff into the Rub' al Khali for one or two weeks at a time and be perfectly satisfied if they return with just one houbara.

Dr Iftikhar showed me round the rest of the farm. As we went out of the gate of the oryx paddock a group of camels were ambling by. Their coats were sparse and the underlying skin was an unhealthy crusty pink. They were extensively affected by mange. Whenever they got the chance they would stop against the corner of a wall or the trunk of a tree and have a satisfying rub. Mange is common in camels and it makes them itch, but the rubbing helps to spread the disease. Dr Iftikhar explained that the camels were passing through the farm. The nomad herdsmen used the farm as a stopping place and every day one or two herds of camel or sheep would rest there, taking advantage of the water and shade for an hour or two while the herdsmen exchanged gossip and took a cup of tea with the Sheik's men.

We entered another paddock, but this one contained only seven minute Arabian gazelles which leaped about in panic as we opened the gate. Iftikhar explained that the Sheik had collected these also. Originally there had been nearly eighty but the disease had hit them, too. Again there were no post-mortem examination reports or preserved specimens. Another paddock contained sheep and goats, but what a difference from the oryx enclosure. The animals were thin and in poor condition. Their food troughs were empty. Many had infected eyes, purulent noses and maggot-infested sores.

'These are a terribly poor lot, Dr Iftikhar,' I exclaimed, picking up a small, almost comatose lamb that lay dying in the fierce heat of midday. 'Riddled with disease and half-starved, I'd say.'

Dr Iftikhar began a verbose apologia. Yes, they were a problem. No, they didn't have enough food. Sadly, no-one seemed to be able to do anything about them. But it was all the fault of a batch of sheep brought in from Saudi Arabia. You really couldn't trust the people over there to eradicate their diseases, and so on. He rattled on and took me by the arm, drawing me away from the miserable flock that were unusually silent, so weak and debilitated had they become.

'I'm sure you don't want to get yourself messed up with these creatures, Dr Taylor.' He brushed flecks of wool and dirt from his natty suit. 'After all, you are here to see the oryx.'

'I'm here to look into the oryx disease problem,' I said, more than a little disgruntled. 'I may be six months late, but at least I may find out something by knowing what sort of sick animals the oryx have as their next-door neighbours. Please arrange for this lamb to be killed now so that I can do an autopsy on the spot.'

I could see in his face that I was disturbing the peace and order of Dr Iftikhar's routine. As for doing autopsies in the field – well! I could almost read his thoughts. Why couldn't this pernickety Englishman disappear into a hole in the ground?

'But we have no facilities, Dr Taylor. It is only a lamb. Lambs die all the time.'

'Of course they do, but they die from something. All I need I have in my bag. Please get me a container of water for my hands.'

When the skinny little body of the lamb was brought I crouched under the shade of a tree and made a crude dissection. It must have been the first post-mortem ever performed on a sheep at the farm. Dr Iftikhar stood some yards off, watching. The chest cavity was full of sticky, honey-coloured liquid. The tiny lungs were affected by dropsy and carried large areas of solid purple inflammation. The lymph glands draining the lungs were enlarged and angry-looking, spotted with bright scarlet haemorrhages. It looked like haemorrhagic septicaemia, a disease of cattle, buffalo, sheep and wild cud-chewing animals which is caused by a bacterium called Pasteurella. I took specimens for analysis and culture. If I could find Pasteurella in this lamb then perhaps I could begin to explain the sudden deaths in the oryx and gazelles. The teeming legions of foraging pigeons would be the obvious carriers of the disease over the wall to the oryx.

In the other farm buildings the earth floors were piled high with mounds of long dead birds, hens, turkey poults and pigeons. Emaciated hens stalked hungrily about, pecking at the remains of their fellows that were slowly rotting into the ground. Every room, cage, hut and pen contained dead or dying birds. Pigeons fluttered everywhere. Many of them were sick, their eyes half closed and the skin of the eyelids, at the corners of the mouth and around the nostrils distended with masses of warts and blisters. Pox virus was rampant. The decaying corpses of turkeys and hens bore the same ugly excrescences. I wondered what Andrew, who has a special interest in bird diseases and has published a paper on pox in falcons, would think of this charnel house. If Sheik Qassin was feeding pigeons to his valuable hunting birds, he must surely be suffering losses from pox attacks.

The farm was literally stuffed with diseased animals. Only the oryx and gazelles were in good condition and they alone showed any evidence of being systematically fed. Carrying samples of the oryx food including fresh and dried lucerne, I was driven back across the seventy miles of desert to Doha. Without dead or sick animals among the oryx there was little I could do to confirm the nature of the disease, but the sources of a hundred and one potentially lethal epidemics were easily identifiable. Haemorrhagic septicaemia was my favourite for the culprit.

On the way back to the city Dr Iftikhar asked me to give my opinion on a case of lameness in a horse at Ar Rayyan, the royal stables. We drove up to an imposing arrangement of white buildings. Round a vast sandy arena were rows of spacious, airy loose-boxes. It was most impressive. We stood in the sunlight as a groom led out a chestnut thoroughbred. It was thin and rangy and had a pronounced limp on one foreleg. I examined the leg and Dr Iftikhar described the history and his course of treatment. It was a case of navicular disease, inflammation of a peculiar but troublesome little bone that lies beneath the horny wall of a horse's (or zebra's) hoof. When we had agreed a plan for further therapy I remarked on the poor condition of the animal. Dr Iftikhar looked embarrassed once again.

'I'm afraid that the horses here have little food. There are sixty of them, blood horses from Britain, Ireland and Germany. But they belong to the ex-Emir.'

'What difference does that make?"

Dr Iftikhar puffed and scratched his head. 'Well, it's a peculiar business. The old Emir was deposed bloodlessly by the present ruler, his younger brother. Now he's in exile. But because its something of a family affair, all his belongings in Qatar remain his property. The new Emir and the rest of the family won't confiscate them, but on the other hand they won't find any money to maintain them. It doesn't matter very much in the case of buildings or motor cars, but unfortunately there are more serious consequences for his horses.'

'Do you mean that no-one feeds the horses?'

'Well, sometimes they get a little, but not often.'

'Why doesn't the Government sell or destroy the horses?'

'Because they belong to the exiled Emir.'

Iftikhar led the way into the well-equipped loose-boxes, in each of which was a horse. They were all obviously of first-quality breeding with fine heads and superb bones. There were greys and chestnuts, bays and blacks but every one was in some stage of plain, down to earth starvation. Some stood like hat racks, their fine skin pulled tight over their skeletons, others lay unable to rise. Some chewed at the sandy floor. Their droppings were a mixture of sand, wood dust and mucus. At least there was plenty of water but of any kind of food there was not a trace in the whole complex. I walked on past box after box, unable to believe my eyes. A stable full of animals that would be worth hundreds of thousands of pounds in Europe were being allowed to starve slowly to death. And I had been asked to look at a case of lameness!

'Doesn't all this eating of sand and earth produce gut trouble?' I asked, literally dizzy with disbelief. 'Surely you get colic cases galore?'

'Yes, we do. That's what finishes them usually. I treat them with pethidine if they're in pain.'

It may have been a bloodless deposing of the old Emir, I thought, but it had meant a cruel death for a collection of innocent animals brought far from the pastures of their birth.

'Is there nothing we can do about it?' I asked.

'I'm afraid not,' said Dr Iftikhar. 'It's very difficult to influence such matters. High politics, you know. Ruling family and so forth.'

I would try to do something about it.

Back in my hotel I decided to go for a swim in the sea before changing my clothes for one of Sheik Qassim's traditional audiences that evening. The waters of the Gulf behind the Alwaha Hotel were shallow, pale blue and highly inviting. As I swam I could see large dark shadows scurrying about on the ocean bottom but without goggles or a face mask I was unable to identify them. Then I saw an Arab wading about in the water, carrying a large tin slung round his shoulders and peering through the water with the aid of an empty jam jar. From time to time he would dive quickly beneath the surface and come up with the biggest pink and brown crabs I had ever seen. So that's what the scurrying shadows were. I swam on, thinking how delectable they would be when prepared in Shelagh's favourite way with the meat dressed with white wine,

129

garlic and capers and roasted in the shell. Suddenly the Arab gave a mighty yell, dropped his tin and his jam jar and lunged off with great leaping strides towards the shore. I wondered if one of his quarry had laid hold of his foot, since the crabs were big enough to pinch severely.

Floating lazily on, I looked down through the clear water at the fuzzy shapes on the bottom and revelled in the cool caress of the sea. One of the dark shapes did not scurry like the others, in fact it was not on the sea bottom at all. It grew bigger. It was swimming towards me, effortlessly and straight as an arrow. It had the strangest head and it was brown on top and dirty white underneath. Suddenly I knew what had made the crab-catcher head so rapidly for dry land, for coming lazily towards me was a full-grown hammerhead shark. These fish, looking like one of the more far-fetched creations of a horror film studio, are definitely known to be man-eaters. The bizarre shape of the head, which is five times as wide as it is long, is unmistakable although its function is a mystery – perhaps these very strong swimmers use it as a sort of anterior rudder. Certainly they are not fussy about what they eat and I had seen them take dead dolphins caught in the nets in Florida. I felt very, very frightened.

On came the hammerhead. Even underwater I could see him now with less distortion. I did not dare turn away from him to swim towards shore, nor did I fancy the idea of standing on the bottom with the water up to my chest. Then, when he was about six feet away, another of the busily hurrying crabs, thank Heaven for a lowly crustacean, came teetering by. With its large, unblinking eyes the shark spotted the creature, and suddenly veered off diagonally downwards. Through the shimmering water I saw it smoothly pick up the crab in its jaws. Scrunch. The crab had disappeared. The hammerhead swirled round in the water, the tip of its tail flashed under my nose and in a moment it had gone, gliding calmly away into deeper water. I made my way to the beach. I did not swim in the Gulf again.

At six o'clock it was time to go to one of the Sheik's regular audiences held twice a day at his town palace or Majlis. At these audiences anyone, from the highest to the lowest in the community, has a chance to exchange a few words with or make a request of the Sheik. With Dr Gotting I drove into the Majlis through an archway guarded by the armed men I had seen at the airport. Inside there were cool courtyards with fountains and orange trees, and cloisters where patient hawks sat hooded on their blocks. We removed our shoes and entered a brightly lit room decorated with the heads of Arabian oryx mounted as trophies. At the far end on a decorated chair sat the Sheik and around him were seated members of the aristocracy and Government ministers. The chair on his immediate right was empty. Here for short periods would sit those with whom he wished to talk or who had a petition to make. Down the sides of the room sat all sorts of other people, the least important and most shabbily dressed next to the door. As we entered the Sheik rose to greet us. The rest of the people in the room also stood. We walked the length of the room, shook hands and retired to two seats halfway along the wall. Everyone took their seats once more. A little whispering was going on and the Sheik would occasionally beckon to some member of his staff who would come to sit briefly at the Sheik's right and talk in low tones. A servant circulated continually with a tray of small handleless cups and an ornate gold pot full of camomile tea. My cup was kept permanently brimming, and I had to learn to shake the empty cup from left to right to indicate that I did not want any more of the rather insipid beverage.

It was a very leisurely business. Shabbily dressed peasants from near the door would seize their chance to sit in the vacant chair and then quickly murmur their request into the Sheik's ear. Rarely was anyone there for more than a minute or two. If the Sheik decided that action had to be taken, he would beckon to an official and give his instructions. Dr Gotting explained that it was at just such an audience that Sheik Qassim had suddenly

131

become alarmed about the condition of the oryx and had commanded him to get professional help from Britain immediately. Although the good Doctor supervised the running of the hospitals and was in no way involved with the veterinary services, he had had to take it in hand. The order might equally well have been given to the Chief of Police or the Director of Oil Production. No matter who is given the order, he has to execute it.

After half an hour and an overabundance of tea Dr Gotting went to the chair and spoke with the Sheik. When he returned he whispered to me that the Sheik had asked him whether I had brought my family with me yet. Apparently he expected me to stay permanently!

'He thinks you are here for good to look after his oryx. He wasn't very pleased when I said you were only here on a short visit. He thinks you should remain ad infinitum.'

Much as the Arabian oryx fascinated me I could not conceive a worse fate than to spend all one's days out on that awful farm in the desert. A few minutes later the chair beside the Sheik was empty again.

'Right, off you go now,' whispered Dr Gotting.

I went across to the chair and sat down. An interpreter came to stand behind the Sheik.

'His Excellency asks what you think of the oryx at Al Zubarrah,' he said.

I realised I would have to get my points over quickly and I wanted also to raise the matter of the horses starving at Ar Rayyan.

'The oryx are very fine,' I began, 'but the cause of the disease cannot be precisely established yet. However I do recommend splitting the herd into two, separating and . . .'

Abruptly the Sheik stood up. Everyone else followed suit as usual. A close member of the Sheik's family, a nobleman in fine robes lined with gold, had entered. Dr Gotting beckoned to me to return to my place. The nobleman kissed his kinsman the Sheik and sat down in the seat that I had vacated.

132

'That's it for today,' murmured my companion.

'What? Do you mean my interview is finished?' I replied.

'Yes, that is his first son and there are a couple of imams, religious leaders from Cairo, waiting to come in. You've had your chance for today. We might as well leave.'

We slipped out of the room. Although I stayed for another seven days taking samples from the oryx and the farm for analysis in England, and although I attended several more audiences, I never got another chance to plonk myself down in the vacant chair. I was always beaten to it.

Although I had not been able to deal with any cases of actual disease in the oryx I was able to suggest measures for tackling the next outbreak and, most important, for getting me the material required for diagnosis. I wrote a long report detailing my ideas for cutting out the spread of disease and improving health generally at the farm, and I wrote scathingly about the horses in the royal stables. Copies were sent to the Sheik and various Government bodies. Then, loaded with samples of oryx droppings, lucerne, hay, blood, barley, and various other possibly useful substances, I returned to England. The customs officer at Manchester Airport extracted the plastic bag containing half a pound of dried lucerne from my luggage, opened it and sniffed suspiciously.

'Bringing rabbit food all the way from the Persian Gulf then, eh?' he said, crumbling some of the leaves between his fingers and sniffing some more. 'Doing some long-distance hay-making?'

'It's not cannabis.' I told him, and showed him my collection of droppings and blood. He believed me.

It was the same customs officer who inspected my bags two years later and grimly withdrew a bag containing five pounds of uncooked foreign meat.

'It's the placenta of a dolphin that aborted in Majorca. I'm taking it to Professor Harrison of Cambridge as a gift,' I explained on that occasion.

'Oh yes,' said the customs officer, recognition dawning on

133

his face, 'you're the bloke who usually has a bag full of antelope crap!'

After my first visit to Qatar I kept in contact with Dr Qayyum and his team and sent out drugs and sample bottles ready for the next outbreak of disease in the oryx. Analysis of the food, blood and droppings had not brought up anything abnormal, but I had had a telephone call from a foreign animal dealer who had heard of my visit to the Middle East.

'I've got a proposition for you,' he said. 'I must get hold of at least three Arabian oryx. If you can persuade the Qataris to part with them, I'll give you £2000.'

'What exactly do you want them for?' I asked.

'You can explain to the Qataris that they are to introduce new blood into the American herd. They'll perhaps part with them if they think it will be good for conservation of the species. Then I'll ship the three to the States and exchange them for an identical threesome which I'll send somewhere else.'

It seemed rather tortuous. 'Exactly where else?' I asked.

The dealer was reluctant to say but I pressed him, knowing that I was his best hope of obtaining such exceptionally rare stock. Eventually he said, 'Actually to Israel. The Israelis are building up a collection of all the animals that existed in the original Palestine. The Arabian oryx is one of them and you can imagine their chances of getting them from the Arabs.'

Not wishing even to dip my toe into the treacherous waters of Middle Eastern politics, I politely told the dealer what to do with his proposition.

It was exactly a year later that the next urgent call came from Qatar. This time there had not been the same inexplicable delay in seeking help, but three days had still elapsed before I was requested to fly out without delay. Six oryx had died and, although no bodies were available for my inspection, tissue specimens and bacterial swabs had been taken. At the farm out in the desert nothing had changed. The clouds of pigeons still filled the sky above the paddocks. Camels and goats wandered at will through the farm and the sheep were in an even more desperate state than before. Again the remaining oryx seemed healthy and in good condition. I examined the bits of lung and other organs that Dr Qayyum and Dr Iftikhar had taken from the dead oryx. It looked like a haemmorhagic septicaemia. I sent portions by air to England and had others processed at the local hospital laboratory.

There were many sick sheep on the farm. Each day there was a pile of new carcasses outside the paddock gates. I walked among the flocks with my stethoscope and listened to the chests of sick and dying animals. The fluid noises and harsh roaring of pneumonia were always to be found. I asked Dr Iftikhar again about the innumerable pigeons.

'Why can't we cut down the numbers of those birds?' I demanded.

'The Sheik will not do it,' he replied. 'He says they are essential for the falcons.'

The results came back by telex from the English laboratory. It was haemmorhagic septicaemia in the oryx and the swabs taken from their tissues had grown pure cultures of Pasteurella bacteria. I was finding the same germ in all the poor sheep that died at the farm, their lungs studded with angry red areas of pneumonia. At least drugs existed to combat the disease.

'I am going to begin a vaccination programme for the oryx,' I told Dr Iftikhar, 'and I'm going to give serum and vaccine to every sheep and goat on the farm.'

The Pakistani looked dismayed. 'It will be necessary first to request permission from His Excellency the Sheik,' he said. 'Without permission, which is difficult to obtain, we cannot inject the oryx; he loves them so much.'

'It will have to be done,' I insisted. 'I'll go to the Majlis to have audience with him tonight.'

It was the fear of injections which had led to the foolhardy practice at the farm of mixing broad-spectrum antibiotics with the food for the oryx. This sounds like a simple way of administering anti-bacterial drugs to nervous or dangerous

135

wild animals, but in a cud-chewing animal the antibiotics kill most of the harmless bacteria in its stomach which are essential for its special type of digestion. The consequences can be serious and often fatal. I wondered whether any of the deaths at Al Zubarrah had been due more to the therapy than to the complaint.

'And unless we do the sheep and goats as well there's not much point,' I carried on. 'Think of the improvement in their value as well.'

'But vaccinating sheep!' exclaimed Dr Iftikhar. 'There are so many!'

'We are going to do it, you and me,' I replied firmly. He looked very miserable.

I went to the evening audience alone and eventually bagged the vacant chair beside the Sheik. Through the interpreter I explained: 'I can help your oryx, Your Excellency, but I need to vaccinate all of them and all the sheep and goats. And to do the oryx I would like to have a strong wooden cattle crush built.'

For a few seconds the Sheik pondered and sipped his tea, then he said a few words to the interpreter.

'The interview is over,' he said. 'His Excellency says you can have what you want. There will be forty men at the farm tomorrow morning to build whatever structure you require. And you can do all the sheep and goats.'

The following day, fortified and refreshed by a pile of water-melons, the forty labourers and I built an elaborate tapering cattle crush against one wall of the oryx paddock. At the end of the crush was a trap designed to hold an individual animal while I vaccinated it. Carpenters cut wood to size, some men dug holes for posts and others unrolled heavy-gauge wire mesh and nailed it to the posts. By midday we were ready to try it out. We carefully drove the herd of oryx into the wide mouth of the crush. As they were pressed in slowly towards the narrow neck they suddenly panicked. In unison they launched themselves at the sides of the crush. As if it were made of paper the whole contraption fell flat before the charging animals. Ten seconds later not a single piece was left standing.

Unharmed and impassive, the oryx gathered in a distant corner of the paddock and surveyed the scene of our fruitless labours. I would have to use the dart-gun. I loaded every syringe I had with a dose of the vaccine and applied a blob of antibiotic jelly to the needle tips. Although the darts were sterile, as they entered the animals' skins they might take in a particle of soil or dust adhering to the hair, and I was not prepared to run the slightest risk of losing any animals from tetanus. When all was prepared I sent everyone including the vets away so that I could move about the oryx paddock quietly and alone, picking off one animal at a time with the minimum disturbance or fuss. That way I could avoid shooting at moving targets. This was important because in each case I wanted to place a subcutaneous injection precisely over the ribs just behind the shoulder. Any reaction to the vaccine in that place would not interfere with movement and would soon disperse. In order not to inject the vaccine too deep I had selected needles only half an inch long which carried fat little collars to control the depth of penetration. One by one I darted the oryx, who were not disturbed by the relatively quiet gas-powered gun. After delivering its contents each syringe fell out of the animal onto the sand and I retrieved it. It was all over in an hour and a half. Within ten days the oryx would be carrying a good level of protective antibodies in their bloodstreams.

I arranged with Dr Iftikhar for him to repeat the process in two to four weeks, then set off to see about vaccinating the sheep and goats by hand.

'Surely we can leave the vaccination of these animals to the farm men,' said Iftikhar. 'I'm sure you don't want to go in with all those hundreds of smelly creatures.'

'I want to see every animal properly vaccinated and dosed with antiserum this afternoon,' I replied. 'I'll do half and you do the others.'

'But the men don't really want to catch the sheep.' Iftikhar was looking positively awkward.

'All right then,' I said, 'I'll catch them and do them myself.'

I went into the sheep paddock with a multidose syringe, grabbed a sheep, vaccinated it and bundled it out of the gate to the watching group of men and Dr Iftikhar. I did another and another. Still the men watched. It was going to take a long time at this rate to do all the hundreds of sheep but I was determined that all susceptible animals were going to be done. Eventually the shamefaced knot of men at the gateway came reluctantly in dribs and drabs into the paddock and began catching animals. Dr Iftikhar filled his syringe and before long we were whistling through the flock at a fine old rate.

Before leaving for England I walked round the whole of the farm again. The pox-infested birds were still everywhere, both dead and alive. Out in the small irrigated fields where the lucerne for the oryx was grown I walked down the rows of succulent green plants and noticed many plastic bags, some containing quantities of white powder, lying on the soil. The bags bore bold skull and crossbones symbols in bright red. The white powder was an insecticide containing the extremely dangerous organo-phosphorus type of chemical. The farm workers had used the stuff and then idly dropped the seemingly empty bags as soon as they had finished with them. In places the white powder was actually caked onto the leaves of the lucerne plants. It worried me. This stuff was fine when properly diluted with water and sprayed, but what if the oryx were fed lucerne contaminated with the neat, concentrated powder? I pointed out the risk to Dr Iftikhar and he had words with the labourer in charge of the fields. There was no risk, said the labourer, as they were not going to crop that area for quite a while. He would see that the bags were gathered up and that the powder was washed off the leaves in future. One month later I received a letter from Dr Qayyum requesting advice on treating animals posioned with organo-phosphorus insecti-

138

cides. Three oryx had eaten lucerne contaminated with the chemical and had developed the typical symptoms of poisoning affecting the nervous system. One of the animals had died by the time he wrote the letter and the other two were gravely ill. Unfortunately the letter took two weeks to reach England and although I immediately cabled detailed advice, once again I was far too late.

Something else once arrived from Qatar. I went down to breakfast to find a small parcel covered with Qatari stamps waiting on the dining table. I opened it and out fell a brain! Stuck to the noisome object was a stained piece of notepaper. After hurriedly removing the thing and all its wrappings to my office I scrubbed my hands with iodine soap and pulled on a pair of plastic gloves. Then I read the letter, which was from Dr Qayyum. The brain was from a dog with suspected rabies and would I kindly confirm or deny please!

With all the careful rules and regulations, quarantine provisions and the lot designed to keep the British Isles free from the horrific scourge of rabies, here was a mass of putrefying material possibly loaded with active rabies virus arriving as calmly as could be on my breakfast table after wending its way through the channels of the Post Office. I telephoned the Ministry of Agriculture immediately. They seemed puzzled as to the correct thing to do.

'None of the rules fit,' said one of the Ministry men to whom I spoke.

'It's not from a British dog so an investigation isn't called for,' offered another.

'You haven't asked for its importation so you can't be held responsible for not getting a licence,' a third reassured me.

'You can't quarantine a rotting brain,' said a fourth, plaintively.

In the end they left it to me to deal with. I was dumb-founded. Nobody in the Ministry seemed to care that I might be about to put Rochdale on the map as the place where rabies entered Britain, possibly never again to be eradicated. I took the brain and all the packing paper, put them in a box filled with carbolic acid and then incinerated the whole thing. If rabies was indeed in that brain, not a virus particle escaped.

Thirteen

On my way home from my first visit to Qatar I made a detour via a zoo at Marseilles in the South of France. The morning after my arrival, M. Villemin, the owner of the zoo, telephoned my hotel to say that he was sending a vehicle and chauffeur to pick me up. After breakfast I went out of the foyer of the hotel onto the busy street. There was M. Villemin in his car, but parked directly in front of the hotel steps was a motor cycle and, waiting patiently on the driving seat dressed in sweater, trousers and peaked cap, was a large and unconcerned-looking chimpanzee.

'Get on the pillion seat behind Henri,' M. Villemin shouted from the car when I appeared. 'He is a good driver.'

The centre of Marseilles is hardly a sleepy Provençal hamlet and the zoo was about a mile or more away. I consider myself a reasonably competent driver in most European countries but the higher mysteries of the logic behind French driving habits continue to elude me. I would not lightly venture out behind the wheel of a tank into that nine o'clock maelstrom of furiously honking Citroëns and wobbling bicycles. But a chimpanzee!

'But does he know the way?' I asked nervously, stalling.

'Of course he does, you can rely on Henri,' was the reply.

The hotel commissionaire came over and reassured me. 'Don't worry, Monsieur,' he said. ' 'E 'as been 'ere to collect guests before.'

I did not dare ask whether all the previous guests were alive and well and living in sanatoria. Instead I walked up to the motor cycle. The chimpanzee looked at me blandly, raised

141

himself and kicked the starter. Brrrm-brrrm, brrrm-brrrm: he revved the engine expertly with one hairy black hand and picked his nose slowly with the other. Brrrrrm-brrrrrm. I put my leg over the machine and sat down on the pillion seat tentatively, keeping some of my weight on my feet and ready to auto-eject at the first sign of disaster. Henri now looked straight ahead. He revved again, short crackling bursts of the two-stroke engine. I put my arms round the muscular waist of my driver and stuck my thumbs firmly into the top of his trousers.

I think it was at this stage that I began to perspire.

Henri looked to his right, stopped picking his nose, revved more strongly and then, when he saw a gap in the traffic, kicked in the gear with a practised bare foot and slipped away from the kerb in a tight turn.

'Put your feet up, M. Taylor,' I heard M. Villemin call as he pulled out behind us into the road.

I lifted my feet onto the rests and found to my delight that we were cruising in a straight line at about fifteen miles an hour straight up the boulevard. It was perfect Highway Code stuff. Unlike the drivers of several of the vehicles on either side of us, Henri knew where he was going and how to go about it. We approached a red light. I tensed. I was definitely perspiring now. The cross-traffic was in full spate. Was it really true that chimpanzees were colour blind? This seemed a novel way of proving the point. Henri slowed down and, like the good motor cyclist he was, maintained our balance at very slow speed by weaving slowly from side to side hoping to maintain some momentum until the lights changed. They did. Brrrrm-brooom-brooooom. Henri took us smartly away with a flick of the wrist and an effortless change of gear.

The next obstacle was a traffic policeman. No problem. As Henri and I approached, the officer smiled, held up the cross-flow and waved us on. Henri crackled past him without so much as a nod or a 'bonjour'. We were getting close to the zoo but would now have to negotiate some narrow streets with

142

several sharp corners. At the end of the boulevard we came to the first turn. Hunched over the handlebars Henri leaned beautifully into the bend. Less accustomed to motor bikes and without the chimpanzee's perfect sense of balance, I rocked awkwardly on my seat and clutched Henri's tummy. The machine wobbled. Uncomplainingly Henri corrected the wobble. I did not dare look round to see if M. Villemin was still following. Henri stared fixedly ahead and I crouched uncomfortably behind the purposefully hunched body. Henri took us nippily along the street, overtook a man pushing a handcart, swerved into the gutter to avoid a dog lying in the middle of the road and then got us back on course by a smart twist of the handlebars. Two more corners, down a hill fast enough to make Henri's saucer-shaped ears flip back and, with a turn into which he leaned over with what seemed to me more than a little flashiness, we arrived in the zoo drive. Henri cut the revs back and we tootled through the grounds to the ape house. Henri braked and brought the bike to a halt. He stood supporting it with his feet while the engine ticked over. I dismounted and walked round to face my driver, who looked at me unblinkingly and began to pick his nose again. It was all in a day's work for a chimp. Just a routine pick-up, nothing to get excited about.

Although M. Villemin had trained Henri to such a degree that he could cope with the murderous Marseilles traffic as well as any human driver and better than most French ones, handling the great apes generally calls for patience, cunning, skill and plain good luck. The discovery of effective tranquillisers for primates at least avoided the unpleasant use of nets and catching bags. As well as panicking the animal these methods of handling were dangerous for the humans involved. I myself was badly bitten by an ape incarcerated securely in a bag made of sacking because although I could not tell which bit of him was which wriggling and protesting under the opaque material, he could glimpse my fingers through the weave of the hessian and sank his canine teeth into them.

Nor were the old methods of control reliable. Most chimpanzees could be conned by waving a plastic snake at them but some, instead of retreating in apprehension, would advance boldly. One keeper tried waving a plastic reptile at a rebellious chimp who had broken into a food store. Not in the slightest taken in, the ape jumped forwards, grabbed the keeper's thumb, spun round and wrenched it off at the root as clean as a whistle. Some keepers of great apes would rely on chemical warfare in times of emergency and squirt ammonia at their unruly charges from plastic lemons which they always carried in their pockets. That was all very well until one was faced by a determined orang-utan. These gentle and most amiable apes would, if roused, do battle unconcernedly when wreathed in choking clouds of ammonia fumes. They seemed oblivious to the irritant and obnoxious chemical and neither coughed nor sneezed nor streamed with tears.

The introduction of phencyclidine and ketamine anaesthetics brought about dramatic changes in the handling of great apes. The drugs could be darted into an ape painlessly or given in a fruit drink. Even so, it is unwise to let a primate see you slipping a Mickey Finn into its favourite tipple. When I first began, several drinks which I had spiked in full view of a curious and wily chimp or gorilla were either thrown back at me or tipped tidily down the nearest drain. No other group of animals is as good as they are at detecting that sort of medical skulduggery!

One morning not long after I had qualified I was called urgently to Manchester Zoo. Adam, the male orang-utan, had escaped from the great ape house. It was the height of summer and Adam had gone to visit the Miniland, an exhibition of miniature fairy-tale villages and model tableaux from children's stories. When I arrived Adam was sitting on the partly demolished cathedral of Nôtre Dame chewing the leg off the hunchback. He gazed at us blandly as he chewed. I approached him slowly, accompanied by Len, his keeper. Len talked soothingly to him: he had looked after the orang since it was the size of a cat. How were we to get Adam back into his

144

quarters? I had phencyclidine in my bag but at that time no dart-gun. Having the dope was fine but how was I going to be able to administer it? Adam threw the mutilated torso of the hunchback at us and grimaced threateningly. He shuffled truculently off, pausing only to pick up one of the three bears and to knock down Don Quixote's windmill with it. Adam made for the open spaces of the zoo gardens. Off to see some action among the crowds, he did not even glance back at us as he lolloped smoothly over the ground. Len, Matt Kelly, the zoo director and I followed anxiously. A mature orang-utan is immensely powerful, as Len had reason to know – an orang had recently sunk its teeth through one of his shoes and bitten off one of his toes. Adam might cause panic among the visitors. He had the muscular power of three full-grown men: what if he grabbed hold of a child?

Fortunately Adam, like most orang-utans, was a shy and undemonstrative creature without the brash exhibitionism of the chimpanzee or the mercurial changes in mood of the gorilla. As he wandered across the flower beds, now trailing an umbrella 'borrowed' firmly but without physical violence from an astounded passer-by, he spied a small wooden hut used by the gardeners. He went in and started to vandalise the interior. At least he was confined. We crept up to the door and bolted it. Adam was too busy smashing plant pots to notice us. What now? How to move the orang from A to B was the problem.

We sat outside and waited and discussed the matter. Len looked at his watch.

'It's almost eleven o'clock,' he said. 'It's his soup time!'

When I had taken over the care of the animals at Manchester Zoo I had introduced the feeding of plenty of meat to the great apes. Best pig's liver, chicken and mincemeat were given daily. Animal protein of this kind is essential for the apes' complete health and indeed it has produced a remarkable increase in the length and glossiness of their coats. All the meat is cooked to avoid risk of infection and the left-over gravy with added vegetables, herbs and cereals, is made into a soup which is given to the animals at eleven o'clock as a mid-morning pick-me-up. The apes seem to appreciate it greatly.

'Can you put some dope in the soup?' Len went on. 'He'll probably take it.'

It was a good idea. Len went off to fetch the warm broth while I measured out a dose of phencyclidine with a syringe. Adam's bright orange eyes watched us through the hut's small window. When Len returned I took the mug of soup and went round to the windowless rear of the hut, away from those orange eyes, and mixed in the sedative. I went back and gave the mug to Len. Adam was now sitting on a pile of shattered plant pots by the window. His stomach told him it was time for elevenses. Len pushed the window open and passed the mug through. Most politely Adam took his soup and drank it, smacking his lips and licking the mug dry as far as his tongue could reach. We watched and waited. Slowly but surely Adam's upper eyelids became heavy. He began to drool a thin thread of saliva and his lower lip sagged. In ten minutes he was asleep and then we carried him, like some pot-bellied and surfeited potentate, back to his house.

Adam and I still meet professionally from time to time. He never produced any offspring during his years at Manchester and the blame was put on him since we could find nothing wrong with any of his wives. Similarly Harold, the male orang at Flamingo Park Zoo, had not been blessed with heirs. We decided to swap Adam for Harold to see if an exchange of mates would remedy the situation. By this time I had a dart-gun and decided to dart Adam, drive him over to Flamingo Park, do the same to Harold and carry him back to Manchester. The orangs could sit beside me in my car.

On the day of the exchange I loaded a couple of syringes with phencyclidine and carefully greased the needle points with penicillin cream to deal with any germs that might be lurking on the dusty skin. Adam was soon lightly anaesthetised and we carried him to my car and sat him on the front seat. The safety belt kept him nicely in position. I set off, with Adam

146

sitting stupefied next to me. He was in a sort of twilight world and with any luck would not start coming round for a couple of hours, long enough for me to make Flamingo Park – just. To be on the safe side I put a loaded syringe containing another dose of phencyclidine on the shelf below the dashboard. This is a wise precaution and I have once or twice managed to stick an injection into the ham muscle of an ape while bowling along the motorway and holding the wheel with one hand. Such irresponsible driving cannot be recommended but is essential when the anthropoid co-driver rouses quicker than antici- pated and reaches for the gear lever as a support or tries to pick his ear with the trafficator control.

I reached Flamingo Park uneventfully with the dreaming Adam. He was still too doped when we put him into the orang house with his two new wives to appreciate the touching way they brought presents of lettuce to their lord and master. When Adam was safely installed I darted Harold, he was carried to my car and without further delay I set off back to Manchester. It was a hot day and Harold turned out to be a trifle flatulent. It became very necessary to wind down the windows. The orang sat comfortably behind the safety belt, his legs dangling over the edge of the seat and his arms in his lap. By the time I reached Leeds it was obvious that Harold's liver was a much more efficient destroyer of phencyclidine than Adam's and that the drug was rapidly being broken down by his system. The first signs were when Harold slowly stuck his arm out of the window and began to clench and unclench his leathery hand in the typical manner of an ape under light phencyclidine anaesthesia. A glance told me that I would have to top him up with a bit more dope in order to reach Manchester, and I decided to stop and attend to him as soon as I had cleared the busy traffic of Leeds city centre. Harold fidgeted slightly in his seat and began slowly to lick his lips. His other hand was now creeping slowly, ever so slowly, around the base of the gear stick. Still barely conscious of what he was doing, Harold drooled while the strong thick fingers of his

147

right hand unpicked a piece of plastic trim with a loud crack. The index finger of the hand, moving as if with a mind of its own, entered the hole it had made and gained purchase on a bigger piece of plastic. Crack! At this rate I would be driving on a naked chassis by the time I reached Huddersfield. There were red traffic lights ahead. As soon as I got through them I would pull up and give him the knockout drops.

I stopped at the lights in the middle of three lanes of traffic. On my near side stood a paper boy on a bicycle, his canvas bag of newspapers slung over his shoulder. He was too busy watching for the green light to notice the fat, red-haired drunk sitting in a car by his elbow. The light changed and I let out the clutch, my eye fixed on a place a couple of hundred yards ahead where I might park briefly. Suddenly there was a piercing yell. I looked in my mirror. Nothing to see. 'Ooooooow! Heeeeeey!' There was the cry again, somewhere to my left and behind me. I slowed down and looked over the head of Harold. Stuck like a fly to the outside of my car was the paper boy. His bicycle was lying some yards behind in the middle of the road. But what was the adhesive that made him cling so closely to the vehicle's side? Then I saw that Harold's wandering left hand had come across the boy's canvas bag when we were stopped at the lights. As soon as we moved off the hand had tightened powerfully by reflex action round the canvas sling of the bag and the lad had been dragged off his bike like a stone from a catapult. I stopped and went round to release Harold's catch. Fortunately the boy was not injured. I retrieved his bicycle, introduced him to the sleeping ape and let him hold my bottle while I prepared more dope. The lad soon recovered his wits and I rather fancy that being unhorsed by an orang-utan made his day. I still wonder whether anyone believed him when he went home and related how, like something out of a crazy gangster film, a car had pulled up alongside him in the middle of Leeds and a fat ugly orang-utan had tried to kidnap him.

If there is one habit which orang-utans have mastered it is

spitting. I have several orang friends who could make those tobacco-chewing expectorators in Western films look positive beginners in the accuracy stakes. Harold, now at Manchester, is pretty good at hitting small targets up to ten feet away but the champion is a male orang at Rhenen Zoo in Holland. He spits with real style both standing upright or when hanging upside down. Indeed I swear he can spit inswingers, so adept is he at reaching intended victims even if they stand behind someone else. Intended victims include veterinary surgeons who have given him medicals and subjected him to similar indignities in the past.

For underhand spitting Jo-Jo, the gorilla at Manchester, held the prize. What he lacked in accuracy he made up for in sneakiness. Jo-Jo's centrally heated, stainless steel fitted quarters had heavy metal doors. It was through a small spyhole in one of these doors that I poked my dart-pistol when gunning for Jo-Jo to anaesthetise him. For several years Jo-Jo had what we felt fairly conclusively was migraine. I closely examined every part of him, taking X-rays, electro-encephalograms and so on, to pinpoint the cause of recurrent bouts of severe headache which he suffered. Of course, all the medical examinations meant dartings, since you cannot handle a 400-pound male gorilla any other way. So Jo-Jo knew that the spyhole in the door was something of a nuisance. The typical procedure went like this.

First I put my eye to the hole to see where Jo-Jo was. I then loaded the dart-pistol while Jo-Jo looked through the hole at me. I could just see one dark shining eye. I returned to the hole to see where Jo-Jo was positioned now and wham! A ball of spittle zipped through the hole and hit me in the eye. Having wiped my face I poked the gun through the hole and squinted down the barrel. There was just enough room for me to see what I was aiming at. No gorilla – Jo-Jo was crouching close to the door below my line of sight. Now he grabbed the metal barrel of the pistol. He could not haul the whole weapon through the small hole, but he had a good try. His next move was to spike my gun before I could get a bead on him. He popped up, opened his mouth and spat long and hard up the barrel of my gun. I withdrew the pistol for on-the-spot de-spitting and Jo-Jo moved back to the hole. As I busied myself cleaning the barrel I felt a blob of warm, sticky saliva hit the back of my neck. First rounds always went to Jo-Jo.

Jo-Jo and his mate, Suzy, first arrived in Manchester as young babies. Gorilla infants are notoriously delicate and easily succumb to germs brought in by human beings. We took every precaution to give them a strong and healthy start, including a ban on any of the great apes being taken out of the zoo to children's parties, fêtes and the like. That cut out the major source of 'flu, colds and infantile ailments. Using glass walls instead of bars for the heated indoor compartments in an ape house also plays a significant part in preventing the spread of bacteria and viruses from the public to the animals. All the keeping staff were regularly vaccinated against influenza and screened for tuberculosis. Tuberculosis still crops up from time to time in the apes and monkeys in zoos that I visit. It is a disease that does not occur in the wild primate but which can cause rapid death once the animals come into contact with man. It is a much more lethal disease in apes and monkeys than in man and if left untreated always results in death. A typical tragedy had occurred shortly before the baby gorillas' arrival when I had had the agonising job of destroying three chimpanzee friends of mine and a pair of gorgeous and valuable silver-leaf langur monkeys which were literally rid-dled with tuberculosis. We discovered that they had caught it from a keeper who was spreading the germs although not feeling ill himself.

Jo-Jo and Suzy were not going to suffer that kind of fate if we could help it. Everything possible was done to prevent the young gorillas meeting up with dangerous bugs. Special measures were taken against cockroaches, frequent visitors to animal houses which can carry poliomyelitis. Like children, Jo-Jo and Suzy also had polio vaccine on lumps of sugar. The air into their sleeping quarters was filtered and treated with antifungal chemicals and their fruit and vegetables were washed to remove traces of any pesticide or other substance sprayed on by the grower. Len, their keeper, virtually lived with them in a small room near theirs in the ape house. There he would prepare their special diet, measure out their vitamin drops, boil their milk and slip in a nourishing egg, whip up their Ovaltine nightcap and select the ingredients for their broth from a larder plentifully stocked with vegetables of all kinds from asparagus to leeks, from string beans to back-eyed peas. Len also spent long periods playing with and nursing the little creatures; of course, a very important part of his job. Their games were simple and boisterous: playing tag, wrestling, somersaulting. The animals thrived and grew rapidly and our precautions seemed to work well. We had no infectious disease, just the development of Jo-Jo's migraine after some years and an allergic rash on his leg that broke out each year when the summer brought plant pollen into his open-air enclosure.

Jo-Jo soon grew into a powerful young juvenile who packed quite a punch when playing with humans. Suzy was gentler and more reticent but Jo-Jo liked nothing better than his daily roustabouts with Len, Matt Kelly or the zoo director, Mr Legge. His favourite wheeze was to saunter past one's legs, apparently intent on other business and ignoring one's presence, but as he drew level he would deliver a beefy clout to the kneecap with a flick of his hand and scurry off gleefully, looking back over his shoulder for the expected pursuit. The bigger he got the more the kneecaps, mine included, began to complain.

The gorillas loved being picked up and cuddled. This was easy when they weighed ten or twenty pounds but later we found the muscular, seventy-pound youngsters who insisted on being rocked in one's arms a bit more of a problem. The trouble was not the ache in the arms as the ape lay dozing cheek to cheek but the crucial point when the nursing and playing

151

had to stop until the next day. Like spoilt children Jo-Jo and Suzy objected petulantly to the humans leaving them to their own devices and would nip firmly at bits of the anatomy or seize hold of clothing with a vice-like grip. At first they were not big enough to enforce their point of view too vigorously, but as time went on this behaviour made inspections increasingly more tricky. I would go into their indoor quarters with Mr Legge and Len, the keeper. To have a good look at Jo-Jo's gums, to see whether his colour was satisfactory, to peer with an ophthalmoscope into his dark and sparkling eyes or listen to his chest with a stethoscope meant first playing the kneecap-knocking game and then, when I could stand no more, letting my playmate drape himself around me for a cuddle. When he was satisfactorily positioned in my arms with bits of him looped round my neck, poked into my ear or lovingly entangled with my hair, I would use a free arm if I had one, or someone else's if not, to remove the necessary instrument from my pocket and to place it surreptitiously on the appropriate spot. The examination over, I then had to rid myself of the gorilla which meant passing him to somebody else, usually Len. The gorillas did not mind being swapped in this way and seemed to think that one cuddler was as good as another. Len would then be the last to leave the quarters. After Mr Legge and I had gone Len would unpick the gorilla from his person and put it on the floor. As it began to protest and snatch for him again he would slip quickly out through the door.

That was how it was at first but as time went on Len did not always make it. He would find himself squeezing dexterously through the door into the passage with two, three or four shiny black arms re-attaching themselves to his clothing, limbs or hair. Increasingly he left bits behind and the rigmarole of breaking off the day's fun became longer and more complex. Came the day when the three of us were in the gorilla quarters for my routine medical inspection and Jo-Jo, now developing the auburn shock of hair on his forehead characteristic of a mature male and rippling his biceps like Mr Universe, decided on a showdown.

The examination on Jo-Jo went without any trouble. He clung to me with an innocent expression on his face and snuffled at my ear. Then it was time to leave him. As soon as I nonchalantly tried to set him down I felt his muscles tighten. He bared his teeth and lost his innocent look.

'You'd better have him as usual,' I told Len.

Len came alongside and Jo-Jo thought about it. OK, he was prepared to move across. Seventy pounds of warm and hairy gorilla slipped from my arms with movements like mercury and made itself comfortable round Len's upper half. As usual Mr Legge and I left the room and Len backed off towards the door. Once there he tried to unpick the ape, but as his fingers tried to release Jo-Jo's grip it either got tighter or simply rang the changes. As soon as he managed to free one hand from a hold on his shoulder, its place would be taken by a foot or, more menacingly, by a strong pair of jaws digging in not quite enough to break the skin but with a mouthful of flesh securely imprisoned. Len struggled and cajoled. Titbits of grapes and bananas and apricots were brought. Jo-Jo was not being bought off. If Len was leaving the room so was Jo-Jo and the gorilla seemed to be adamant that as far as he was concerned the Siamese-twin relationship would last forever.

'Let me have a go with him,' said Mr Legge. 'Perhaps he'll let me put him down. Anyway I'm perhaps a bit more nimble than you, Len.'

He went back in. Yes, Jo-Jo was quite happy about another change. The look of innocence returned to his face and he transferred his affections to the zoo director. Now it was Mr Legge's turn to move with his burden until he was just inside the door and then, cooing soothingly and stroking Jo-Jo's head with one hand, to try to loosen the ape's hold with his other hand. Jo-Jo pretended to be snoozing peacefully but his iron-hard black nails dug into Mr Legge's clothing with a sudden sharp movement. I swear he was peeping out between closed eyelids. Nothing doing. The gorilla stuck like a malevolent limpet. Half an hour went by and it was time to try another change. Matt Kelly was called in. Jo-Jo went to him like a lamb but when Matt tried to divest himself of the animal he lost some hair, a pocket and all the buttons from his shirt front. He did not lose the gorilla. I was in a quandary. Transferring the gorilla was easy but at this rate we would soon run out of gorilla holders or ape donees or whatever one likes to call them. Dope seemed to be the answer but using the dart-gun or giving tranquillising injections might stimulate Jo-Jo to take it out on the current holder before dropping to sleep, and gorillas can bite hard and rip viciously with their fingers. We would have to do it without the infliction of even a minute amount of pain, which meant that the only way to adminster the drug was by mouth. In the food store I injected a knock-out dose of phencyclidine into the pulp of a banana without actually peeling the fruit. Jo-Jo likes to peel his own.

Back in the ape house Matt was sitting glumly on the floor, almost totally submerged by the loving heap of gorilla that clasped him. There is a rule about giving doped bananas to apes or doctored sausages to wolves or hollowed-out loaves of bread containing medicine to suspicious hippopotamuses: always proffer first a sterling, pristine, untampered-with and impeccable article of the same kind. Having established your credentials with number one, you then emerge in your true colours by nobbling number two. With this in mind I offered a normal banana to Jo-Jo. He took it, peeled it with one hand and his teeth (the other hand was maintaining its hold on Matt's right ear), ate the pulp with relish, licked the skin and threw it down. Now I produced the Trojan horse, or rather the Trojan banana. Again Jo-Jo took it, peeled it and prepared to thrust it into his mouth. Then out of the recesses of his mind came either a generous thought or, more likely I suspect, an inkling, just an embryonic inkling, that malpractice was afoot. With a gentle pouting of his lips and a soothing cooing sound Jo-Jo rammed the fruit of the banana firmly between Matt's lips. The head keeper spluttered and gulped but Jo-Jo was insistent that Matt was going to have his banana. I was horrified. If Matt swallowed the doctored banana pulp he would be unconscious within ten minutes and, worse, might suffer for days afterwards from the reported side effects of erotic fantasies and burning sensations in the extremities.

'Spit it out, for God's sake!' I shouted. 'Don't swallow any banana, Matt!'

Matt spat for dear life. Jo-Jo seemed distinctly surprised at the ingratitude and tried to poke bits of the mushed pulp back between Matt's teeth. Matt continued to puff out furiously, rolling his eyes at us as we stood watching helplessly. Suzy came over and helped clean up the mess. She picked the spat-out bits off Jo-Jo's hairy chest like a wife carefully sponging the soup stains off her husband's dinner jacket. Not a bit of the banana did Jo-Jo eat nor would he accept any further pieces of food. Eventually, for it was by now well on into the evening, it was decided to try to relieve poor Matt by doing yet another change, this time back to Len again. The transfer went smoothly but still Len could not get out of the room without his ape.

'I've heard of having a monkey on one's back,' he remarked glumly, 'but I've got a gorilla on my front!'

At last it was decided to leave Len in the gorilla quarters. A comfortable chair was brought in and a transistor radio was left playing outside the door. When Mr Legge went back at midnight Jo-Jo was still comfortably, immovably, in situ. Len tried to doze. It was seven o'clock the following morning before Jo-Jo finally fell into a deep, forgetful slumber and Len was able to lower him gently to the floor, to steal out of the room and lock up.

Never again did we go in with the two gorillas. When I needed to examine them I used the dart-gun and a tranquilliser. But we all remember affectionately the happy times we had playing tag with a pair of baby gorillas. Like children, it's a pity they have to grow up.

155

Fourteen

Of all the trips abroad on which my work has taken me, the one which may yet have the most far-reaching results came about when, after years of fruitless applications for a visa to visit China, I was eventually invited to spend two weeks studying animal acupuncture and inspecting zoological collections in that country. At that time few Western zoologists had been given the opportunity to see the Chinese animal collections, many of which contain species never exhibited in the West. I was anxious to see some of the very rare creatures that inhabit China's most inaccessible regions and to find out whether and to what degree the science of acupuncture was being applied to animals, particularly undomesticated ones.

With Gary Smart, one of the directors of the Royal Windsor Safari Park, I flew out to Peking. We arrived in bitterly cold weather, and in the middle of the night, at the forbidding, Stalinesque Peking airport, where we were met by Mr Lo, a delightful, slightly-built young man who was to be our guide, interpreter and political mentor. He told us we could go where we liked and photograph anything and explained that, although he had not handled a veterinary scientist before, he had carefully prepared a handwritten phrase book of words which might be needed by him during our discourses. It was crammed with every conceivable veterinary word from anaplasmosis to Zonules of Zinn, each with the corresponding Chinese ideogram.

'That, Dr Taylor,' he said, smiling broadly, 'will come in useful when we go round the zoos and hospitals. But first, as a good friend of China, you will want to see our progress in light engineering, agricultural communes, heavy industry, textile production and so forth.'

We felt obliged to murmur our assent. For three days we inspected light-bulb factories and sheds where Peking ducks were force-fed by machines, we were sung to by infant schools and toured secondary schools where every class had some special item of entertainment ready for us, we looked at tractor exhibitions and blocks of flats, we had tea and sweets with little old ladies who told us how cruel landlords used to be, and we drank gallons of delightful green tea with innumerable revolutionary committees, each member of which described a particular aspect of progress in birth control, the manufacture of bricks, shipbuilding or the eradication of all traces of Confucianism. But not a zoo, not a wolf nor a snake, not a monkey nor a panda did we see. We became increasingly anxious that the continuous socio-political hurly-burly might take up the whole of our visit. Then, far more pleasantly, began a series of visits to the great and glorious relics of the old China, the Forbidden City, the great wall, the Ming tombs and palaces, temples, monasteries and gardens. It was all immensely fascinating, but still we saw no zoos. At last, our patience wearing if not thin at least somewhat slimmer, we felt that we had served our apprenticeship in Anglo-Chinese friendship and made forceful representations to be shown the things that we had paid many hundreds of pounds to come and see. At last we set foot in our first Chinese zoo park, in Peking.

The zoo was stuffed with animals and birds that we had never seen before. There were giant Tibetan donkeys, the most dangerous animals in the zoo, we were told, when they are in the mating season. A north-east Chinese tiger far out-stripped the record size given in the *Guinness Book of Records*. There were reptiles and birds found only in remote corners of that vast country, and elephants and rhinoceros only recently discovered in their own Chinese forests. We spent a long time admiring the fabulous golden monkeys from the snow-covered north. These unique primates with bright blue faces, snub noses and long golden hair were the most handsome monkeys I have ever seen. Then there were the giant pandas, an adorable group of youngsters lying on their backs in the sun chewing sugar cane and bamboo.

All the animals seemed very healthy and contented but when at the end of our tour of the zoo we had the usual formal meeting with the revolutionary committee that runs it, I could find out little about their veterinary services. They declined to show us the veterinary laboratory as being unworthy and inadequate and they said that acupuncture was never used on the zoo stock. I asked for samples from the giant pandas, which I was keen to examine for parasites. There was always the chance that one would find some new and unnamed species of worm or fluke in the droppings of so rare a creature. Plastic bags full of droppings from each of the pandas were promptly produced. At the end of my visit I carefully carried them back to England, only to find on detailed microscopical examination that not one of the samples contained any sign of a single unwanted guest. My daydreams of being remembered by posterity through some obscure maggot bearing my latinised name were dashed.

After Peking we visited Shanghai and Canton zoos. At each the picture was the same – a priceless stock of mainly Chinese animals, a polite but firm refusal to give information on medical care, and a complete lack of interest in buying from or exchanging animals with the West. As for selling animals to European zoos it was politely explained that as the stock belonged to the people only the people could give permission. It was not altogether clear how the people went about voicing their opinions. No-one cared to comment on the pandas given to certain Western heads of state nor on the sensible exchanges of animals which had recently taken place with Whipsnade Zoo in England.

I was determined to see acupuncture being practised and insisted that Mr Lo should organise it, since I was being frustrated in the primary aim of my Chinese trip. First we were shown dental clinics where patients sat in long rows of chairs receiving routine attention to their mouths. Some had opted for what we would call orthodox local anaesthetic injections to numb the pain. Others were receiving treatment under acupuncture anaesthesia, and these patients had one or two fine stainless steel wires protruding from their hands or arms. Next we were taken to an outpatients' clinic where minor ailments such as headache, lumbago and muscle sprains were being dealt with. In a small room we found a crowd of people of both sexes, standing, sitting or lying on benches. They positively sprouted needles all over the place, from heads, necks, arms, backs, legs and toes. Not a drop of blood could be seen oozing anywhere. Later I saw a baby delivered and a lung lobe removed using the same techniques. In each case the patient was conscious and able to talk with the surgeons during the operation. But I still had to see acupuncture used on animals.

One day Mr Lo arrived at our hotel to say that I was invited to the Central Veterinary Clinic in Peking, where an operation had been laid on. We drove out to the clinic, a complex of single-storey buildings covered in anti-revisionist slogans. The revolutionary committee of veterinarians welcomed us with the usual tea party and hour of political instruction before we got down to business. It was explained that although they used acupuncture anaesthesia in around 200 major operations on cattle, horses and mules each year, they had not got any large animal needing surgery on the day of my visit. To my dismay, although I must admit I felt unwilling to try and stop them, they proposed to operate on a perfectly healthy old horse and remove a piece of its large intestine.

First they gave me a carefully prepared lecture, illustrated with pictures pinned up on the wall, on the precise anatomical landmarks used for finding the correct acupuncture spot for each operation. It appeared that the clinic was using the method as a matter of routine for surgery of the head, chest

159

and abdomen, although they reported only fair results in removing sensation from the limbs below the elbow or knee. Research, they said, was continuing into animal acupuncture anaesthesia: the operation that I would see that day would need only two needles, whereas a year before they would have had to use fourteen for the same job. Research and refinement of the technique for locating the needle points precisely by using a sort of galvanometer that detects changes in the electrical resistance of the skin at these points, together with the diligent application of Chairman Mao's thoughts, had rendered twelve needles redundant.

We went into a rather odd operating theatre that resembled a Pennine cow byre and all donned white gowns, caps and masks. The place was poorly equipped and badly in need of painting but they did have a useful-looking, hydraulically operated large-animal operating table. A tired old grey mare was led in. She was hobbled to the table in the verticle position and when secure was gently revolved until she was lying on her side. The anaesthetist produced two long acupuncture needles which had been sterilising in a pan boiling away on a gas ring and indicated the points which had been described in my briefing. For complete anaesthesia of the left side of the horse's abdomen and bowels she was going to put one needle into the leg foreleg above the knee and the other into the same leg but below the knee. Swabbing the chosen sites with alcohol, she pressed the needles in. The one above the knee was pressed diagonally downwards through the flesh until it had almost transfixed the limb and was tenting the skin on the inside of the leg. Mr Lo moaned as he stood beside me.

'Dr Taylor, I am going to be sick,' he said, turning away. He was certainly going green above his mask.

For the horse the insertion of the needle was probably no more painful than having a deep shot of local anaesthetic and it lay calmly enough. When the needles were exactly in position wires from an alternating current generator were clipped to them. Knobs were turned and dials were set on the machine.

Small muscles in the leg near the acupuncture needles began to twitch and flicker.

'Now we wait for ten minutes,' said the anaesthetist. 'Then the surgeon can begin.'

Ten minutes passed. The horse lay blinking and supping water through a tube from a kettle. The foreleg muscles continued to twitch but otherwise there was nothing to suggest that the animal was anything but totally conscious and in command of all its senses. The surgeon picked up his scalpel. I clenched my fists under my gown. He was going to have to open the flank for a good twelve inches in one continuous incision biting deep through skin and fat. Rather you than me, old boy, I thought. It was impossible to conceive that those two needles and the electric box buzzing away by the horse's head could have removed all feeling of pain from an apparently unrelated area several feet away. Nothing I had learnt in those long days at university in Glasgow, taking formaldehyde-pickled horse corpses to bits under the eagle eye of the anatomy tutor, had suggested any link between the foreleg and the belly. I was a prisoner of my Western training. What do we really know about the nervous system, particularly the elusive network that we call the autonomic? I was to come to believe that it was in this microscopic infrastructure of communication and command that the secret of acupuncture lay.

The scalpel pressed down onto the flesh and with a single elegant stroke the horse's side was unzipped down to the muscle layers. It did not bat an eyelid. I was watching intently for any sign of tensing or other reaction to the sudden pain of the knife, but there was nothing. The surgeon deftly opened the muscle, then sliced through the most sensitive layer of all, the peritoneum. A horse's peritoneum is thick and jam-packed with nerve endings. Surely now the old grey would wince or struggle? No, it just supped on at its kettle.

The loops of intenstine were now visible. The surgeon pulled gently and then vigorously on a loop. Oddly enough, the bowel and its attachments have no nerve endings that can detect cutting or even burning, but they do contain lots of endings that scream blue murder at the slightest tugging, stretching or twisting. That is why horses suffer such pain from the griping distensions and distortions of the bowel in colic, pain that can literally shock them to death. This old grey seemed totally oblivious to the pulling. Expertly the surgeon took out a portion of the bowel wall and stiched up the incision, then smoothly and rapidly he closed the various layers of the operation wound. Half an hour later the skin was closed. The anaesthetists switched off the electric machine and withdrew the needles. The table was returned to an upright position and the old horse was released. Steady as a rock, and dropping a healthy pile of manure on the way, she walked outside into the yard and began to eat corn heartily from a trough. I was most impressed.

Over the next few days I spent as much time as I could with the vets at the clinic. They had no experience of working with zoo animals, and as dogs and cats are regarded as unproductive creatures and are rarely seen in China (they are as rare as flies, which have been almost completely eradicated in China; during two weeks in the country we saw no dogs, one cat and two flies) they could give no advice about using acupuncture on carnivores. However, charts of the acupuncture points on horses, cattle and humans, together with sets of needles and even little plastic men and animals on which to practise, are widely and cheaply available throughout China. The man in the street and the 'barefoot doctors', the medical auxiliary workers who go into the countryside to take medical attention to the peasants and the peasants' animals, are encouraged to become proficient in this cheap and highly portable means of wide-ranging therapy.

China convinced me that there is a place in Western medicine for the development of acupuncture. If I worked with small animals such as dogs and cats, I would experiment with the needles on certain conditions which are still difficult to tackle thoroughly by orthodox methods. Nervous diseases, fits, paralysis, arthritic conditions and skin diseases seem ideal areas for investigation. But how to use the technique on my patients, the zoo animals? By studying the charts of the cow and the horse and the man which I had brought back from China, together with the set of 'barefoot doctor' needles and a small electric machine, I realised that the needle insertion point which treats a specific type of disease or produces anaesthesia of a particular area is in the same corresponding anatomical position in each of the three species. For example the point on the human hand between the base of the thumb and the index finger, which affects the teeth, is anatomically identical to the position of the outside of the cow's foot or on the top of the horse's cannon bone which affects the teeth in those species. In difficult cases which were not yielding to conventional treatment I would try transposing the acupuncture points of the horse, cow or man onto my zoo animal patients. It would be difficult with uniquely shaped animals like dolphins, and I have since learned that American vets have so far had no luck in identifying the acupuncture areas in these creatures. Still, the striking improvement in many cases of dolphin disease where the animal has been pricked with injection needles carrying perhaps only vitamin shots suggests that it is not always the medication that does the trick but that unwittingly the hypodermics may have hit the bullseye on an acupuncture point.

Shortly after returning from China I had my first suitable case for acupuncture. Eddie, a young giraffe at Royal Windsor Safari Park, had been dogged with chronic recurring arthritis of all four ankle joints ever since he had damaged the joints repeatedly during a rough passage through the Bay of Biscay on his way to Britain as a baby. Eddie's joints were a mess – enlarged, thickened with scar tissue round the joint capsule and prone to flare up frequently into a painful, laming, inflammatory condition. He had had all sorts of treatment from poultices and cortisone to courses of gold and new anti-arthritic drugs. Nothing worked for long. I decided to give Eddie five twenty-minute courses of acupuncture at weekly intervals, using the points on his body anatomically equivalent to the ones which the Chinese used for polyarthritis in cattle.

Eddie was enticed by succulent oak branches into a restraining pen where he was unable to turn round or back away. With the aid of a ladder I climbed up the side of the pen and selected the two points over the rib-cage which I hoped would do the trick. I disinfected the skin and pushed the thin needles in about one inch deep. Eddie did not seem to care: he was used to injections and these needles were far finer than the ones used for administering drugs. I clipped on the two wires leading to the generator which was powered by a tiny transistor radio battery. Tense with anticipation I turned on the control switch. A little red light began to flash in the box. I adjusted the frequency control according to the instructions I had received in China, and the superficial muscles in the skin between the two needles began to twitch. Eddie continued to munch oak leaves. Twenty minutes later I switched off, withdrew the needles and climbed down the ladder. Eddie limped away.

The giraffe's condition appeared unchanged, but three days later the giraffe keeper reported a definite improvement in Eddie's gait. I was not prepared to hope that it was because of the acupuncture. One week later I repeated the treatment. Eddie was undoubtedly walking much better and I had a sneaking suspicion that his joints were not quite so grotesquely enlarged. The next week I was certain. Eddie's joints were on the mend. By the time the course of treatments was complete the giraffe's joints were almost down to normal size, better than we had ever seen them since he had arrived, and he walked gracefully without a trace of a limp. Now the question was whether the arthritis would relapse after a time just as it had done following all the other forms of therapy. We waited. One, two, three weeks went by. Two months passed and still Eddie's joints were holding up. He had never been sound for so long. After four months we decided that it was fair to claim that he had made a remarkable recovery quite different from the temporary improvements seen in the past.

It left me itching to try the technique on some more knotty cases in exotic animals, but my second acupuncture patient turned out to be my elder daughter, Stephanie. Going home one evening I found her miserably complaining of toothache. Remembering the dental clinic I had seen in China and the ease with which the acupuncturists had numbed the teeth via a readily locatable point on the hand, I prevailed upon her to let me use my magic box and needle on her. Reluctantly, but remembering my frequent enthusiastic progress reports on Eddie, she agreed. Two minutes after I had popped in the needle she announced that the toothache had gone. Whatever the explanation of the mechanism behind acupuncture, I admit that in her case suggestion may have played an important part. But when I see Eddie cantering in the sunlight with that fluid motion so charming and so typical of giraffes, his ankles slim and free from ugly knobbles, I am certain that nobody suggested anything to him.

Doctor in the Zoo

The Making of a Zoo Vet

One

Fifty yards away I knew by the high-pitched bleep-bleep coming from my car that someone, somewhere, was looking for me. I unlocked, switched off the bleeper and called up the radio telephone operator.

"Call for you from Holland, Dr. Taylor," she said. "A dwoniker has escaped from an animal dealer near Utrecht. He wants you to go over straightaway with your dart-pistol to anaesthetize it. Over."

"Roger, wilco," I replied, according to protocol, and drove home wondering about the meaning of the peculiar message. "Shelagh," I called to my wife as I walked in the door, "what the dickens is a dwoniker?"

Shelagh had no more idea than I did. I called up the operator again to check the name of the beast. Yes, she was quite certain. A dwoniker was on the loose in the land of windmills. As we made our way to Manchester Airport Shelagh and I went over the possibilities concerning the identity of the mysterious animal. Brand new kinds of animal are discovered every year, and it is not all that long ago since as large and spectacular a creature as the okapi was first reported, but I thought it unlikely that the dealer had stumbled across a completely new species. Assuming I was right, the dwoniker might be a beast that I had never heard of, the name of something that had been mangled in the process of transmission by phone from Holland to England, or the Dutch name for something mundane like a deer or a llama. I plumped for the last alternative. "It's a typically Dutch word," I stated confidently. "Bet it's a rhinoceros gone berserk." Although "dwoniker" did indeed have the ring of a Dutch word, my knowledge of the language was in fact limited to the three words for "yes", "no" and an unmentionable part of one's anatomy.

Shelagh was convinced that the answer lay in the name being scrambled by the telephone operators. "Think of some animals' names that are similar to 'dwoniker'," she advised, "something that sounds roughly like it." We tried, but the best we came up with was duiker, the English name coming from the Dutch for a genus of small African antelopes.

The more I thought about it, the more I came round to the idea that duiker was right. But if one of those fleet-footed, minuscule creatures had done a bunk, it would be incredibly difficult to pursue it, stalk it and fire an anaesthetic dart successfully at it in open countryside, even assuming I could find it in the first place. I had chased escaped red deer, ten times the size of duiker, enough times and been lucky to get a momentary glimpse of them after hours of searching. Nor did I know much about duiker. I had seen them at London Zoo but most other collections in Britain did not exhibit them. This would be my first encounter with one: that was about all I knew. I hoped that these small, frail and probably highly expensive individuals would agree with my anaesthetics if I was lucky enough to get within darting range. God forbid that they should be one of that "awkward squad" among antelopes for whom certain knock-out chemicals paralyse the heat-control centre in the brain so that the unconscious creature suffers a rocketing rise in temperature that can easily and fatally cook the vital central nervous system.

At Amsterdam's Schiphol Airport the animal dealer, Mr. van den Baars, was waiting. As we walked to his car I forgot that the real identity of the "dwoniker" still hung in the air. "Where is the duiker, exactly?" I asked.

"Duiker, what duiker? Oh, do you mean dike?" said

van den Baars, slightly puzzled.

"The duiker, the one that's escaped."

The Dutchman laughed. "I really don't know where you got that from. My duiker are all safely tucked up. No, the problem is with two onagers that have slipped out of my quarantine farm."

Onagers! Two onagers. "Dwonikers". Listening to the dealer's rapid, accented English, I understood how the radio telephone operator might easily have created a mythical beast. At last I had the solution to the mystery and knew my quarry: a couple of onagers, the rare and valuable wild asses of Central Asia which always reminded me of sandy-coloured and rather unspectacular mules.

"They've been sighted on a water meadow about a mile from the farm," said my companion. "It's open country and they're grazing quietly, or at least they were."

We swept along the motorway past the neat, dull townships outside Amsterdam with the evening sun flashing off the black water of the narrow canals that ran everywhere. Onagers were also a new species for me, but they were nice-sized members of the equine family. I had doped a good number of horses and zebras and even the odd Przevalski's horse, another wild species. I was carrying drugs which could be used safely on all the equines, although some needed comparatively bigger doses, pound for pound, than others.

Mr. van den Baars stopped the car in a narrow lane and pointed across a low hedge. At first all I could see were acres and acres of green grass in one gigantic field. Then I spotted the onagers. They were right in the middle, looking like two creamy-coloured mice from where we sat and cropping happily at the lush pasture in the golden light. "There they are," said the Dutchman, "and here come Piet and Kees with crates on the tractor. I'll stay here in the car. What do you plan to do?"

I squinted into the distance. There was no cover anywhere

near the onagers. I would have to try the disarming, non-chalant approach. "I'll go alone to see if I can dart the pair," I said. "Keep your men back here till I wave. Then send them over. Shouldn't be much problem, if I can get within forty feet. But if they start to run. . . ." I shook my head. With night coming on and so much room to manoeuvre, the onagers could stay out of range until I had to give up. I wished I had a dart-rifle, for in that vast field my pistol seemed about as potent as a peashooter.

Loading two darts with anaesthetic, I climbed over a gate in the hedge and ran down a bank onto the billiard-table surface of the meadow. I marched off towards my prey, cocking the pistol, screwing the gas-control knob to maximum pressure and keeping one finger on the safety catch. The sun was an orange semicircle on the horizon. I realized that I was working several feet below sea level. As I came nearer to the grazing onagers one of them looked up, munching, pricked its ears and alerted the other. From 250 yards away they stared at me. Now for my display of cunning, a simple device which I had found effective three times out of ten and idiotically useless the other seven. It relies on my ability to impersonate a harmless rustic out for an evening stroll with nothing but innocent thoughts in his head. The yokel ambles along and pays not the slightest attention to the odd hippopotamus or aardvark—or onager—that might cross his path. So bucolic a fellow, gazing at the sky, humming to himself, is the very opposite of the predatory human, the pursuing keeper or beady-eyed veterinarian, whom such creatures can spot from a mile away. It is essential when using this ploy not to approach the animals head on. I shuffle along on a course which will take me at an angle across their bows and not too close to them.

This is what I did as I came closer to the onagers. My dart-gun was hidden in my arms folded idly across my chest. I seemed, I hoped, to be deep in thought, thought far removed from onager hunting, as I flicked at the occasional tussock of grass with my toe, watched birds fly by and sang a low, gentle song. Having taken a furtive glance at the onagers to establish their position, I gazed steadfastly at everything else and studiously avoided being seen looking at them. I was quite pleased with my performance. "Dum de dum dum," I carolled softly. I was reducing the distance slowly but steadily. I picked a stem of grass and chewed it like rustics are said to do. Great acting— I reminded myself of the young Olivier. "Dum de dum dum." It must have been plain that if there was one thing I was not interested in, that thing was wild asses. "Dum de dum—aaagh!" With a great splash, the rustic found himself up to his knees in water and sinking deeper as his shoes hit mud. I had wandered into a narrow, straight-sided dike running across the meadow with banks so close together that it was almost impossible to see from twenty yards. Dripping, I struggled out and looked around. The onagers were still standing peacefully, eating and keeping an eye on me as I tried with one hand to wring some water out of my trouser legs. Yes, they must have been thinking, that's the village idiot for sure. They shook their heads and chewed on.

I resumed my quiet ramble but kept a sharp eye open for more dikes and ditches. I found them. It became apparent that the whole area was neatly subdivided by water channels in place of fences or hedges, and each time I discovered one I was almost on top of it. The harmless peasant had to do some jumping, but I was getting almost within range of my quarry. Eventually I judged I could risk standing still and glancing out of the corner of my eye at the two onagers. They were watching me but were obviously not alarmed. The range was thirty-five feet, I guessed. Close enough. I released the safety catch, followed the flight of a heron against the sky, let my face turn slowly with the bird until I was looking at the onagers, and unfolded my arms. Humming disarmingly, I took aim down the barrel of the pistol and pulled the trigger. Plop! A dart embedded itself in the plump haunch of one of the animals. Swishing its tail, it trotted off a few paces and looked round at its flank. By then I had turned my back on the onagers, apparently unconcerned but in fact hurriedly loading my second dart. Slowly I turned again. The second onager was staring at me uncertainly, ready to beat it at the first inkling that I was up to any skulduggery. It watched me bring the pistol up, sensed danger but made its move to wheel and flee too late. A red-tasselled dart thwacked into its shoulder muscle.

Both animals were injected and should be unconscious within five minutes. I waved furiously towards the road where van de Baars and his helpers waited. By the time they arrived, the onagers should be ready for the crates. Once they were loaded, all I would have to do would be to reverse the anaesthetic with a stimulant antidote and my work would be done. The onagers began to stagger and to trot round with the peculiar high-stepping gait that equines show when an anaesthetic begins to make the world spin before their eyes. Then, suddenly, they did what so many animals do when darted with potent anaesthetics—they went straight for the nearest hazard. Be it zebra, deer, antelope or domestic horse, if there is barbed wire or a rocky hole or a marsh or a pool of water in the vicinity, a half-doped creature seems more often than not to be uncannily drawn towards it.

The two onagers high-stepped their way towards the nearest canal. With a frantic dash I managed to catch up with the closer of the two and grabbed its tail to try to brake its progress. No use. The onager blindly pulled me along behind it. I tried hauling the tail to one side to steer it away from trouble, but the wild ass was too powerful for me. With a great eruption of green water, my onager plunged into the canal. Seconds later its mate did the same twenty yards away. Now I had two expensive and rare creatures about to lose consciousness in five feet of water. Both seemed likely to drown.

I looked desperately towards the road. Van den Baars's men were just driving the tractor with the crates through the field gate towards the narrow, grassy bridge across the first dike. "Come on, schnell, schnell!" I shouted, hoping that they understood German and could hear me at that distance over the roar of their engine. The head of one of the onagers, eyes glazing, rested against the muddy side of the canal. The other was repeatedly dunking its muzzle. It was almost fully unconscious. There was only one thing to do. I jumped into the canal alongside it and grabbed the heavy head. Slithering frantically on the soft mud bottom, I tried to hold my balance and keep the nostrils above water as the onager pitched all its weight onto me. Straining, I pulled myself from under the animal and tugged its muzzle until the tip of it just rested on the bank. The other onager was going under. I dragged myself like a dishcloth out of the water, squelched quickly along the grass and then leapt into the canal again to grasp the second beast's head. "Schnell, schnell!" I kept yelling.

After what seemed like years, the men arrived, jumped off the tractor and dashed over to me. "Get the boxes off the tractor, quick!" I gasped. "I can't hold the head up much longer." I was going to have to reverse the anaesthetic with the animals still in the water. The three of us could not lift the heavy, unconscious onagers bodily out of the vertically sided waterway, but if I could bring them round enough to help themselves, maybe between their efforts and ours we could get them out and box them before they were awake enough to disappear over the horizon and start the hunt all over again. Underwater I fished in my pockets for plastic syringe, needle and antidote. There was no hope of sterilizing or disinfecting anything. The two asses and I were all covered in slimy water from top to toe.

Getting my head under the space between the lower jawbones of the onager, I managed to support the animal's head painfully on top of mine, thus freeing both my hands to load the syringe. That done, I punched a clenched fist into the base of its neck somewhere under the canal surface and raised the jugular vein where it emerged from the water. A minute after I had inserted the needle and pressed the antidote in fast, I felt power returning to the onager's muscles. It lifted its head unaided. Looking quickly to see that its mate was still breathing above water, I told the men the next step. "I'll go under, grab one foreleg at a time, bring them up and shove them on the canal bank. Then you position the forefeet and haul on the neck. With me behind and the animal getting thrust back in its hind end, it should clamber out."

They nodded. I dived under the cold water; up to that moment I had not noticed how chilled I was. Groping blindly under the stocky body of the wild ass, I found a foreleg and hauled it up to the surface. The men reached down to help. I repeated the procedure, then waded round to the onager's rear. Slapping it on the rump and hauling its tail forward, I encouraged it to move. The drug was now almost completely reversed. With a great heave, the beast lunged over the edge of the canal, the men clung onto its neck, and before it could fully regain its senses it was bundled into one of the waiting crates.

I refilled my syringe and for the fourth time that day did my impersonation of a cumbersome water sprite by jumping into the water by the second onager. We went through the same routine. The reviving animal scrambled out and was pulled towards the crate. This time, as it went over the edge of the canal with me manipulating the tail, it lashed out smartly with one of its hind legs. The unshod but solid hoof caught me squarely on the chest and I crashed backwards under the water for yet another thorough immersion. Picking myself up from the mud beneath the water, I wondered momentarily what on earth had made me choose a life which led to floundering in the depths of a Dutch canal with water weed over my eyes and up my nostrils.

When both onagers were safely restored to the quarantine

farm I darted them again, this time with long-acting penicillin, for fear that my insanitary injections in the canal
might have introduced germs along with the needle.

"Now, Dr. Taylor," said van den Baars as I stood
shivering in my underpants and put on my spare clothes,
"perhaps you would like to warm up with a glass or two of
our good Holland gin. You've certainly earned it. I must
thank you most sincerely—on behalf of the dwonikers."

Two

The first steps along the road to that muddy Dutch dike were taken as a young schoolboy with an absorbing interest in everything which flew, swam, crept or crawled. Wandering the fields and moors of the Pennines around my home in Rochdale, near Manchester, I would find no end of creatures obviously in trouble, especially sheep. Unable to rise, often with inflamed and swollen vulvas, frequently being eaten away by blowfly maggots, these pitiful animals lay alone on windswept hillsides or at the bottom of quarries, or struggled in moorland streams. It was no use trying to find the owners of the sheep. The moors are vast and the flocks wander for miles, gathered in only once or twice a year by shepherds who miraculously know where they are likely to be. Besides, the farmers did not bother to do anything for these fallen individuals even when they came across one. "'Twon't do no good, lad," they would say, turning their back on the animal's misery and trudging off. The moor was common land and the grass free food. Losing a few sheep from disease or foxes or thieves was part of the game. They still made enough to live by.

School homework would be forgotten as I crouched in the rain over yet another sodden woolly body, thumbing through a book called *Veterinary Counter Practice*. This slim volume was written to help chemists give first-aid advice in their shops to pet owners. It was illustrated by Edwardian engravings of bearded men in frock coats solemnly holding unprotesting and improbable cats with linen-draped heads over bowls belching medicated steam, and of ornately coiffed ladies using what looked like armoured gauntlets to thrust pills down dogs' throats. Certainly it was the Gospel on veterinary matters as far as I was concerned. I did not know that I was looking at sheep dying of gas-gangrene brought on by difficult lambing, with livers riddled with fluke parasites or with bloodstreams lethally deficient in calcium, none of which was mentioned in my book. I just covered the animals with my jacket, treated their inflamed parts with Germolene ointment, picked the maggots off them and forced Dad's brandy between their lips.

I do not think a single one of my sheep patients ever recovered. Once, twice, sometimes three times a day I would go out to them and sooner or later I would find them dead. On one black occasion I came across a ram that had fallen into a quarry but was still alive. The jagged ends of its shattered femur poked a full four inches through the skin, alive with industrious bluebottles. Trembling and sick with fright, I killed my first patient, suffocating him with my jacket wrapped tight round his nostrils and mouth. He took a long time to die. I walked home dizzy with remorse and did not sleep at all for two nights.

In addition to the Germolene and brandy, my box of medicaments included vitamin tonic and tincture of arnica, a stinging brown herbal preparation which was my grand-mother's cure-all. Grandmother seldom walked out on the moors with me, but was my ally, mentor, co-conspirator and assistant in all my surgical work at home on small beasts. She was a spirited, bustling woman with features the colour of pale honey and homely as an oven-bottom muffin. She knew alcohol, tobacco and cosmetics to be works of the Devil and had stormed out of church in mid-sermon when the new curate had revealed himself to be an evolutionist. Sturdily built, with grey gleaming eyes in a round face, she ate little other than a sort of unbleached tripe, a diet which she never appeared to find monotonous and which she augmented on

Mondays with cold fatty mutton and mint sauce. The small boys of the neighbourhood held her in great respect for the way in which, if she were so minded, she could strike a brilliant shower of sparks from the cobblestones in our back street by clipping them expertly with her iron-soled Lancashire clogs. Lots of the lads, myself included, could kick atoms of fire from the stones like this as we lounged outside on a summer evening, but none of us could approach the effortless pyrotechnic display put on by the old lady as she passed us on her way to or from the tripe shop.

There was a second reason why the small boys held her in great awe. Along with the strictly seasonal hobbies of "swaling" (burning the dead grass on the moor edges), "conkering" (duelling with horse chestnuts hardened and threaded onto pieces of string in which the object was to split one's opponent's nut away from its string), cricket, and whipping tops along the flagstones, we all kept mice. The problem was that getting hold of tame mice was almost impossible during the war years, and there was a serious dearth of the small rodents in the hutches, pockets and private hideaways of the boys in our street. Grandmother solved the problem. Somehow she found out that they kept mice, both white and chocolate coloured, at the Rochdale gasworks, presumably to test for gas just as canaries were used in coal mines. One Saturday morning she led a band of us down to the gasworks. We each carried some form of small container, a tin or a cardboard box. Ecstatically, we came home with mice; Grandmother knew the man who had the key to the room where the mice were kept. Normally a surly individual, he was genial in Grandmother's presence and chuckled as he put one or two of the velvety little creatures into each of the containers thrust urgently under his nose. After that breakthrough, we tried visits to the gasworks alone, but without Grandmother it never worked. They had none to spare, they did not keep any mice, the man was too busy. But for Grandmother, persuaded by a gaggle of imploring six-

and seven-year-olds to make a detour from her Saturday trip to market, mice were always forthcoming.

Hardworking and practical, she was at the same time highly sentimental. She paid me threepence a week to sing for her each Sunday evening a sugary ballad entitled "I'll Walk Beside You" while my mother accompanied me on the piano. This excruciating ritual regularly brought tears to Grandmother's eyes (and had the same effect, though for different reasons, on the rest of the household); mercifully it ceased when my voice began to change.

In her youth Grandmother had been a seamstress, and she insisted that I learn to sew and knit, arguing that the art of surgery on which my heart was firmly set was just cutting and stitching, and that neatness in weaving threads in and out of living flesh could be developed on pieces of flannel, silk and worsted. I spent hours grafting squares of cloth together under Grandmother's grey, hawk-like eyes and had my knuckles painfully rapped by one of her thick metal knitting needles whenever I grew careless. Her wisdom was confirmed years later at university when the Surgery Professor, watching the students clumsily practise their first simple operations on the chill, unbleeding bodies of already dead animals, urged us to darn our socks and sew on buttons at every opportunity. "Less beer and wenching and more needlework, gentlemen," he would roar as we cobbled away at the corpses.

Grandmother and I made a good team. She was adept with the only anaesthetic we had, a freezing spray of ethyl chloride. With one hand she would hold the struggling form of a thrush I had found fluttering and tumbling frantically through the undergrowth, and with the other would direct a stream of the numbing liquid onto the bird's shattered wing bone. As hoarfrost formed on the bloodstained flight feathers, she would tell me to begin splinting the limb with matchsticks and strips of sticking-plaster, her eyes following the movements of my fingers through a pair of gold-rimmed spectacles.

My parents tolerated well enough at first the toads convalescing in the bathroom cupboard, the paralysed owl that sat on top of the grandfather clock in the hall and the rabbit road-accident victims that either regained vitality or inexorably wasted away in the emergency wards I established in empty zinc washing tubs. But as the number of patients grew, so did the problems. The owl on the hall clock stopped the ancient timepiece when I forgot one day to replace the sheet of newspaper on which he squatted and his droppings slipped through a gap in the wooden casing and completely clogged the brass works. With the greatest difficulty Dad cleaned them up, but the clock never worked properly again. Still, if any member of the family raised the matter of the luckless clock, Grandmother would fold her arms, heave up her bosom and tetchily remind all present that it was her clock, that it suited her very well and that it never had kept good time: a preposterous statement that all knew, but none dared say, was the very opposite of the truth. With the grumblings silenced, Grandmother would slip me a solemn wink.

When the war came, our house's old coal-cellar was converted into the family's air-raid shelter. Its ceiling was reinforced by bracing beams and pillars, and bunk beds and supplies of tinned food were put in there. In fact, Rochdale was never attacked and the family did not seem to make use of the shelter during the infrequent air-raid warnings. I soon saw how this could be turned to my advantage, for there had been more trouble with my parents over my veterinary activities. My father, going into the garden to inspect the rows of glass cloches under which he grew radishes and lettuce, had found not only that his ripe, fresh salad had been requisitioned for essential victualling of the rabbit wounded in the zinc tubs, but also that two recuperating old hedgehogs were actually bedded down within the line of cloches. Grandmother to the rescue again. She stood between my irate father and myself and defended her beloved seven-year-old grandson. "Enough of that, Frank," she said to my father, wagging a stern finger. "There's a war on, you know."

That was all she said. The power was in the way she said it. I can still remember clearly the sheer force of her words as she stood, arms akimbo, grey eyes unblinking. Nothing could have sounded less unreasonable or more obvious: with a war on it was time for every English man and woman, and every English rabbit, owl and hedgehog, to stand shoulder to shoulder in the common cause.

Next day, as Grandmother replanted Dad's garden with salad seeds, I took her into my confidence and outlined my idea of putting the more contentious species of mammal and bird in the apparently unused air-raid shelter.

"Your mum won't have it, dear," Grandmother murmured as we discussed the possibilities. "I know we don't often use the shelter, but suppose we do, some time?"

I argued that it was most unlikely that we would and that, apart from the old lavatory in the yard, I had no alternatives. Grandmother eventually agreed to help me but suggested that I bring my patients into the room via the chute which had been the means of delivering coal from the street when the coal-cellar was being used for its original purpose. In this way I would avoid the front and back doors and the attentions of other members of the family. It was a sound idea. My accomplice waited in the big room next door to the coal-cellar, bottling fruit, squeezing clothes through the mangle in front of the high open coal fire or doing a bit of whitewashing. With my patient in a sack or wrapped in my jacket I lifted the heavy iron grate from the coal chute at pavement level and slid down into the new hospital ward. There on the bunk beds I had the boxes, tins, jars and cages that held the sick and infirm. When the coast was clear, Grandmother would slip in and we would get to work.

The air-raid shelter hospital survived a first discovery by my young sister, Vivienne, who stumbled on it one day but was bought off by Grandmother, who gave Vivienne a little locket in exchange for her silence. Shortly afterwards, however, an air raid over Manchester led to Rochdale having a long alarm call on the sirens. The sound of bombing could be distinctly heard in our house that night and my parents decided we should all sleep in the shelter. Piling through the doorway in their pyjamas, the family found the place of refuge already fully occupied by things furry, scaly and feathered. Worse, my father discovered that I had used almost the whole cache of tinned corned beef on feeding the hedgehogs, and my little sister was bitten through her night-dress as she sleepily sat down on the bottom bunk and on the orphan fox cub to whom it belonged.

Grandmother miraculously soothed everyone's shattered nerves and fearlessly admitted opening the tins of corned beef for me, but then and there my long-suffering father decided to convert the lavatory in the yard into a recognized and approved wild animal hospital. The problem with the lavatory/hospital was that there was no room for Grandmother and me to do any actual work. That still had to be done elsewhere. Our favourite place was the kitchen. The light was good and that was essential, particularly for our regular hedgehog clinics. Together we would set about painting with chloroform the bloated blood-sucking ticks clinging to the bellies of our prickly patients. After waiting a few moments for a parasite to loosen its hold, Grandmother would stand back while I, as head surgeon, picked it off with tweezers. The trouble with hedgehogs, particularly sick ones, is that they often carry a hefty load of fleas around with them as well. The warm kitchen seemed to encourage these prodigious jumpers to leave their hosts, and on one potentially disastrous occasion my mother found scores of energetic little varmints leaping about on some pastry she was rolling out. Grandmother seized one, cracked it between finger and thumbnail and pronounced it to be a mosquito. Since it was late January, she had to add that it was an unseasonably early mosquito, but after that we began to use DDT powder on the animals before putting them into the hospital shed. Grandmother always made sure my mother was out or busy somewhere else in the house before we began hedge-hog clinics. We used the kitchen table and spoke in low voices.

When things went well, Grandmother would hum gleefully and give me a hug. Just having me to herself pleased her enormously and, although she undoubtedly loved the animals we dealt with, her principal reward I think was to feel that in some way she was helping to lay the first tiny foundations of what we both wanted me to become—a veterinarian. We would never dream that I might do anything else or that I might not be able to qualify for veterinary school. "Why," Grandmother would tell her cronies, "one day David's going to treat tigers." She was dead right.

When it came to goldfish, newts and frogs with skin diseases we at first did not do very well. I painted their ulcers with creams and antiseptic lotions but the water quickly washed these away. Time after time I had to bury my failures in the garden.

"I've an idea," Grandmother said one day, as she watched me dispose of the most recent victim, a goldfish. "Go and get me the paste I use for my false teeth, David!"

I went upstairs for the ointment that Grandmother, locked in the bathroom, used in the mysterious ritual of her toilet each morning.

"Now," she said when I gave her the tin of tacky grey stuff, "next time we have a goldfish with one of those nasty sores, we'll paint on the arnica as usual but then, before putting him back in the water, we'll smear on some of this denture paste. It's funny stuff; as soon as it gets wet it sets like wax. That's how I keep my teeth in, young feller. Here—try a bit."

I took a little of the grey paste and put it on my tongue. It was tasteless but I could feel it changing its consistency and sticking tight. I ran my tongue along the top of my mouth but the paste did not come off, and it was still hanging around when I went to bed that night. When I found the paste still unpleasantly tacky on my gums the following morning I began to realize the possibilities of the stuff. Now all we needed was a suitable case.

Some weeks later a friend brought me a lovely big frog. He was green, glistening and impassive as he sat on the palm of my hand, gulping. One of his front toes was swollen and had a parboiled appearance. Serum oozed through the skin. I showed him to Grandmother. "The false-teeth stuff," I reminded her. "This is our chance."

Grandmother was enthusiastic. "Get the paste from my room," she instructed. "We'll put it on over some comfrey ointment."

Comfrey ointment was only one of the herbal preparations whose virtues Grandmother preached. As well as arnica tincture, she taught me how to use quinine, senna and ipecacuanha wine. I was supervised in applying iodine and gentian violet and sticky kaolin poultices. Sometimes we would take animals with respiratory troubles and go out to seek the municipal road-menders with their smoking tar-boilers. Grandmother would tip the wide-eyed workmen a shilling as we stood letting an armful of sniffling hedgehog breathe in the pungent vapour for a quarter of an hour. "What's good for whooping cough in children will be good for hedgehogs," she would say confidently.

Grandmother held the frog gently while I smeared soothing, dark-green comfrey ointment on the inflamed toe. Then I covered the whole of the delicate foot with the false-teeth paste and placed the frog in a large glass jar with a couple of inches of water and a stone to climb on. I was pleased to see the paste stick to his foot as he paddled about. Next day it was still holding the comfrey ointment in place. Grandmother seemed very pleased and patted my head. Three days later we wiped away the paste and the ointment and looked at the toe. There was no doubt about it; the swelling was going down and the toe looked healthier. I repeated the double application, returned the frog to his ward and presented him with half a dozen fat bluebottles that I had caught for him. The frog and Grandmother made veterinary history, for the toe healed completely in a week, a record for frogs attending my clinic, and we released him in the pond of a nearby park. I still use Grandmother's denture paste on dolphin and sea-lion wounds.

Grandmother also hit on a novel way of treating tortoises and similar creatures that had taken a tumble or received blows hard enough to crack their shells, exposing the soft tissues underneath. Nowadays I happily cut away great windows in tortoise and terrapin shells to do operations; the window in the shell is repaired with modern epoxy resins and glass fibre and heals perfectly in a few months. When Grandmother and I were in practice, we had no such thing as epoxy resins and plastics, but she was on the right track. I must have been about twelve years old when she came up with the notion.

"It occurs to me," she said one day when we were surveying the septic, irregular hole in a terrapin carapace caused by the bite of a cat, "that to protect the soft stuff underneath once you've cleaned it up, we should seal the hole in the shell properly. Get the Bulldog kit."

My Bulldog kit for repairing punctures in the tyres of my bicycle consisted of a small tin containing sandpaper, glue, french chalk powder and discs of inner-tube rubber. I fetched it. Inner tubes, fine, I thought as I returned with the kit, but terrapins?

But there was no arguing with Grandmother. "Now, my boy," she said, "cut out the diseased flesh." She sprayed a fine stream of freezer on the spot. "Dab on the arnica." I did as she directed. "And now go ahead as if the terrapin was just an ordinary tyre puncture."

The terrapin pulled in his head with a faint hiss, apparently resigned to reincarnation as a bicycle. I sandpapered the edges of the hole in the shell, dusted them lightly with the chalk, applied the sticky glue and pressed on a rubber patch of the appropriate size. A perfect job.

Grandmother beamed. "Now," she said, "judging by the size of the hole and knowing how long it takes one's fingernails to grow half an inch and allowing for the fact that terrapins are cold-blooded and likely to heal slower than mammals like us, I reckon you ought to be able to take a peek in about a month."

The punctured terrapin, with the black patch looking like a trapdoor covering his machinery, re-extended his head and legs when he was certain that he was back in his vivarium and not likely to find himself caught up in the Tour de France. He looked unconcerned and began nibbling a tiny pond snail.

The patch held underwater, and each day I checked the edges to see they were secure. As the days went by, "Black Spot" seemed destined to be a good deal luckier than the name I had given him. One month later to the day, I brought the terrapin into the kitchen. Even Grandmother held her breath as I snipped the rubber patch with her nail scissors. I peeled the rubber back and we bumped our heads as we bent for a closer look. I let out a gasp of delight; the shell had knitted together completely and healthy new carapace covered the hole. "Black Spot" did not allow himself to get excited as Grandmother and I hugged one another and laughed with relief—we took our work very seriously and shared our occasional successes with no less intimacy than when we commiserated with one another over our frequent failures.

"Grandma," I said, "one day they'll award you the Nobel Prize for Medicine."

I had total faith in Grandmother's knowledge, and only slowly did this state of affairs reverse itself. By the time I went to university she was laid low with chronic heart disease and would not take a pill or a drop of medicine prescribed by the most eminent of specialists until her grandson and one-time partner had given the OK. She was immensely proud when I made it as a veterinarian. She hung my degree scroll above her bed and lived for me to go and talk about the old days and check the latest advice of her doctor.

Some years later I tackled my first giant tortoise case, one of the massive and rare 300-pound Galapagos tortoises at Belle Vue Zoo, Manchester. Not having had experience of the immense contractile power of their hind-leg muscles, I had let the beast trap my hand securely within the shell where I had been injecting into the soft skin of the groin. I wonder what Grandmother would have to say about patching up monsters like this, I was thinking as the keepers dragged on the rapidly disappearing leg that was pinioning me. I would tell her about it when I visited her that evening, now bed-ridden but alert as ever. I could imagine her softly wrinkled golden face breaking into a wide grin as I reminded her about "Black Spot" and compared him with his huge Galapagos relative.

The telephone rang. The head reptile keeper took the call and then came over to me.

"Dr. Taylor," he said, "bad news, I'm afraid. Your father rang to say that your grandmother has just passed away."

Three

Thanks to Grandmother's encouragement, my passion for animals stayed with me through school and university, and at university I found myself being drawn more and more towards the care of the exotic species, the wild, sometimes rare animals who, it seemed to me, demanded veterinary work of the most challenging and the most rewarding sort. After graduating in the late 'fifties I took a partnership in a veterinary practice in my home town of Rochdale, Lancashire. Rochdale is a grey, lustreless town of around 100,000 souls lying beneath the damp western slopes of the desolate and rocky Pennine moorland, with the big industrial centre of Manchester situated on the flat land twelve miles to the west and surrounded by smaller towns and villages, all of which saw their heyday in the industrial revolution and the reign of King Cotton, when the moist climate of Lancashire was so perfect for the spinning of yarn before air-conditioning and humidifiers were dreamed of. Above Rochdale's cobbled streets rose a forest of tall mill chimneys, but what sorts of animals were to be found in those drizzly streets, in the shabby smallholdings and on the bleak, windy moorlands? Certainly none of the wild, exciting creatures of which I dreamed: tigers, buffaloes or armadilloes.

A typical veterinary practice in Rochdale consisted of a mixture of household pets and farm animals, and it was on dogs involved in road accidents, sows that got into difficulties when giving birth and sheep struck down by mysterious lethal epidemics that I learned the arts of surgery, obstetrics and medicine. It was useful, rewarding experience in a general practice like hundreds of others in the north of England— but there was something else, something of vital importance to a young vet who had already developed a consuming interest in exotic species. Among the clients of the practice I had joined was the large zoo in Manchester, Belle Vue. There were other practices nearer the zoo but the connection went back to the nineteenth century, when Rochdale was the veterinary centre of that part of England. The vet in the practice who had for several years done all the work at Belle Vue was Norman Whittle, and with him I had visited cases at the zoo as a student and had first gained some idea of the problems of exotic animal medicine. Now that I was qualified, surely I could achieve my ambition and get to grips myself with the diseases of the wild animals in the zoo in Manchester. But how? The zoo director had a good working relationship with Norman Whittle and trusted him. If an elephant was sick or a python poorly, it was Whittle he sent for. What possible good could Taylor, the new boy, do? There was apparently no escape from my predicament. I could not get in to do the work because my experience was virtually nil, but unless I did achieve a breakthrough and treated some zoo animals I could not begin to get the experience.

Wednesdays began to assume an immense importance in my life, for Norman had his half-day off each week on Wednesday afternoon and I was on call for Belle Vue. This might be my chance, I thought, but for months I was disappointed. Unless the zoo needed him urgently they would leave a message asking Norman to call on the Thursday morning, and in the rare event of an emergency, Edith, our receptionist, would manage to contact him wherever he was and that was the end of his half-day relaxation. It was most frustrating; my one chance to deputize for my senior partner was if he was out of contact on a Wednesday afternoon or away, on holiday abroad for instance, but on these occasions Belle Vue's animal stock seemed to be strictly on their best behaviour and paragons of blooming health and vitality, right down to the weediest chipmunk in the small mammal house.

Then it happened. It was Wednesday afternoon. Norman Whittle had gone to the coast and was not expected back until late. The zoo director, Mr. Wilson, rang. Edith explained that Norman was away. Yes, OK then, was the reply, if it had to be Dr. Taylor, Dr. Taylor it would have to be. But hurry! One of the chimpanzees had lost a thumb. I jumped gleefully into my battered old Jowett van and set off.

It had all started over the asparagus. Each day a rich variety of fruits and vegetables was sent up to the great ape house at Belle Vue from the wholesale market in the city, depending on price, availability and what was in season. Out of the day's selection Len, the senior ape keeper, would build up a balanced and attractive diet for his collection of chimps, orang-utans and gorillas. A slim, phlegmatic individual with grey eyes blinking behind spectacles and a chirpy Manchester accent, he had to make sure that the apes received essential protein, vitamins and roughage. Whenever possible he included delicacies which his charges could enjoy for the sheer fun of eating—grapes, pomegranates or peaches. An odd case of eggplants or avocados left unsold at the end of the day would usually end up at the zoo, and on this particular day a crate stuffed with tender asparagus bunches had arrived. Len took a few bunches down to the ape house to see what his chimps would make of them.

Robert, the big male chimpanzee, shared quarters with two adoring females, Sapphire and Chloe. Robert was a highly successful chimp Casanova who had sired a number of healthy infants at Belle Vue. As his reputation for a reliable, no-nonsense approach to the business of breeding grew, he acted as surrogate husband to a number of females sent in from other zoos. Whether they were ugly or pretty, placid or cantankerous, intelligent or somewhat simple-minded, it did not matter to Robert. He accepted all comers with equal decorum, and the erstwhile barren females would leave after a few weeks' amorous holiday in Manchester, indubitably and uncomplainingly pregnant. As well as being a most gallant and gentle begetter, though, Robert was also a gourmand; in fact he was downright greedy. Woe betide anybody who came between him and his victuals. If he fancied something tasty he had to have it, and none of his companions dared indicate that perhaps Robert's eyes were too big for his belly.

When Len gave a bunch of the tender white and lilac asparagus shoots to each of the three chimps who stuck their arms through the bars, it was the first time that any of them had seen this vegetable. Robert shuffled through his bundle of succulent stalks, sniffed the buds, took a bite and found them exquisite. Sapphire and Chloe were doing the same. Robert gulped down his share and craved a second helping. Sapphire's had all gone but Chloe still held a few pieces; like Gladstone, she believed in the virtue of thoroughly chewing her food. Grunting, Robert shuffled over to Chloe and imperiously thrust a hairy hand towards the remaining asparagus stalks. Chloe whipped them smartly behind her back and screeched at the importunate male, her lips curled back and her white teeth chattering. For a second or two Robert was nonplussed—he was used to getting his own way without resistance. He put on one of his menacing looks and pushed his face close to Chloe's. Eyeball to eyeball, unblinking, Robert glared one of his most meaningful glares, a glare which in the past had never failed to bring mischievous adolescent chimps and timorous keepers to heel, and which had quelled many a nagging old matriarchal ape. Chloe did the unthinkable; she bit his ear, neatly punching a small but painful hole through the middle of the flap. Astounded, Robert backed off half a pace. This was too much! With a short, sharp rush he threw his 150 pounds at Chloe, bowling her over and grabbing with both hands at the stalks she was tenaciously clutching. Struggling and screaming, she refused to let go as Robert pulled her clenched fist towards his bared teeth. His enormously strong index finger could not winkle its way into her palm, nor could his conical yellow canine teeth prize open her grip. Thwarted, Robert was driven to desperate measures, and with a single easy scrunch of his jaws he bit off Chloe's thumb; it was sliced off as cleanly as a severed stalk of celery. Chloe at once released the remains of the asparagus. Robert quickly gobbled them down, then picked up the amputated thumb, sniffed indifferently at it and threw it out of the cage in the direction of Len, who had watched the drama helplessly.

Those few sticks of asparagus resulted in Chloe being maimed for life, although she learned to make do with nine instead of ten digits in no time at all. They were also the reason why I was bouncing in the Jowett through grimy streets of small terraced houses and steaming fish-and-chip shops, on my way, alone, to my very first unaided zoo case at the age of twenty-two.

The twelve-mile drive to the zoo gave me time to think. The message had said something about a thumb being lost by a female chimp. I knew little else at that stage. Still, fingers were like toes and I had treated dozens of cases of domestic animals which had lost toes or had had to have them surgically amputated. The operation was comparatively simple. Bandaging the injured zone after treatment presented no complications, and I had long ago mastered a handful of little tricks using lacquer, sticky tape, repellent aerosol sprays, leather bootees or plastic bags to protect dressings against the teeth, claws and persistent ingenuity of indignant tabby cats and frantic poodles. Yes, I reassured myself as I wound my way through the traffic, fingers were indeed like toes.

Then the snags started to occur to me. Tabby cats and poodles, even for that matter cows, were all fairly easy to anaesthetize. There was always a fond owner or burly farmer to hold the creature while I injected the anaesthetic. Dartguns were still years in the future. Who was going to hold the chimp? Again, my arts of wound dressing had been developed in animals which had no manual dexterity. Might not a wily ape remove whatever dressing I used in little more time than I took to put it on? It dawned on me that I did not know the best dose for chimpanzees of the one anaesthetic that I might have to use: barbiturate. At the time all my other anaesthetics were either gases like ether and halothane— and I could hardly walk up to a 150-pound great ape, slap a mask on its knowing face and ask it to count backwards from one hundred—or other injectable knock-out drugs which were old-fashioned, risky or corrosive. Barbiturate, the latest anaesthetic for veterinary use at the time, was at least safer but one needed to know something about dosage. Supposing I lost my first zoo patient! I gulped. It was a prospect too awful even to contemplate. Take it easy, I told myself, what am I worrying about? Drip it into the chimp's vein a little at a time until the desired level of sleep has been achieved. That way, providing I don't rush it, I'm bound not to exceed the safety limit.

Two miles to go. I tried not to think about the anaesthetic problem; the dripping-in method would be just the thing. But hold on a minute, the slow drip into the vein is all very well, but what is the chimp going to do during the seconds or even minutes when she begins to sense the first hint of dizziness, when she sees double or the room gently begins to spin? She's going to have ample time, if you don't knock her straight out, to part company with your carefully implanted intravenous needle and play havoc with any homo sapiens in the operating theatre—particularly the anaesthetist. Less than confident now, and for a fraction of a second cursing my stars for arranging that the thumb should take leave of its owner on a Wednesday, I swung into the zoo entrance. The commissionaire peered suspiciously through my side window and beckoned to me to wind it down.

"Yes, sir," he growled, "what can we do for you?"

I tried to shake off my apprehension and put on a professional face. "It's the vet," I replied loudly.

"You're not Dr. Whittle."

"No, but I am the vet." And then, as an afterthought—
it sounded rather grand—"To see the chimpanzee, an
emergency." The gates were opened and I drove into the
grounds.

As I stopped the van outside the great ape house, the
face of Matt Kelly, the head keeper, peered from the door.
Grabbing my bag I climbed out of the van. My heart was
hammering in a mixture of excitement and dread. This was
it. Another face appeared at the door as I approached. It
was Mr. Wilson, the zoo director. Just my luck, I thought,
to have this pair of Celts to deal with on my first zoo case.
I had met both of them at the zoo with Norman Whittle
when I was still a student. Kelly was a tough, experienced
and shrewd Irishman and Wilson an acerbic Scot with a face
like a walnut. Both knew a lot about animals, were intolerant
of fools and amateurs and did not seem much impressed by
veterinarians in the zoo. Students, it had seemed to me,
were held by both of them in some contempt, and both of
them undoubtedly considered me still very much a student
where exotic animals were concerned. It was true, but
dammit, I had to begin somewhere. The trouble was that
they knew this was my beginning, and I knew they knew. I
crossed my fingers under the handle of my medical bag.

"Good afternoon, Mr. Wilson, Mr. Kelly," I began, "Dr.
Whittle's away and out of contact, I'm afraid, so you've
got me." I gave a rather tentative jolly laugh.

The two zoo men greeted me stonily. "Yes, well, come
and have a look at Chloe," Wilson said, and led the way
into a corridor flanked with a number of intricate barred
gates that opened onto small cells lit solely by electric bulk-
head lights. It was like walking along one of the gangways
at Alcatraz. All around me the chimpanzees and orang-
utans set up a deafening din, screeching, rattling and beating
food dishes against the walls. One big male chimp burped as

I passed him and pressed his face close to the bars. I smiled at him and put out my hand to tickle one of his knuckles clenched tight round a bar.

"Careful! Don't do that!" hissed Kelly, walking behind me. "He'll have your arm off if ye don't watch out! That's the feller that took the thumb off this afternoon."

I looked at Robert the maimer, inside for life. He gazed at me intently, eyes never blinking. As I continued on down the passageway, I felt a warm moist patch soaking through my trousers. Robert had urinated on me through the grille.

Chloe sat alone in her sleeping quarters, banging a stainless steel drinking dish on the floor with her good hand. The other, mutilated hand she held high above her head so that all the world could see the damage wrought by the evil Robert.

"That's it," said Wilson, pointing. Kelly said nothing. Both men stood looking blank. They did not seem to be anxiously awaiting my words of wisdom. I looked hard through the bars. The diagnosis was clear and simple: the thumb was off. So far so good. Now for the next stage: treatment. There were some drops of blood on the floor but the hand did not seem to be actively bleeding at present. It looked as if Robert had performed his amputation rather neatly straight through the bottom knuckle joint, so there was no surgical operation for me to do, but he had left a rather irregular edge to the skin. Ought I not to straighten that up, stitch up the hole and put a dresssing on? And was there not a risk of infection? Chimpanzee mouths normally contain a rich variety of nasty microbes, some of which can cause serious diseases when given the chance to invade healthy flesh. Yes, it looked as though I would have to do something.

I decided to broach diplomatically the subject of how to get to grips with Chloe. "Hmm," I murmured wisely and subtly. "Hmmm." I hoped the "Hmmm" was of a tone, pitch and duration perfectly calculated to suggest not that

197

I was at a loss but rather that such cases were well within my province. Wilson and Kelly said nothing and stared blankly on.

"I see," I continued, again trying to convey optimism and confidence rather than sterile perplexity. Still they said nothing; they were forcing me to the point where I would have to make a positive suggestion for treatment. I decided to approach the nettle obliquely before grasping it. "What's she like?" I asked. It was a suitably vague question.

Wilson frowned. "D'you mean what's she like to handle?" he snapped.

"Er, yes," I replied brightly.

"Can't," said Kelly lugubriously. "Can't."

"Well, I think we ought to stitch up the hole if we can, dress it and give her a shot of antibiotic," I went on. "What would be the best way, do you think?"

A distinctly aggravated look appeared on Wilson's walnut face. "Can't," he said. "There's no way of doing it."

I had to say my piece. "Is there no way you can hold her long enough for me to get some barbiturate into her vein?" I asked in my politest voice.

Both men broke into a burst of humourless laughter. "Catch hold of her? Chloe? Impossible. Impossible." Wilson's nae-nonsense Glasgow accent seemed stronger than ever. "How do you suggest we do that?"

The ball was back in my court. "Well, if you've no way of trapping her, and we've no way of getting a drug in by injection, the only thing is to try doping her food."

"No chance." This time it was Kelly's turn. "She's fed up for today, won't take any more. Anyway, Chloe's as sharp as they come at spottin' doctored food."

If I had to wait until the next day, and then still use the imprecise and unpredictable way of introducing barbiturate in the food, I would have lost valuable time. Infection might have set in and the stitches might not be so certain of holding. What would we have done if the animal had been haemorrhaging severely? Waited until she was so weakened by blood loss that she had no more will to resist?

I stood looking in at the wounded chimpanzee. The case was a supremely simple one, the type of therapy obvious, but there was nothing I could do. The zoo director and the head keeper knew that I would be unable to make any positive, constructive contribution; they must have known it when the call had been put through to my office. With a first personal taste of gnawing impotence, I began to realize the futility of veterinary medicine as applied to zoo animals. It seemed in those days before the invention of the dart-gun that the zoo vet had only two alternatives: to inject, dose, lance and anoint only small, relatively non-violent creatures such as lizards and turtles, whose problems were obscure, unstudied and baffling to the veterinarian familiar with the workings and ways of domestic animals; or to stand at one side of the bars and guess what might be wrong with the choleric gorilla or tiger that lay on the other side, obviously ill or injured but just as obviously an ungrabbable and ungrateful patient.

Chloe was one of the latter cases. I knew that with some animals it had been possible to immobilize them for treatment by using sheer brute force, casting nets over them and then having seven or eight of your heaviest men sit on the captive until it was almost suffocated or someone was severely bitten through a gap in the rope mesh. Even if such humane barbarity worked, the effect on animals and staff was utterly demoralizing. The end result was a terrified, exhausted patient, still virtually unexaminable. No point in taking his temperature; it was roaring up in panic. No chance of feeling with one's fingers for the liver abscess or ball of cancer that might lie in the abdomen; the body wall was held hard as iron. And even if one could get the bell end of the stethoscope into the right position without it being bitten off, the galloping heart was masking much else which might be significant. I was not going to begin by treating my first zoo case that way.

There was nothing more to be done for Chloe except to give the zoo director a broad-spectrum antibiotic which could be added to her fruit drinks for a week or so. The three of us retraced our steps. Robert was still hugging the bars of his cell closely. I looked at him as I passed, keeping close to the opposite wall of the passageway in the hope of staying out of range. Was there in his gaze the merest hint of mockery? He grimaced and stuck his tongue behind the barely parted rows of yellow teeth. "Tsk, tsk, tsk," said Robert.

The two zoo men and I went outside and stood for a moment before I climbed back into my van.

"Well, thanks anyway for coming," said Wilson.

"Yes, it should heal up without any trouble," Kelly reassured me. "Oi've seen these chimps do terrible things to one another. It's amazin' what nature can do. Healed up in no time at all. Baboons, too—wounds ye could put your hand into after fightin'. But they heal up with no bother in a couple o' weeks."

"Well, I'd like to have sutured Chloe's hand," I replied. "Perhaps one day we'll have ways of doing such things easily enough."

I still wondered why they had bothered to send for me in such a hurry in the first place, since they did not seem the slightest dismayed by my non-performance. Having just achieved my dearest ambition, my first zoo case, I found myself driving home to Rochdale in a black depression. Could it be that after all I should stick to cattle and horses?

That evening I told my wife about my uncertain debut with Chloe, Mr. Wilson and Matt Kelly. Shelagh and I had met while we were both still at school and had courted for six years while she qualified as a therapy radiographer and I carried through my veterinary studies. Her green eyes and strong determination bear witness to her Irish ancestry, and she has a deep love and understanding of animals of every kind; I had seen her move earthworms from footpaths with the concern of a devout Hindu lest they be trodden upon and injured, we had wrestled together over many a dying animal brought to our doorstep, and we had worked side by side over pregnant ewes needing Caesarians in the middle of the night when I had no anaesthetist or surgical assistant available. Her optimism was unflagging and her judgement of the right approach to animal patient and owner impeccable.

"Don't worry," she said reassuringly, "you've not lost Chloe. There will be other times. One of these days you'll show 'em! There'll be new ways of getting at these animals and then you'll get the upper hand. Men like Kelly and Wilson have been in the business all their lives. You know the problems you've had with old-fashioned Pennine farmers in the six months since you first started in practice—they didn't want the young feller with the new-fangled ways, laughed when you sterilized the skin before injecting a cow down with milk fever, wanted you to cut the tails of tuberculous cows to get out the 'worm' that was sucking the meat off the beasts' bones—you're getting over all that with time and battling on. Same with the zoos. You've got to keep reading about exotic animals, keep going if you get the chance. One good success can make all the difference."

Shelagh was right. It would be a long haul before I could ever move about the zoos with the same growing confidence in handling every kind of case, together with the right psychological approach to the owners, that I was developing in general practice. The idea of one day working solely with exotic animals seemed the most tenuous of dreams. Even Shelagh doubted whether we would ever be able to achieve that.

On the day after my first visit to Chloe, I also tackled Norman Whittle about the affair. Norman was a quiet, elegant individual ten years my senior, with a fair moustache and, if the term can be applied to animal doctors, a superb bedside manner.

"Why do they bother to call us at all when they know there is little we can do?" I asked him.

He smiled. "Quite simply to cover themselves. To cover themselves for the sake of the Board. Happens to me all the time. Something ill, they fiddle about with it as best they can for a few days until it looks as if the poor sod's going to die, then they send for the vet. If there's going to be a corpse, they've got to be able to report to the Board that 'the vet was called in but the animal expired'. As for Chloe, she wasn't likely to die, but the same principle applies. A high-value animal they can't get to grips with and so, just in case something goes wrong, or if a visitor reports the presence of a nine-fingered ape to the RSPCA, they've got to be able to say that the buck was passed to the vet."

"So what you're saying is that we're professional fall guys for the zoo?"

"Yes, essentially. OK, so we supply them with drugs they can put in the food of animals with diarrhoea and vitamin syrup for things that look out of condition or down in the mouth, but basically we go so that on the monthly reports it can read something like 'Despite veterinary treatment, x number of mammals, y number of birds and z number of reptiles cocked their toes.' "

"Don't you feel you do some good for the zoo animals, though?"

"In a few cases, yes—calving a giraffe that's in difficulties, lancing an abscess on the occasional elephant—but they're few and far between. Mostly I haven't any way of knowing what's wrong with these creatures and they, people like Matt Kelly, know I don't know. I don't think zoos in general have much time for vets."

"But they need us to rubber-stamp the losses?"

"Afraid so."

Not only was Matt Kelly right about Chloe's hand—it healed perfectly without any infection or discomfort and within three weeks the skin had closed the gap completely—but I knew that Norman's analysis of the relationship between zoos and vets was basically true as well. Perhaps it was partly the profession's fault for paying too much attention in the past exclusively to domestic animals. Not many years earlier, veterinary education had concentrated almost solely on the problems of the horse. Gradually, as the automobile seemed likely to be more than a nine-day wonder, farm animals and then later the dog and cat received a more appropriate proportion of a student's time. Even today the handling, diseases and therapy of exotic creatures are squeezed into a total of one or two hours' instruction out of a five- or six-year course in some veterinary schools. When I first treated Chloe not even that amount of tuition was available.

The more I thought about Norman's remarks the more crystal clear it seemed to me that I had to have three things if I was ever going to progress in zoo medicine. First I had to look into new ways of getting drugs accurately inside the bodies of creatures too dangerous or too nervous to be injected by hand; secondly I needed powerful, compact, safe sedatives and anaesthetics for every possible class of exotic patient; and thirdly I would have to learn everything I could from old-timers like Kelly at Belle Vue about the lore of zoocraft, about moving among and handling difficult and dangerous animals. Matt Kelly might not know the exact location of the sinuses of Rokitansky-Aschoff in a rhinoceros's liver, or the dental formula of a binturong, but he knew a hell of a lot about the care of wild creatures. I must pry some of it out of him.

Four

For a long time after the incident of Chloe's thumb, Norman Whittle's Wednesday afternoons, vacations and odd days in bed with influenza came and went with the same monotonous absence of disease at Belle Vue. Freezing snaps accompanied by choking yellow fog on November Wednesdays never seemed to provoke the acute lung emergencies in giraffe or antelope that sent Norman dashing out in like weather on every other day of the week, and in summer the milling crowds of visitors who fed the elephants with mouldy sausage rolls, umbrellas or cigarettes, or threw contraceptives, pins or bits of glass into the monkeys' cages, seemed to be on their most civilized behaviour whenever Norman was away and unavailable to deal personally with the resulting cases of colic and acute enteritis.

There was just one source of practical experience: the trickle of wild and exotic animals that ran fitfully through my daily work with farm animals and domestic pets. Even in darkest Lancashire there were folk who preferred keeping slow lorises to Siamese cats or who had a penchant for pythons. If their pets needed medical attention, more often than not they telephoned Belle Vue Zoo, who referred them to us. It was not much compared to the experience with real zoo animals that I longed for, but it taught a callow young vet a thing or two the hard way—and sometimes more about humans than about animals.

Most numerous among my exotic patients at this time were parrots, the choleric, beady-eyed individuals that perch behind the bars of numerous pubs in Greater Manchester, sweetly and ever so gently take peanuts placed on the capacious bosoms of the landladies whom they adore and, cursing raucously, try to take the fingers off all other members of the human race who come within reach. Without exception, these birds of glorious plumage and lengthy life-span dislike me and, as I count a fine collection of old scars on my hands, I am not sure that I am very partial to them. Parrots were small beer, I thought, but the beer soon turned distinctly sour.

Thus it was after I had been working with Norman Whittle for about a year that I met Charlie, a fine blue and gold macaw with claws overgrown as a result of twenty years without exercise behind the bar of a Manchester pub and a surfeit of fattening sweet sherry, his favourite tipple. Would I kindly trim his toenails? Certainly. The macaw glowered darkly in his carrying cage, which had been set in the middle of my surgery table. His owner, the pub's landlady, stood smiling proudly at her "cheeky little Charlie". She was a large lady with a bosom like the prow of a galleon and with peroxide-blond hair rolled tightly in curlers.

"Er, can you hold him for me?" I asked. Cheeky little Charlie turned his head to one side and fixed me with a malevolent, red-rimmed eye. A low, sinister, grating noise came from his scraggy throat and he thoughtfully honed one half of his beak against the other.

"Oh goodness, no, my dear," exclaimed the landlady. "Charlie's a darling little boy but he won't let me handle him. He'd tear me to bits. And he hates men." I reflected that I had known more promising cases. I had yet to learn the art of mastering parrots by using a piece of stick and a kung-fu-like flick that renders them harmless and unhurt in the twinkling of an eye.

Charlie rocked slowly on his perch from one foot to the other, like a boxer limbering up for a fight.

"Well, can you at least entice him out of his cage?" I

asked. I was not going in to fight, so how about him coming out and settling this thing man to man?

"Well, he might come out for his favourites, after-dinner mints. He adores those. He sits on my shoulder and takes one that I hold between my lips. He's ever so gentle!"

It turned out that we had no after-dinner mints between us and I sent Edith, my receptionist, across the road to buy some; I would learn in time that a zoo vet carries a variety of delicacies in his medical bag along with the drugs and instruments; one's essential first-aid kit must include after-dinner mints for a wide variety of monkeys, parrots and small mammals, clear mints for wallabies, sugar lumps for elephants and small cheroots for aoudads and other members of the goat tribe.

"Now," said the landlady when we had the mints, "I'll put a mint between my lips, Charlie will come out, and while he's nibbling it perhaps you can clip his toes."

The macaw acted absolutely according to phase one of the plan. As soon as he spied the sweet he waddled along his perch and out of the door of the cage, and sat squarely on his owner's shoulder hard by her ear. With one golden eye he watched her place the mint between her lips and with the other he kept me under unblinking observation. Like a ventriloquist's dummy, he reached round the woman's cheek and began to nibble the mint. Slowly I sidled up and, feigning nonchalance, began to raise the clippers towards the parrot's long toenails, which were perfectly displayed against her dress just below her left shoulder. Six inches, three inches, one inch; I was getting closer to the curved talons. They certainly needed chiropody, with some grown almost to full circles. Somewhere inside them was a core of flesh with nerves and blood. I must avoid cutting into that area and simply trim back the dead, overgrown portion. But how could I tell exactly where the core of each shiny, black, opaque nail was? I would have to compromise to begin with and snip off just a little bit, see how that looked and then maybe take a sliver more.

As I reached the first claw and gingerly touched it with the tip of my clippers, Charlie kept his eye fixed firmly on me but continued to crunch at the mint without budging. Very gently I slipped the toenail clippers over the end of the first claw. Suddenly Charlie decided he had had enough. Something dastardly was afoot, and he was not going to stand by and let it happen. In order to lean forward and launch a pre-emptive attack on me and my clippers he would have to have a more secure base to perch on, so with the black claws of his left foot, Charlie dug through the landlady's dress and deeply into the flesh of her shoulder. The poor woman spat out the mint and uttered a piercing shriek that set the waiting dogs in the reception room barking and howling. A nimble tactician, Charlie was determined to bring his steely bill into close combat with the foe, but to stop himself from pressing the attack too far and too fast, with the result that he might fall off his defensive position, he needed another good secure hold for his right foot. The object he sought was right there—his owner's ear. Charlie grabbed it tightly and dug in his curly nails. The lady let out a second, more raucous shriek and clutched the parrot with both hands, whereupon he bit a plump finger and drew blood. More shrieks.

All this flurry of action had taken only a few seconds, during which time I had seemed to be transfixed, incapable of action, but now I moved forward. Impotently waving my clippers, I tried to separate the struggling mass of feathers, hair, claws and fingers on the landlady's shoulder. Scrunch, scrunch—I was painfully bitten on two fingers. Wild-eyed, ruffled and squawking, Charlie launched a new attack on my clippers. Clang! His gaping black beak punched sharply forward and knocked them from my grasp. They slipped neatly down the inside of the landlady's dress.

With the enemy now in complete disarray, Charlie was still in command of his redoubt. The ear, bright red and resembling a crushed strawberry, remained under requisition for essential military purposes, and he had given up not one inch of ground on the left shoulder. He had sacrificed a few green feathers and in the excitement of battle had elected not to desert his post to go to the latrine but to obey the call of nature just where he stood. It improved neither the lady's appearance nor her morale.

"For God's sake, can't you do something?" she yelled. "Get the little beggar off me!"

Charlie bit the back of one of her scrabbling hands. When I tried again to grab him he reinforced his hold on ear and shoulder, whisked his beak to and fro and deftly removed a piece of nail from my left index finger.

I looked desperately round for something to help me. A towel hung by the sink; perhaps I could use it to keep his deadly beak occupied long enough for me to unpick him from his owner and get him back into his cage. The nails would have to wait. I grabbed the towel, tossed it over the bird and stood back. Somewhere underneath, Charlie wriggled, screamed, chewed and blustered furiously.

"Don't worry," I gasped with some relief, "I think we've got him now."

"He's still got my ear, though!" the landlady wailed as the towelled mass on her shoulder threw itself about.

Before picking up the entrapped parrot it would be prudent to ascertain where the beak-bearing head end was. I took a pencil and gently prodded the stuffed towel. With a crisp crack the pencil was split into two and fell apart; I had found the head end. Without losing more time I grabbed hold of the part that was probably the plump little belly and tugged hard. The parrot tugged hard at the lady's ear. Her shrieking resumed. Feeling in need of reinforcement, I took off my white surgery coat and threw that on top of the towel, completely covering the woman's head. As best I could I felt for the parrot's head, held it and set about releasing the grip on the mutilated ear. The landlady put both her hands on the hidden bird and allowed me to try to detach the claw dug into her shoulder. When I got beneath the towelling I found that the other claw was now also firmly attached to her shoulder. Charlie was no pushover.

Suddenly I realized that I was touching the very things that had been the cause of all the bother: the overgrown nails. I carefully lifted a corner of the towel and looked at them. There they all were, side by side. A perfect opportunity! With the vicious end of Charlie still gurgling and spitting somewhere higher up in the folds of material I might well be able to do my stuff—if I had my clippers. Then I remembered that they were still lying somewhere in the décolletage of the buxom lady who stood before me, my white coat draped over her head and both hands clasped to a jumble of protesting towelling on her shoulder.

"Er, I can do his nails very well now," I began. "I've got his claws out perfectly. Can you hold on like that for a few moments more?"

"Yes, but get on with it. My ear's hurting like hell. Little beggar. Get on with it!"

"Er, well, my clippers . . . you've got my clippers in your . . ."

"I know. Get them out. I can't hold him much longer!"

"I'll have to put my hand down your dress, madam. . . ."

"Of course you will. GET ON WITH IT!"

Squeezing my fingers together rather as if I were preparing to lamb a ewe, I entered the talcumed valley and probed downwards in search of my instrument. When my unwilling hand was completely within her dress and I was beginning to worry about just how far down I was going to have to go, I mercifully felt metal lodged behind some item of twangy underwear.

"I'm awfully sorry about all this," I was saying in embarrassed confusion as I pinned the clippers between two fingers and began to extract them. Then the surgery door opened and Edith, the receptionist, came in. My hand was

209

still down the front of the landlady's dress.

"Just cutting the parrot's toenails, Edith," I explained brightly.

Edith was a non-conformist lay preacher, and I often wondered whether she treated her Maker with the same brisk and relentless efficiency which could be a source of terror to both slow-paying farmers and ham-fisted young veterinarians. She glared icily through her spectacles and backed briskly out again. Meanwhile I had re-armed myself with the clippers and started to trim the bird's claws. Following my plan to cut back a little at a time, I pruned them bit by bit to what seemed a more reasonable length. When I had finished I noticed that the end of each nail was showing a little blood. It was only the merest drop but I had obviously cut back just a fraction too far. I dabbed each nail with a styptic liquid to seal it up neatly.

At last Charlie, almost apoplectic with rage, was securely back in his cage. The landlady adjusted her dress, I put some antiseptic on her abused ear, bandaged her wounded fingers, sponged her down and talked soothingly about what lovable if naughty little fellows these parrots were. She seemed reassured and even grateful, and if anyone's dignity had suffered wounds from our experience, it apparently was not hers.

To my dismay, Charlie's owner and his vet did not bear the only physical wounds from our encounter that morning, for Charlie had not been gone from my surgery for more than ten minutes before his toenails began to bleed again. It was only after ten days and considerable care that the intermittent bleeding completely stopped. On subsequent visits I learned to handle him more deftly, and the experience also taught me something about cutting the sensitive nails of other Charlies to come.

There were plenty of them, for Manchester parrots seemed particularly prone to overgrown toenails, to diarrhoeas that resisted treatment because the unco-operative birds steadfastly refused to take their medicines, to coughs and sneezes that resisted treatment because the un-co-operative microbes causing these complaints just as steadfastly ignored my medicaments, and to baldness. The baldness was self-inflicted—the parrots persistently plucked out all their feathers (except the ones on the top of their heads, of course) until they became pink-nude, pot-bellied and scrawny-necked. They reminded me of bellicose minia-ture Colonel Blimps emerging from the Turkish baths. I could find no itchy skin parasites or nutritional deficiency to cause this craze for full frontal exhibitionism.

My failure to counter what seemed sheer cussedness on the part of my malevolent parrot patients was underlined by the raucous cursing that they heaped upon me week after week as I surveyed the results of my impotent efforts to grow even one single plume on their old men's bodies. What irritated me about the nudists was their sheer cheek; having extracted almost all its plumage, one of these in-furiating creatures would sit on its perch, tilt a choleric, red-rimmed eye in my direction—and then shiver. Of course you'll shiver, you dum-dum! I wanted to shout in my frustration. If I had had the temerity to write a con-sidered dissertation on the Diseases of the Parrot, it would have consisted of but two sentences, written in blood on the finest parchment: "Parrots are incontinent, wheezing asth-matics in need of chiropody and tungsten-wire whole-body toupees. They get well if they feel like it, or they don't."

Nevertheless, I had to carry on. Dump the parrots and there might never be any condors or cassowaries or King penguins. And I had to do something to reassure the doting owners that Rochdale was the Mecca for infirm and irascible parrots. Although my treatment of their pets' ailments seemed to be meeting with a singular lack of obvious success, I decided that at the very least I could thwart the parrot nudist brigade in its efforts to commit suicide by self-refrigeration. I was damned if I would let these birds have the last laugh by developing hypothermia or pneumonia or frostbite.

First I gave instructions for all such patients to be confined day and night for one or two weeks at least to rooms where the temperature never dropped below 80 degrees Fahrenheit. Then it struck me that parrots really did appear to be old-fashioned sort of fellows; the analogy to Colonel Blimp really did stick. Where more genteel birds such as doves might get tipsy now and then when feasting on fermenting berries in the fall, parrots have the leery, rheumy eye of the hard-liquor drinker who prefers the grain to the grape all the year round. If the incontinent wheezers spurned my antibiotics and sulpha drugs, let's see how they fared on a drop of the hard stuff. As soon as I began to prescribe minute tots of rum or brandy for all my sick parrots I began to have successes. My knowledge of disease in exotic birds had not advanced very much, but a combination of the Turkish bath and hard-liquor regime for nearly all my cases resulted in more and more incontinent birds passing normal stools, the wheezers beginning to breathe more easily and some of the Kojak types even growing a soft covering of grey down and later the colourful plumage that was their rightful attire. As time went on the booze-'em-and-bake-'em therapy persuaded quite a few parrot owners that Dr. Whittle's partner had a knack with their favourite bird.

I also earned the rather more demonstrative gratitude of a lady almost as exotic as her pet. It all began when the surgery telephone rang as I was showing out yet another parrot owner who was looking forward to giving his wife the perfect excuse for taking out the brandy bottle as soon as he got home.

"Hello," said a sultry voice as I picked up the receiver. "Is that Dr. Taylor?"

"It is," I replied. "Who's this speaking?"

"It's Miss Seksi. I expect you've heard of me. I'm the speciality danseuse at the Garden of Eden."

This surprising statement did not perplex me as it might have done, for I knew of the Garden of Eden, a sleazy Manchester night-club from whose doors there wafted a permanent smell of stale beer, yesterday's cigars and cheap perfume.

"What can I do for you, Miss, er, Seksi?" I asked. Edith looked up sharply from her book-keeping.

"Well, it's very confidential. Private, if you know what I mean."

"I see, but how can I help? Do you wish me to visit or will you come to the surgery?"

"Well, if you can be sure it's all confidential I'll come with him to the surgery if you'll give me an appointment."

"Er . . . come with who, Miss, er, Miss Seksi?"

"My Oscar, of course."

Who or what was her Oscar? I doubted if she had won a Hollywood Academy Award and decided Oscar must be a friend or husband. Well, I thought, she must realize I'm not a people doctor. We had had cases of Pakistanis and displaced persons from Eastern Europe queuing patiently for hours among the dogs, cats and budgerigars in the waiting room, only to find when it was their turn that we did not extract human teeth or issue National Health Service sick notes. This lady sounded one hundred per cent English, but she still wanted me to treat this chap Oscar. Then again, I thought, I had had a few human patients. There was the window cleaner who regularly had our fiery horse linament for his arthritic knee, many a farmer swore our medicaments were the most likely to cure the ringworm he had contracted from his calves, and I had dealt with all sorts of problems from impetigo to impotence among the hill-farming folk of the Pennines, who found it easier to talk to the vet, sitting over a cup of tea in the farmhouse after calving a cow, than to the doctor in his surgery in town.

"But, er, are you and Oscar bringing the animal?" I asked Miss Seksi.

"I work with Oscar. Oscar is my python."

"Oh," I said, grateful that at any rate part of the mystery had been solved.

A confidential consultation, with no nurse and no assistant present, was arranged for the ailing Oscar for three o'clock, and I waited in intrigued anticipation. Punctually at three, a taxi pulled up outside the waiting-room door and Edith ushered in a startlingly painted lady of Junoesque proportions dressed in an imitation tiger-skin coat that seemed to be afflicted here and there with remarkably accurate imitations of sarcoptic mange. She teetered on six-inch stiletto heels, lugging awkwardly in one hand a large canvas bag. As she sat down she dabbed the perspiration from her face and touched up the paintwork expertly. Then she switched on the multi-volt smile that had been designed to cut its way through cigar smoke, wolf whistles, rude remarks and embarrassing silence with the ease of a disposable scalpel. Her first words to me were "Bloody heavy, he is, poor little darlin'."

Undoing some cord tied tightly around the neck of the canvas bag, Miss Seksi switched off the head-splitting smile and plunged an arm inside. Slowly she withdrew a glistening, plump snake, an anaconda that must have been every bit of twelve feet long.

"There he is," said my client. "Poor, poor Oscar; I'm really worried about him."

"What seems to be the problem?" I faltered, looking down the undulating length of Miss Seksi's partner as he gently wound himself round her shoulders and waist. His weight seemed normal and there was a healthy fluorescent glint as the light caught his rippling scales. Oscar was trying to disappear inside Miss Seksi's fur coat. Already the first six feet of him were making her torso bulge and warp beneath her coat as if she were made of rubber; in a moment my

214

patient would have gone completely to ground. Remembering Charlie the parrot and the fate of my toenail clippers, I firmly resolved that I was not going in there after him. Instead I grasped twelve inches of Oscar's tail end, flexed my biceps and stood firmly with my legs apart. Oscar, like all such non-venomous constrictor snakes, was ninety per cent muscle. He continued to contract his powerful twelve-foot body as I held staunchly onto his tail and refused to be pulled inside the perfumed recesses of Miss Seksi's tiger-skin coat. The result was predictable. If I was not going to release the tail and if Oscar continued doggedly to go places, there was only one thing left that had to give way: Miss Seksi. The contracting snake pulled her right into me. "Dear God, keep Edith out of here at this moment!" I prayed, as I stood nose to nose and thigh to thigh with the lady from the Garden of Eden. Oscar wedded us like Scotch tape; as he threw a loop or two around my wrist, I wondered who was holding whom.

"The, er, the problem," said Miss Seksi from two inches away, "the problem is personal. It's his eyes." She breathed a cloud of Chanel No. 5 and onions into my face. "If you can reach my handbag, Doctor, you'll find the card; you'll see what I mean."

Still clutching my bit of Oscar with one hand, I clicked open her handbag with the other, fished vaguely about inside it and pulled out an oblong card.

"That's it," she said. "That's the card from the clinic."

I had no idea what she was talking about. "What clinic?" I asked.

"The venereal disease clinic." She lowered her voice confidentially and looked at the door to make sure it was firmly closed. "I think Oscar's got it."

"Got what, venereal disease?"

"Yes. You see, Oscar and I are in the burlesque business. We've appeared in Paris and Beirut, haven't we, Oscar?" Oscar's head had emerged from below Miss Seksi's coat and, with flicking tongue, he had begun to investigate my shoes. "Yes, we've been very well received, Oscar and I. Very exotique, very good money."

"But how do you and Oscar work together?"

"I'm a speciality danseuse ... exotique ... you know."

"A stripper?" I hazarded.

Miss Seksi gave me a five-second, full-power burst of the smile. "Yes, but not low-class, my dear," she said. "Seksi's my stage name; actually it's Schofield."

"Please go on, Miss Schofield."

"Well, during our act I do a very exotique speciality dance as Cleopatra. See what I mean? That's where Oscar fits in."

An embryonic glimmer of light began to spark in my brain. We bumped foreheads.

"During the act—it went down *awfully* well in Beirut— I disrobe to exotique music" (Miss Schofield emphasized the *tique* each time she uttered her favourite word) "and the climax, when I'm in the buff—you know what I mean, Doctor—is when I commit suicide."

"So Oscar is Cleopatra's asp?"

"Exactly. Oscar is the asp. Rather exotique, don't you think?"

If Cleopatra really did shuffle off this mortal coil with the aid of a reptile it must have been one of the small venomous Egyptian snakes, possibly a cobra, but certainly not a 65-pound South American constrictor.

"Yes, Doctor," went on Miss Seksi. "My agent thinks it's a really dramatic finale, with Oscar twining all round my body."

"I see, I see," I interposed quickly.

"Now. The thing is, Doctor, I've had a touch of, er, VD. The clinic gave me cards to hand out to anybody I might have had what they call contact with. I've dished out the cards, of course, though I couldn't care a fig for my boy

216

friends—they're all pigs. But Oscar, he's my partner, my little darling. He's everything to me."

"Why do you think Oscar might have picked up an infection from you?"

"His eyes, Doctor, look at his eyes. I'm worried sick by them. It's his work, Doctor. He's got it from me, I'm sure." Miss Seksi was becoming tearful. We were still so closely entangled that any sobbing on her part was likely to soak my tie.

"Trouble is," she continued, "the clinic wouldn't see him, even though I told them all about him, how he worked with me. That's the National Health Service for you! So that's why I came to you."

"Let's get ourselves sorted out and have a look at his head," I said. My own head was spinning. Whatever it was that did not look right with his eyes, it certainly could not be VD. That disease of humans does not affect other mammals, and in reptiles like Oscar it is out of the question. Although, I reflected, I could not be positive that no scientific paper had ever been published stating categorically that anacondas and their like were immune to the gonorrhoea microbe.

Eventually Miss Seksi/Schofield unravelled the snake and I took a relieved step backwards. For the first time I had a good view of his head. "Look at his eyes, Doctor!" his owner wailed. "They've gone like that in less than a week!"

Both the anaconda's eyes were indeed abnormal. Instead of being limpid dark jewels they were blind, milk-white blobs. Looking at them carefully through the magnifying lens of an ophthalmoscope with its intense beam of light, I was able to make out the eye lying beneath the milky film.

"When did Oscar last shed his skin?" I asked. I had not seen this eye condition in snakes before, but an idea was forming in my mind.

"About a week or ten days ago. Came off as clean as a whistle."

"And round about then you first noticed his eyes?"

217

"Yes."

Snakes' eyes are completely covered by a non-moving transparent third eyelid. As the rest of the skin is shed from time to time as the animal grows, the old outer layers of the third eyelid are sloughed too. Or rather they should be. I was convinced that the "VD" infection of Oscar's eyes was the old third eyelid which had not fallen off with the rest of the skin. It was a sheet of tough, dead tissue covering an otherwise healthy eye.

While I prepared to try and restore the sight of the un-complaining trouper there and then, his owner became tearful again. "If he's blind, I won't be able to work with him any more," she moaned. I did not quite see how vision was essen-tial for Oscar's act. "How can I replace him? I just couldn't get another like him. It would mean back to my Florence Nightingale routine—and at half the salary." The wailing increased as I dropped a little paraffin oil into each of the white eyes.

"Hold tightly onto his head, please," I instructed. Oscar began once again to intertwine us both, and I felt his rear end drag me into another bout of intimate contact with his mistress. The latter was now red-faced and sweating as well as weepy. Even her mask of make-up was beginning to erode.

With a pair of fine-toothed forceps I gently began to tease up the edge of the white film covering one of the snake's eyes. Bit by bit, and using more drops of oil as I progressed, I slowly freed the crust. A dark gold glint showed that Oscar's eye lay uninjured underneath. At last the entire piece of dead tissue came away. Oscar eyed me, unblinking and inscrutable. I set to work on the other side of the head and soon the second eye was clear as well. The "VD" had gone. Putting down my instruments, I struggled out of Oscar's coils and stood back to survey my handiwork.

Miss Seksi was open-mouthed in astonishment and delight, gurgling and smiling real, unprofessional smiles. Releasing Oscar's head and letting him roam where he would, she came over and hugged me. "Doctor, how can I ever thank you?" she purred. Then she imprisoned me in a python-like embrace and planted a big, soggy, bright red kiss on my forehead, just as Edith came back into the surgery.

"Ah, you're just in time, Edith . . . " I said.

"So I see," she interrupted drily.

" . . . to help get Oscar back into his bag."

Between us we untangled the now clear-eyed anaconda, and Edith saw Miss Seksi out.

"We can do without that sort," she said, coming back into the room where I was sterilizing the forceps.

For all her stagey manner, Miss Seksi had enlivened my afternoon, and there was nothing artificial or overblown about Oscar: he had provided my first experience of what I later found to be a common problem in snakes.

"Oh no, we can't, Edith," I replied.

Five

Although it was now almost two years since I had joined Norman Whittle in his practice, I seemed to be no nearer the solid diet of zoo cases that I craved. Without a background of zoo-animal experience I was frequently forced into tight corners where my ignorance was nakedly exposed. It was not just the difficulty of diagnosing a whole new range of diseases in animals that figured nowhere in orthodox veterinary education—there were times when I could not even put a name to the species of creature that was borne, dragged or prodded into the consulting room. Animal owners often do not take kindly to the veterinarian working with pet cats and dogs who has forgotten the name of "Fluffy", "Poochie", "Garibaldi" or whatever in the time between visits, even though these may be years apart. The position was considerably trickier when a furry brown creature about as big as a ferret and with large orange eyes with pinpoint pupils was proudly plonked down on the table and the owner said, "Horace, this is Dr. Taylor. Be a good boy now," and then continued, "I've brought Horace down from Carlisle, Doctor, because the zoo told me your practice could get rid of this skin disease that's been bothering him for months."

Having travelled 110 miles with this whatever-it-was, the smiling owner of Horace would not be impressed if I started off by asking what sort of beast I was dealing with. He was absolutely certain I knew. I looked at the Horace and the Horace gazed gently back to me. He seemed docile enough as he moved slowly around the table top. Anyway, he had to be a mammal because he was hairy.

220

"He's got these small bald patches on his head, Doctor," the proud owner announced.

I looked at the Horace's head; it was mongoose-like, with small ears and a pretty damp nose about the size of a chihuahua's.

"Well, well," I began hopefully, "it's not often we see one of these." The idea of this artful gambit was to lead the owner into giving me the clue I needed by agreeing that crunchlappets or flummerjacks or whatever the thing was were indeed getting rarer.

The owner of Horace did not fall into my rhetorical snare. "No, Doctor," he replied, "but Mr. So-and-so says that Dr. Whittle's practice did wonders with his when it was sick." Impasse.

I looked at Horace's feet; they were finger-like and reminded me of a monkey's. Although there was not much sign of anything to grab hold of I decided to stall for time by first stroking Horace and then picking him up so that I could get a better look at the diseased areas. He diffidently sniffed my fingers as I approached him. To my horror, as I stroked him I felt his backbone. Horace had a backbone like all mammals, but what chilled me as I ruffled through his fur was that the spines of his vertebrae appeared actually to be jutting out through his skin; my fingers were pressing directly on his spinal column! He seemed plump enough and there had been no talk of an accident—why on earth should Horace's owner be worrying about bald patches when there was something much more dramatically significant happening to his beloved pet's back? Perhaps I could get through the examination, diagnosis and treatment without actually knowing what Horace was. No, that was a hopeless idea. I was a fool—I should have admitted my ignorance as soon as Horace arrived.

At this juncture Horace decided to bite me. He did it once, precisely and powerfully, on the index finger which I was using to feel his spine. He then gazed gently at me once more as I jerked back my hand with a yelp and stuck the bleeding digit in my mouth.

"Oh my, Horace," exclaimed his owner, "that's a naughty boy. Still, I suppose you get lots of those in your job, Doctor, dealing with the likes of him."

My finger was bleeding copiously and hurt like hell, but at least Horace had given me the chance I needed to save my ridiculous dignity. "I'll just nip and get a Band-aid," I said and slipped smartly out of the consulting room.

In thirty seconds I had plastered up the punctured finger and shot upstairs to my collection of zoo books. Somewhere in there, God willing, I would track down the Horace animal. Feverishly I flicked through the pages of an encyclopaedia of the animal kingdom. Horace's fingers seemed to be the crucial feature, but then I remembered his strange protruding spine. Not a monkey and yet not really like one of the small carnivores such as a stoat. There was nothing like him in the mongoose line. I turned to the raccoon family—maybe Horace was a cacomistle, whatever that looked like. I found the photograph of the cacomistle. Yes, the face was similar but the ears were too big and the clawed feet were most un-finger-like.

Hoping I would remember the appearance of a cacomistle should one ever be brought to me, I hurried hopefully on to the chapter dealing with the pro-simians, that strange bunch of individuals who lie halfway between insect-eating carnivores and monkeys. Horace certainly had some of the typical appearance of an insectivore, as well as those monkey-like fingers. Bingo! As I looked at the appealing faces of these most distant cousins of Man, the aye-aye, the tree-shrew and the rest, I suddenly found myself faced by an illustration of Horace in glorious colour. "Long time since I was bitten by a potto," I said gaily as I opened the door of the consulting room.

Pottos, the caption to Horace's picture stated, have horny processes on their spinal columns that project through their skin, so at least my fears about what had appeared to be Horace's exposed backbone were set at rest. He was my first pro-simian patient, though, and of pro-simian ailments I knew not a thing, but by taking scrapings and swabs of his bald patches for analysis I would try to find out what was causing the hair loss.

About a week later, Edith handed me the laboratory report on the scrapings I had taken. It started, "Your sample from a ?dotto??? (what breed of cat is that—or is it a joke?) . . ."

I would have to become accustomed to folk thinking that I was some sort of nut addicted to practical jokes. I would learn to wait patiently while the person answering the phone at a pharmaceutical company scoffed disbelievingly when a vet from Rochdale ordered some special tropical drug for bilharzia in baboons, or when the international cable operators stopped me in mid-dictation of some urgent message containing phrases like "Suggest your penguins have got bumblefoot" with a "Come off it, mate, is this an April-fool thing or something?" Years later I had to threaten an operator with legal action if he did not type out my cable about a deadly serious matter which concerned not a potto, nor indeed any kind of wild animal, but a footballer. The star player of the famous Real Madrid soccer team in Spain had contracted a unique fungus infection of his knee bone; he might well never play again. The fungus infection had never previously been recorded in humans, but the Spanish doctors knew that I had been involved in treating various kinds of fungus infection in zoo animals. They contacted me via my friends, the directors of Madrid Zoo, and I cabled what information I had concerning the fungus. I suppose one can excuse the disbelief of the cable operator as I began to dictate: "Concerning the footballer's kneecap, I know of one case of an otter in Africa and one possible hedgehog . . . ." Eventually the cable was accepted, and I like to think that the otter and the hedgehog helped that soccer star to play again.

The rest of the lab report on Horace the potto read: " . . . is positive for Trichophyton sp.—Ringworm." I handed the report back to Edith and sighed as I wrote a prescription for Horace's owner to pick up that would in time completely clear his pet's ringworm. Even if a potto was unusual, his skin disease was anything but. Would I never be let into the zoo?

After two and a half years of treating cats and dogs, pigs and cows, with the occasional potto or python to bring me tantalizingly close to zoo work, I was all ears when Norman Whittle casually broke some news one winter's day as we both stood warming the seats of our pants in front of the gas fire in our little office. "There's a new director been appointed at Belle Vue. Name of Legge. Got a first-class reputation as a naturalist and particularly with fish."

Could this at last be the opportunity for me to begin doing some of the real zoo veterinary work? A new director could well mean a brand new approach to the management of the animals. The zoo had recently been taken over by an international hotel and leisure group, there were rumours of new animal houses to be built and new species to be exhibited. It sounded like the perfect chance for a young, green veterinarian to get in at the beginning of a fresh chapter. I tackled Norman about it at once.

"You know how I feel about exotic animals," I said, "but I don't seem to be getting anywhere with the odds and ends, the parrots, bush babies and monkeys, that come here from time to time. I learned more when I went with you as a student to Belle Vue."

Norman knew what I was going to ask him. "Zoo work," he said, screwing up his face pensively and rocking back and forth on his heels. "Do you think there's a future in it?"

"I'm absolutely certain there is."

"As I've told you before, we don't know much about what we're doing down there, David. Can't handle most of the animals. Guesswork, inspired guesswork, most of it. It's the

224

know-how of keepers like Matt Kelly that counts. They call us in as a formality."

"But it's one of the biggest zoos in Britain; there must be a vast amount of work for us. What about nutrition, preventive medicine, fertility improvement? There must be limitless scope for things that only a vet can do. And with a keen new director. . ."

"You may be right, but I don't go very often, you know. In the past they've called me only when they've got themselves into a sticky hole. We're the last resort."

"But if they don't appreciate veterinary work in the zoo, we should get involved deeper, show them, force them to see the value. The new company and new director mean a chance for new attitudes."

Norman sighed and slowly shook his head. "We don't know enough about these creatures. We haven't the tools. You know how it is; if a gorilla gets a bad eye they ask some specialist in humans from the eye infirmary to look at it. He comes along if and when he can spare the time, but he's used to humans who don't break both your arms and chew the top off of your ophthalmoscope if you try shining bright lights in their sore eyes. So the specialist loses interest and the case isn't followed through. A bunch of human surgeons from the university come to take blood from the lions, and three lions die because the anaesthetist doesn't have a clue what frightening things morphine does to cats. So they try again, this time using a barbiturate, and another one never wakes up. It's rather depressing. You'd find it very hard to break into that sort of set-up."

The story of the dead lions I had heard before. It made me angry then and the thought of it still does.

"Doctors be damned," I said. "It's the veterinary surgeon who should be in charge of the health of every one of those animals in Belle Vue."

My partner laughed but there was sadness in his eyes. "You're right, but you'll have a rugged time trying to convince some folk. Most of the time, with things like rhino and giraffe, I'm completely in the dark. The best I can do is to treat zebras like horses, giraffes and camels like cattle, lions and tigers like domestic cats."

"But that leaves out most of the animal kingdom. What about reptiles, primates, things like tapirs and elephants and porcupines?"

Norman shrugged. "Hobson's choice. Follow first principles."

"And animals die."

"Yes. And I have to admit that even at post-mortem I can't usually be sure why a creature gave up the ghost. Now and again I can do something positive, but mostly it's terribly frustrating. Anyway, remember we are a mixed farm and small-animal practice—don't you think the zoo could well be more trouble than it's worth?"

Norman's last sentence chilled me. I did not care to hear him even hinting that we might consider pulling out of zoo work. It was my only chance of penetrating the world of wildlife medicine. He—we—must not lose heart. Fearfully I asked, "Would you seriously think of dropping the zoo?"

"Well, it's twelve miles away, the city traffic's getting worse, all the rest of our work is round Rochdale, there are practices nearer to the zoo than us."

I felt my pulse quicken. If Norman went on in this vein his next words would surely be the renunciation of the one thing that I felt made our partnership special: the collection of strange and wonderful beasts in Belle Vue that fascinated me so powerfully. The very possibility made me shiver. I made up my mind immediately: nailing my colours to the mast with brass studs that hold firm to this day, I said, "Let me take over the work at Belle Vue. I want to make something of exotic medicine."

Norman smiled again and slipped on his white coat. It was time for surgery. "OK," he said, "that's fine by me."

At last I was going to do the zoo work; now all I needed was for the zoo to ring and report a sick animal. I made sure the other members of the staff understood that it would not matter whether I was on or off duty, I must be informed immediately the new zoo director called. God forbid that it should happen when I was in the middle of a difficult calving out on the moors!

A week went by. My visiting list consisted solely of dogs, cats, cows and pigs. Another week came, and another, and still whenever the telephone jangled it was the same sort of request: "Got a heifer here with a bloated stomach that's tight as a drum," or "Our old bitch is drinking day and night and gone off her legs." Just when I was beginning to wonder whether the Belle Vue stock had been given a bunch of remarkably effective amulets as well as a new director, the message I had been waiting for came in. A young camel that was being raised on the bottle was having problems with its mouth. Could the vet please attend?

I was delighted as I set off for Manchester. Here was an animal made for my opening performance: easy to handle and with few anaesthetic problems. I reckoned I knew a thing or two about mouths. Camels' teeth resemble cattle's, and I had pulled out dozens of those. Tongue infections, ulcers, oral forms of cancer, foreign bodies: I had no qualms about dental work and I had covered, so I thought, the whole field in pet and farm animals as well as the odd new-world monkey with so-called South American primate disease, which deforms the facial bones and scatters the growing tooth buds in bizarre disarray. I hoped camels were not prone to some esoteric mouth complaint afflicting them and them alone, murrain of the Pyramids or Gobi Desert tooth rot or some such pestilence, about which I had not read but which was common knowledge among Egyptian camel drivers and head keepers like Matt Kelly.

The road from Rochdale to the zoo in Manchester ran past an unbroken succession of terraced houses with sooty brick facades, cluttered corner shops that sold everything from a yard of elastic to sweet Cyprus sherry from the barrel, and towering mills with massive iron and brass mill gates and names like Bee and King emblazoned in white on the sweating red brick of their chimneys. It was an easy, familiar journey for me. As a small boy and later as a student I had often taken the yellow and orange double-decker bus that ran to the city and then rattled out by tram to the zoo, which stood behind high walls in a wilderness of mean streets, coal mines and railway sidings. This was the unloveliest part of the city, where sparrows sported uniformly sooty black plumage, where the vagrant and ubiquitous pigeons limped along dripping gutters with swollen, arthritic joints and gouty feet, and where the sulphurous fogs of autumn condensed on the clouded-glass windows of the tap rooms of the Engineers Arms and the Lancashire Fusiliers. Today the mills, the dreary dwellings and the churches standing shuttered and forgotten in yards of weeds and broken glass went by unnoticed. I was going to the zoo as its official vet.

Within the high walls of Belle Vue the jungle began. In the grey desert of Manchester there existed this oasis where wild creatures from every part of the globe were to be found. Just beyond the box office on the busy main road, a stone's throw from the mighty pit-shaft wheel of the Bradford colliery and within spitting distance of the London Midland and Scottish railway yard, were Africa and Asia, the impenetrable green of the Mato Grosso and the endless horizon of the steppes. There was no more than an acre of meagre, consumptive-looking grass in the whole park, and that was planted on a bare one-inch layer of soil overlying ashes. In spring the air reeked of engine smoke and in November it stung the eyes. Yet here lurked leopard and lion, eland and elephant. Here as a boy I had scaled the walls, despite the broken glass on top, to gaze down gratis on the tigon, that curious and long-lived hybrid donated a quarter of a century ago by some maharajah, and to make faces at the bears until pursued by irate keepers. It was a magic place for me, and it seemed unbelievable that at long last I was going "on safari" professionally (at the princely fee of eight shillings and six-pence per visit) among the enchanted beasts behind the high walls.

The zoo was built when the reign of Queen Victoria was at its zenith, when Britain ruled the waves and the flower of the Indian Empire was still in full bloom. It was thought appropriate to design the buildings in the style of Mogul India which the England of the Raj had found so much to its taste, so the animal houses were built with windows, roofs and doorways in which the sensuous curves of Islamic art were wedded firmly to the heavy, worthy Victorian ways of working wood and iron. To the crowds who came from the cotton towns by train on a line that ran right into the zoo grounds, the sea-lion house in its heyday must have seemed like a delicate pavilion transported from the palace lawns of Mysore, the sort of place where, but for the drizzle and the smog and the clank of trams from the road, one might take tiffin among the jacaranda blossom with the Colonel's lady. Gardens and long rose walks were laid out between the animal houses, artificial lakes were dug, trees and bushes were planted, and among the bushes nestled the onion domes and minarets of ornamental mosques and palaces done in stucco.

In these pleasant surroundings the Victorians could prom-enade and admire the wild animals held behind massive bars or beyond deep pits. When they tired of the animals they could listen to brass bands in one of the several concert halls, eat in cafés, drink in pubs or amuse themselves on carousels and coconut shies in a fairground—all within the same high-walled park. The park had its own brewery and bakery inside the grounds and the facilities for great banquets, balls and fireworks displays. As I drove through the grounds on my way to see the sick baby camel, the light growing dim with the approach of evening, I could imagine what Belle

Vue had been like a century before. The crumbling remains of the ornamental mosques peeped out of rhododendron bushes, defying the damp and the attrition of small boys' feet who clambered over the "Keep Off" notices to reach the muezzin's turret. Despite dry rot, peeling pale blue paint, a hundred years of sea lions' splashing and the dank smell of herring impregnating the wooden Mogul arches, the pavilion still stood and there was a tiny bit of one of the rose walks, too. The thick bars were gone, new animal houses had been built of concrete and fine steel, the railway stopped far short of the park and the brewery was derelict, but here and there among the modern things like the speedway and the children's playground, an arch, a dome, a pierced screen or a fragment of curled iron winked out, conjuring up a lost age of stylish self-assurance.

The young camel to which I had been called turned out to be a friendly two-humped (Bactrian) female. As I arrived Mr. Legge and Matt Kelly were feeding her from a bottle. I introduced myself to the new director while Kelly stood silently by, frowning in surprise at my appearance. Ray Legge was a slim, pale, military-looking man in his mid-forties, with dark hair and moustache, an aquiline nose and a warm and generous smile. He was neatly dressed and moved easily, with the precision of the rock climber that he was. When he spoke, it was in the crisp, public-school accents of the army officer that he had been. Quite a dramatic change from his predecessors in the post.

He pumped my hand energetically, threatening to pulverize my knuckles. "Jolly pleased to meet you. As you know, I was at Chester Zoo but I've concentrated on aquaria over the past few years, especially Blackpool Tower aquarium. I'm a fish man really, but my mammals and birds will be brought up to scratch in the next few months. Now, let's show you this camel."

Kelly the head keeper held the animal with an expression of weary scepticism at this young vet who was all book-learning and had no idea of zoo animal management. As I inquired what seemed to be the trouble, he quietly gritted his teeth and did an impersonation of St. Ignatius Loyola staring heavenwards in a baroque painting. He had a ruddy, puckish yet handsome face and a close-cropped head that appeared dice-shaped, cubic with slightly rounded corners, the whole set on a short, stocky body. Matt had put the fear of God into me when I was a student with his apparent omniscience, a sleeveful of zoological tricks and the autocratic bearing of a sergeant-major. Now his powerful hands held open the camel's jaws.

"She isn't suckling strongly," said Legge, "and there's this white coating developed in the mouth."

I looked inside. Sure enough, the entire internal surface of the mouth was covered with a milky white membrane. "That's thrush infection," I pronounced immediately, "the fungus you see so often in human babies. You have been sterilizing your feeding bottles properly, haven't you?"

Matt Kelly cleared his throat, went redder, but said nothing.

"Yes, Matt boils the bottles before each feed," replied the director. "Can it be serious?"

"No, not usually. We'll soon have that right. Hold on a minute."

I went to my car and brought back a bottle of gentian violet solution. While Matt held the camel's mouth open again, I used a small brush to paint the bitter purple liquid over her gums, teeth and lips. The animal screwed up her face at the taste and bubbled out a foam of purple saliva, staining Matt's hands. Gentian violet does not wash off easily. Matt's face was now plum-coloured and I feared his teeth-gritting might shatter every tooth in his head.

"Right," I said, "that'll do the trick." Confidently I said my farewells and set off home with the conviction that I had made the best possible start.

Two days later the zoo telephoned again. It was Matt

Kelly. "This here camel, Dr. Taylor," he said in his light Dublin brogue, "oi don't think your purple paint's done one bit of good. She's worse." And then, as if he had already decided the patient was in such a critical state that anything more I might do could not make things any worse, he added, "Ye can come down if ye like." Damn, I thought, he talks as if I'm invited to pay my last respects.

The camel was indeed worse. The white membrane was still coating much of her mouth and the animal's general condition and vitality were deteriorating alarmingly. More of the white fungus was coating the bowels and the vagina. I had never seen thrush, a usually mild, yeasty fungus, on the rampage like this, but my training at university had paid scant attention to the germ. It was regarded as an opportunist, secondary bug of little menace under normal circumstances. Yet this camel was very definitely ill. Could the thrush alone be doing that? Much later I would learn that thrush can be rather a tough and sometimes fatal infection for birds and dolphins, but at the time I felt sure the camel case was more complicated than I had first suspected.

Matt raised his eyebrows when I began to mutter my doubts about the case. "Sure, oi thought all along she wouldn't make it," he said. "Bottle-reared animals haven't the resistance." He adopted an expression of tired patience.

Suddenly something came back to me. Fungi. Yeast fungi. Yeasts, the kind of things that are used in making bread and beer. The yeasts thrive in the bread dough and, during the brewing, on sugar. Sugar, that was it. Somewhere I had read that people with excess sugar in their urine, in other words diabetics, are more susceptible to yeast fungus infections.

"I'm going to take a urine sample, Mr. Kelly," I announced. Matt stared. He had never heard of such a thing being done to a camel. Still, I could imagine him ruminating, young vets do strange things like that when they don't know where the devil they are.

With much difficulty I passed a catheter into the camel's

bladder, drew off a few teaspoons of urine and dipped one of my glucose test strips into the sample. It turned deep blue— the camel was diabetic. "Sugar diabetes, Mr. Kelly," I proclaimed excitedly. Matt scowled. "Now I want some blood."

The blood test's abnormally high sugar level confirmed beyond doubt the cause of the camel's disease. The thrush was secondary and could probably be eradicated by anti-fungal drugs, but the question of how to handle the diabetes was a tricky one. I talked it over with Ray Legge.

"It looks as if she'll need a daily injection of insulin," I warned. "We'll start off with the fairly long-acting protamine zinc kind and fiddle about with the dose until she's just free of sugar."

It was not a very encouraging prospect, possibly having to give shots to a camel for life. I knew a number of dog owners who were used to jabbing their diabetic pets each day with insulin; the animals tended to develop small knobbles all over them and felt like pineapples.

"Couldn't we give anti-diabetic drugs in her food?" asked Ray.

There were at least two kinds of oral drug which were proving effective in some human cases at that time, but they had failed to reduce the sugar level and control the progress of the disease in almost all animal cases. I explained this to the zoo director and we decided to embark on the course of insulin shots. Matt Kelly was armed with a bunch of syringes and needles, and I showed him how to adjust the dose according to the colour of the test strip after it had been in contact with the urine.

"And where do oi get the urine from?" Matt inquired. "Oi can't stand waitin' behind the craytchure all day long hopin' it'll pee!"

"Of course not," I replied. "All you need do is spot a damp patch on the concrete where she's passed water and dab your test strip in that."

Matt looked at his collection of medical paraphernalia with the enthusiasm of a bilious leprechaun. Crawling about over the floor blotting up camel-juice indeed! Just what he had known would happen if novices like young Taylor started interfering.

The young camel began to put on weight and condition over the next few days as Matt gave the insulin and the anti-fungal treatment annihilated the layers of yeast fungus. Things were progressing admirably. Then, on the ninth day, the youngster refused to feed and took on a drawn and depressed look. The sugar content in the urine rocketed upwards. When Ray Legge went into the hospital on the morning of the tenth day he found the little camel lying dead. Miserable, I drove over to perform the necropsy. The pancreas, the organ which produces natural insulin normally and also serves a number of other vital functions concerning digestion of food, I found to be a shrivelled, almost non-existent piece of tissue. What there was of it was inflamed, red and yellow. Matt Kelly silently returned to me the unused syringes, test strips and injections. So much for veterinary science.

Despite this early setback, Ray Legge set off to a cracking start at Belle Vue. He supervised the building of one of the finest aquaria and reptile houses in the country and then designed a modern great ape complex complete with isolation rooms, a self-contained kitchen and food store for Len, the senior ape keeper, and underground tunnels leading from centrally heated, glass-fronted indoor quarters to circular open-air play pits again protected from the germ-bearing visitors by armour-plated glass. In these new buildings I was going to spend much of my time in the next few years, for it became a mutual, unspoken arrangement that I would visit the zoo regularly at least once a week and not just when I was called. Exciting new inhabitants for both completed residences had been purchased by the zoo, giant tortoises and alligators for the one and a pair of young gorillas for the other. These would join the existing reptiles and apes from the old reptile and great ape houses.

Ray was a stimulating and sympathetic person to work with: a talented artist and sculptor in wood and stone, he had a sensitive and humane approach to zoo animals wonderfully combined with the never-ending curiosity of the born naturalist. To hear him talk, his time with the British Army in India during the war had been one glorious natural history ramble, finding new fish, rare insects or strange plants wherever he was posted. During the Cyprus crisis, when he instructed troops hunting Eoka terrorists in the arts of mountain climbing, he found the greatest excitement in pursuing the nimble lizards of the Troodos Mountains under the concealed rifles of General Grivas's guerrilla snipers.

But it was with Matt Kelly that I had to build some sort of bridge if I was to carry out my resolve to learn something of his zoocraft. This most renowned of British head keepers had worked for many years at Belle Vue and before that at Dublin, which at the time had an unrivalled reputation for the quality of its lions. Matt was no naturalist, no lizard chaser, no smooth utterer of Latin names, no scientist; he was simply the perfect head keeper of his time. An out-and-out practical zooman, he was born with that "feel" for his animals which is to be found in good shepherds and in farmers who rear plump beef cattle efficiently and with apparent ease, not by any high-falutin knowledge of food analyses, digestibility factors or other scientist's jargon, but by observation, experience, personal attention to individual feeding and plain, inborn talent. Also, in the same indefinable way that natural seamen sense impending changes in the weather, Matt had a nose for trouble. Long before it was obvious to others, he would start to fret about the rhinoceros or the ostrich or any other of the numerous creatures that he knew so intimately.

"Matt," I said one day, shortly after the death of the baby camel, "you know I learned a lot at Belle Vue as a student. Now, doing the veterinary work myself, I'm going to need your help in showing me a whole lot more of the things a vet doesn't know."

Matt seemed pleased with my approach. A wide grin, showing broad white teeth like a chimp's, split his face. "Sure and we'll see what we can make of ye, Dr. Taylor," he replied.

Things, little things, immediately began to go wrong. If there was a wrong way to do something, some particularly obtuse, disastrous or all-fingers-and-thumbs way to do it, I did it. There was the cardinal sin of zoo keeping which I quickly committed—leaving a gate unlocked. Matt and I had been looking at the Barbary sheep as they sprang from rock to rock round the artificial mountain in their pen. Bald, scurfy areas on their coat suggested mange. I would arrange to have them trapped, take skin scrapings for examination and dip them like farm flocks. Ping, ping, ping. Surefootedly on their tiny hooves they leaped from one minute ledge to another with infinite grace. Then, just as surefootedly, one of them went ping, ping, ping out through the gate into the zoo grounds. The last in, I had not bolted the gate behind me. Red-faced, I chased after a fuming Matt Kelly as we pursued the agile creature like two decrepit satyrs on the trail of a wood nymph. Out of the zoo grounds we went and onto the main road that leads to the city centre. The Barbary sheep was gaining ground; the way it was galloping along one might have thought it was making for the docks and hoping to dash aboard a freighter due any moment to sail for its native North Africa. Eventually, with the aid of Ray Legge, keepers and sundry other citizens who had been informed of or had actually witnessed our puffing, cursing dash towards the town, the creature was cornered in a coal merchant's yard. Master of rocky pinnacles and sandstone cliff faces, the Barbary sheep found that the scree-sloped black pyramids of coal did not provide firm footing. Scrabbling vainly to reach the sooty peak of one mound it slipped relentlessly backwards and was caught.

Covered in coal dust that stuck firmly to our clothes and sweating skin, Matt and I returned to the zoo. "Jeez, ye made me purple a few weeks ago, Doctor," he lamented, clicking his teeth, "and now ye've made me black!"

Our next joint foray concerned a monkey that had been fed the most potentially deadly titbits. Every zoo attracts a tiny proportion of nuts, dangerous eccentrics and vandals among the crowds of paying public. I can understand the impulses that make folk ignore the "No Feeding" signs and pass potato chips or boiled sweets to elephants or monkeys; I detest it, but see the motivation involved, when drunken louts climb over the walls on a Saturday night after the pubs close and, in the fuddled spirit of bravado which this most primitive of mammalian species exhibits at such times, knock hell out of defenceless creatures like penguins or wallabies or peacocks. But I do not understand, cannot in my wildest dreams explain, the workings of the mind of the human who passed a bunch of thin, new, stainless-steel razor blades through the bars to a monkey. The monkey liked the look of the shining metal wafers and, so that his fellows could not purloin them, put them safely away—in his mouth. Like anyone who has received a present of which he is rather proud, the monkey just had to keep taking them out from time to time to admire and shuffle through them, and it was while he was inspecting his treasure in this way that his keeper spotted the blades and raised the alarm. Quick as a flash, the monkey put his fascinating little collection back into his cheek pouch.

When Matt and I arrived the monkey stared innocently at us. No blood ran from his mouth. His fingers appeared uninjured. Razor blades? What razor blades? his eyes seemed to say. Like some Indian fakir, he had so far avoided doing himself harm by manipulating the blades delicately with his soft tongue and velvety cheek lining. But how were we to retrieve them? I still had no speedy, safe monkey anaesthetics. If we netted him, might he not slice up the inside of his mouth in the fracas?

"What do you think, Matt?" I asked my mentor. "How do we get the bloody things out without carving him up?"

Matt thought for a moment; then, with an air of relaxed confidence, he said, "Get me a sweepin' brush."

I found a brush for Matt, who slipped into the cage through the trapdoor at the back. The monkey darted to a far corner well away from him and prepared to do battle. It was obvious the head keeper was going to try to pin him in the corner with the brush. OK, the monkey was clearly thinking, we would see about that, and he tensed his powerful leg muscles, ready to leap out of the way of the imminent onslaught. With all the space available, the monkey must have reckoned that by jumping rapidly round from bars to branch to ledge to bars again he could wear out this lumbering human with his unwieldy brush in a war of attrition that might, as far as he was concerned, last all day. My forecast of the outcome, inexperienced as I was, agreed with that of my little simian friend; if I had been a betting man, I would have laid my money on the monkey.

Both of us were barking up the wrong tree. Matt's battle plan was quite, quite different. Without warning the stocky Irishman began to shout and swear at the top of his voice. Every oath invented in the isle of saints and sinners came blasting out. His face contorted with rage and he waved the brush vigorously about, clouting it with resounding bangs on the walls of the cage. It was an unholy din, but he did not make one move towards the monkey, nor did he bring his weapon within feet of the startled animal's crouching body. To the monkey it must have seemed as though the head keeper had gone mad. Any second this Fury would bring the flailing brush smashing down on his puny frame. With wrath like this he would not be just pinned and caught, he would be smashed to smithereens! This was going to be no game, but a matter of life or death somehow to keep out of range of the murderous maniac. He was going to have to run and run and run.

When running for your life you discard all inessential baggage so, watching for the first thunderbolt, the monkey picked the razor blades out of his mouth and dropped them on the floor. Matt stopped shouting, put down his brush, replaced the expression of mock rage with one of twinkling satisfaction and gathered up the slivers of steel. "That's the way ye do it, Dr. Taylor," he said. "Now we can bag him and ye can check him over if ye like."

I was very impressed. Catching the monkey in a sort of butterfly net did not take long, then the captive was transferred without ceremony to a sack for carrying across to the hospital. When we arrived there the bagful of monkey was put on the table and I prepared to do my bit. I would sedate the monkey with a small shot of barbiturate so that I could examine him. I had the choice of injecting through the sack—an unhygienic procedure—or fishing the animal out, putting a full nelson on him and doing it elegantly in arm or thigh. I decided to extract him, but which end of him was where? There were three or four moving lumps in the wriggling sack, but were they arms, head or buttocks? I reckoned that one spherical lump must be the head and seized it firmly through the sacking. It was not the head—it was the other end. A second later the dagger-like fang teeth of the genuine head end lanced through the sack and sliced my left index finger almost in half. As I tried to stem the bleeding and prepared to go down to the city hospital for suturing and tetanus injections, Matt gave me the word. "Never try grabbin' a monkey in a bag like that again, Doctor. Remember his eyes are pressed close to the coarse sackin' stuff. Ye can't see where he is, but sure as hell he can see ye."

Painfully I acknowledged my dumb stupidity and went off to the Manchester hospital, where the house surgeon declined to use one drop of local anaesthetic as he cobbled together my sliced extremity. (My colleagues in human surgery do not realize how easy their primate species are to handle; try doing the same on a young chimp, for example.) He also cauterized the wound deeply and painfully with silver nitrate, neglected to give me any antibiotics and consequently produced a throbbing infection.

It was when the finger was at last settling down and my hand was once more available to do surgery on my own behalf that Ray Legge informed me that one of the zoo's golden pheasants had a lump on its eyelid. When I examined the bird there was no doubt that the hard, yellowish swelling was a tumour, but not very difficult to cut out. I decided to take the bird back to my surgery in Rochdale and do the small operation under gas anaesthesia. Matt Kelly came along with me.

With its striking art-nouveau plumage of scarlet, green, gold and black, the golden pheasant is one of the handsomest birds in the world and definitely among my favourites. Like many other species of pheasant, the male sports a particularly gorgeous flourish of tail feathers, and it was on one such exquisite avian dandy that I was operating. All went well as I cut out the growth with scalpel and forceps and Edith puffed air and a minute quantity of halothane gas into the syrup tin containing the head of the slumbering bird. Matt watched and seemed moderately impressed. After stitching the wound with fine nylon thread, I told Edith to stop the anaesthetic and stood back to admire my work. The bird drowsed peacefully on the operating table. Then, as is the way with birds coming out of anaesthesia, it suddenly blinked its eyes open, flipped itself up onto its feet and fluttered off the table before any of us could move. Rapidly gaining strength, and finding itself in surroundings quite different from its native Tibetan forests or its range at Belle Vue, it dashed merrily round the room, knocking over light pieces of equipment and provoking the cats who sat in wire-mesh boxes waiting their turn for surgical attention. Edith and I gathered our wits and set about retrieving the energetic post-op patient.

"Careful!" shouted Kelly, crouching down in the posture of a rugby full-back about to tackle his man. "Leave him to me! I'll get him as he comes round!"

But we took no notice and scuttled in hot pursuit, while Matt waited to bag the pheasant as it dashed towards him on its next lap of the room. Anxious to impress the head keeper with my animal handling expertise, I ungallantly elbowed Edith out of the way, put on a spurt and made a determined grab.

"Leave him to me!" Matt yelled again, but I had caught the bird—or so I thought. With a firm grasp of the careering pheasant's proud tail feathers, I applied the brakes and the long plumes came to a halt. The pheasant, to my horror, dashed on, straight into Matt's arms. Now bereft of its full complement of the tiger-barred plumes which in the complete bird make up an arching tail of just the right artistic length, the pheasant was exposing a stubby, yellow-pink butt end reminiscent of a Christmas turkey on Boxing Day.

"Dammit, look!" groaned Matt, his teeth grinding as he struggled to contain more picturesque Irish turns of phrase while Edith was present. "Look at the bird's ar . . . posterior!"

Although unhurt, the bird looked most undignified as it squatted in Matt's folded arms. Both of them, I thought, looked at me with a red and reproachful eye. There was no way of making up for my mistake, no glue nor subterfuge could save my face. It would be many months before nature restored the pheasant's fine cockade and covered the evidence of my ineptitude.

Matt's sour expression confirmed that I had done it again.

"Never catch hold of a bird loike that again," he instructed as he made for the door and I stood glumly, still clutching my wretched bunch of feathers like a schoolboy caught in the act of picking the neighbour's strawberries. "And give me those feathers," he added, holding out a hand. "Dozens of schoolchildren ask me for such things." I could imagine him handing this lot out and saying in his fruity brogue, "And these were pulled out of a golden pheasant by a clumsy young vet. Can ye imagine that?" I was not building much yet in the way of bridges with Mr. Matt Kelly, that was certain.

At least Ray Legge was encouraging and tolerant as I stumbled my way painfully through the minefield of practice among creatures too dangerous or too difficult to handle safely, who presented symptoms that bore no resemblance to anything I had seen in cat or pig or carthorse. I also had to contend with techniques of animal self-defence which I had not met before, from the torpid sloth who is anything but slothful when slashing rapidly and accurately with its front claws, to the coatimundi who, if you pick it up by its tail and hold it safely at arm's length, will athletically climb up its own tail and summarily deal with you. It shares this contortionist ability with the opossum, Matt instructed me. It came as a relief sometimes, though one which I would have vehemently denied at the time, to return at the end of a day of "guess-agnosis" at the zoo and get stuck into a surgery full of common or garden domestic pets with complaints that seemed like old and trusted friends, where drugs acted predictably and surgery was a romp round anatomy as familiar as one's own back yard.

Matt Kelly continued to supervise my enthusiastic meddling with a melancholy reserve. My wrong diagnoses were shown up when I performed post-mortems. The square-faced Irishman would click his teeth as I prodded around inside the cadaver of an antelope that I had considered to be afflicted with liver infection but whose diseased lungs were manifestly the cause of its death. "Knew it hadn't much chance," he would opine as I began to mutter the Latin name of the condition and hopelessly try to baffle him with science. "Seen it before, oi have, Dr. Whittle and oi both. Knew the powders ye gave him would do no good." Matt would shake his head and reflect aloud on the good old days when yoghurt, cider vinegar, honey and molasses had been the elixirs of life in the zoo and everything from axolotl to zebra had apparently expired only from advanced old age.

It seemed that the only common fact about exotic species was their unwillingness to exhibit symptoms that had much logical connection with the diseased portion of their bodies. In the evenings I would complain to Shelagh as I ate my supper about how a hippopotamus with chronic pneumonia of both lungs had breathed apparently evenly and without difficulty right up to the point of death and had not been heard to cough one single, soft cough. And about how monkeys that I found to be riddled with tuberculosis had played, fought, eaten, mated and harassed their keeper until struck down within the space of five minutes as if smitten by thunderbolts. "It's as if the zoo animals have some tacit conspiracy to give me a hard time," I would ruminate as I tackled my steak pudding and peas. "Maybe Norman Whittle was right. It doesn't make much difference whether I do anything or nothing, the outcome is inevitable."

"Nonsense!" Shelagh would reply. "You've got to learn to walk before you can run. And after all, it was your idea to go in for zoo animals."

With more homilies on the general theme of having to break eggs to make omelettes, she would brew me a mug of coffee and I would go into the lounge to spend an hour or two reading books or journals on exotica. Although there were as yet no books available on zoo medicine, occasional papers were being published here and there by scientists

243

working in Africa, in laboratories and in places such as the mighty San Diego Zoo. For a few minutes in the evenings I could escape from my problems with Belle Vue and Matt Kelly and learn what veterinarians were doing in sunnier climates. Even San Diego, it appeared, did not have it too easy, and the Prosector's Annual Report from London Zoo, a detailed record of the toll of creatures dying from disease and accidental injury, grimly reflected my experience in Manchester. The crying need was still for a range of powerful but safe sedatives and anaesthetics which would enable all of us to examine and treat living exotic creatures more thoroughly. On top of that, we needed a sure way of delivering the drugs to wild and dangerous critters over distances ranging from a few feet to tens of yards. Until we had such weapons in our armoury I would have to go on collecting hair, droppings, urine and other possibly useful stray material from sick animals in the hope of getting enlightenment from the Test (rather like a soothsayer pondering the entrails of a sacrificial chicken), while Matt Kelly stood stolidly by with an expression on his face which said quite clearly that scientific mumbo-jumbo could never take the place of good old-fashioned zooman's know-how.

Six

One way Matt Kelly demonstrated his inborn zooman's skill brilliantly was in knowing exactly when it was safe to go into a cage or den with a seriously ill animal, even a dangerous one. He had an eye for picking the earliest moment when, providing I did what I was told, I might get away with injecting an ailing lion, lancing an abscess on the butt of a blood-poisoned and uncaring bear or snatching a quick feel of a tigress's swollen belly without losing a limb or my life in the process.

My first such venture was a David-in-the-leopard's-den episode involving a cat that had picked up the miserable running cold symptoms of feline influenza, no doubt from some mundane domestic puss who had wandered through the big cat house at night in search of stray morsels of meat. Feeling and looking just like a human on the first day of an acute attack of 'flu, the leopard lay in his cage, sneezing miserably, drooling ropes of saliva and blinking blearily through inflamed and watery eyes. I was most impressed when Matt produced his keys and unlocked the cage door.

"Oi think we can go in," he said. "Stick close behind me all the time." I nodded. "All the time," Matt repeated as we crept warily through the door and closed it behind us.

The leopard sneezed, snuffled and snorted where he lay in the straw, but appeared not to notice us. "Oi'm goin' to grab his tail," Matt whispered. "Keep behoind me and jab your injection into it." Tail injections in domestic animals are considered to be utterly beyond the pale, but in zoo animals one sometimes has to give thanks for whatever bit of the patient's anatomy the Good Lord provides. I had my syringe and needle full and ready.

Matt walked quietly over to the leopard, with me shadowing him a full six inches behind. Bending slowly down, he picked up the leopard's tail and pulled. The leopard, miserable as he was, just had to react to such provocation. Growling, he dug his claws through the straw into the wooden floor and glared back over his shoulder at his tormentors. Matt continued pulling. "While he's like this, if oi keep pullin', he can't get his head round and into me," he grunted.

Suddenly the grip of the leopard's claws on the floor gave way and the animal skidded back towards us. Angered now, he slewed his front half round and lashed out with his front claws. Matt continued to pull the tail and started to skip backwards. "Oi've got to keep the tail at full stretch," he said more loudly as I skipped backwards too, trying to match my footsteps with his to avoid our legs tangling and both of us tumbling over with an increasingly irate, probably headachy leopard on top.

Back we went and back came the cat. The more he struggled, the faster we went. As we came near a corner, we backed off at an angle. Our strange paso doble, or rather paso triple, continued round the cage. We just could not afford to let the leopard catch up with the end of his tail.

"Roight, now," said Matt eventually, puffing with the exertion of the dance, "reach round me and stick it in!"

It was not easy, tripping energetically backwards, with Matt's bulk blocking my view of the rear half of the spitting 'flu victim, to reach round and stick the hypodermic needle under the skin of the tail. I looked round Matt as we danced, chose my point and thrust forward my syringe. Matt's shoulder obstructed my line of sight again. I prodded blindly towards the position I had chosen. "Bejasus," yelled Matt, "ye've jabbed me hand!"

Startled, I pulled back my needle. Luckily I had not begun depressing the plunger, but the back of Matt's neck had gone the colour of smoked salmon.

"Again, again, try again," he shouted testily, "but for Gawd's sake look where ye're goin'."

Still trotting backwards behind the now-sweating head keeper, I steadied myself with one arm round his waist, craned my neck awkwardly to the right, spotted the tail once more and launched a second attempt. This time I struck home and was greeted by the manhandled leopard with a throaty roar of outrage. "Done," I declared. "What do we do now?"

"Keep goin' till we're next by the door," replied Matt, "then ye back out. Oi'll throw him forwards and follow ye." It was our last circumnavigation of the cage. When I was in position I retreated from the dance floor and crashed with relief through the doorway. With a skilful flick of his strong wrists Matt threw the leopard forward and away from him. Before the animal had time to gather himself for a riposte, Matt had joined me outside the cage and banged the door to.

Puffing, the head keeper wiped his forehead and sucked the red spot on his hand where I had punctured him. "Not bad, young feller," he said, "not bad." I was delighted. That "not bad" from Matt was worth a thousand guineas to me. "But ye'll have to practise your Oswaldtwistle Barn Dance." He reminded me about it the following Christmas when, at the annual Belle Vue party, he took the floor for this English north country dance where partners go three by three. Not a bad dancer, Matt.

My successful injection of the fully conscious savage beast produced a euphoria which was to last all of twenty minutes. Walking back from the big cat house, Matt and I passed the ape house. In the sunlit open-air cage was a fit-looking three-year-old chimp with eyes as bright as buttons.

"Who's that?" I asked the head keeper.

"That's Lee, son of Katja and Robert, a grand little feller."

I stood for a moment to admire the chimpanzees. Lee seemed positively entranced by me; his eyes never left me. Could it be, I thought in the afterglow of my feat of derring-do with the leopard, that he senses in me something of Dr. Dolittle? Maybe I have got that special way with animals. Lee stared on. True, he did not seem to be quite catching my eye, but there was no doubt that something about me was riveting his attention.

I vaulted the metal barrier designed to stop the public from doing what I was about to do and went closer to the cage. My confidence knew no bounds. Lee continued to gaze adoringly at me but seemed to be fascinated by my chest rather than my face. The reason rapidly became clear as he pushed an arm through the bars of the cage and with a lightning-fast movement snatched at my shirt, an expensive pink one lightly embroidered with glossy whorls in light brown, of which I was rather fond. With one single, precise yank, he pulled the garment clean away from my body. I stood unhurt but dumbfounded, naked from the waist up. In the background the Irishman began to scoff loudly as Lee shuffled off to the back of the cage with his prize and tried it on for size. It was not a very good fit, but that did not seem to bother him at all.

"My shirt," I exclaimed pointlessly. "My shirt."

"Ye've seen the last of that," chuckled Kelly. "All the tea in China couldn't get it away from him; oi've told ye before about goin' close to primate cages." He had. One of the first lessons I had learned when walking along the narrow central corridor that divided the sleeping quarters of Belle Vue's monkey house was to keep dead on the middle line, or grey, brown, black or greenish little arms would snake out and pull my hair, give me a thick ear or steal any detachable object such as fountain pen or stethoscope. Now my shirt was very definitely Lee's. For long after you could still see the remains of it lovingly hoarded in his bed, fragmented and less recognizable, but Lee appeared to treasure it even more than I ever had.

I felt rather exposed setting off home half naked, as Matt grinned and said something to Len, the head ape keeper, about "young boyos with more larnin' than sense".

"Hello, Tarzan," said Shelagh with a giggle as I walked into the kitchen, "tea's ready."

It would be wrong to give the impression that everything I attempted in the zoo fulfilled Matt's gloomy predictions by ending in disaster. Cracked toenails on elephants did well on the hoof oil I prescribed, and I had cleared a llama or two of lice—but Matt Kelly had ,been getting similar results on zoo animals before I was born. Maybe he had used automobile engine oil on the elephants' feet and simple flowers of sulphur to destroy the llamas' parasites, but they had worked almost as well and nearly as quickly as my up-to-date drugs. To break into the business properly and become a zoo vet in Matt's eyes I would have to do better than that. I consoled myself with the thought that the director, Ray Legge, seemed to appreciate my efforts. Perhaps it was because, as an aquarist, he too was learning in this hotch-potch of a captive jungle.

We learnt together on one emergency which happened on Matt Kelly's day off. Some mindless member of the public had thrown a ball of string over the wire into the big cat enclosure, and a puma had decided to play with it. It was fun! When he tapped it, it rolled along the grass. A thwack from a paw and it spun through the air. The puma pounced on it and gnawed it, pretending it was a rabbit that he had cleverly stalked and finally seized in one irresistible attack. The ball of string began to unravel. The big cat licked idly at the imaginary body of his prey and a loose end of string stuck to his tongue. All cats' tongues have harsh, abrasive upper surfaces on which prickly cells point backwards to help the animal lap up liquids efficiently. The puma continued licking when he felt the string in his mouth, and the movement of his tongue inevitably pushed it farther and farther backwards. Like the incurving fangs of a snake, the scales on the tongue provided a one-way ratchet, making it difficult if not impossible for the creature to spit out what had been taken in. The puma felt the string at the back of his throat and pawed vainly in an effort to dislodge the tickly thread. The string stayed put, so the puma started to lick and swallow to try to put an end to the irritation. The end of the string disappeared. The puma licked and swallowed. The unravelling ball of string became smaller as inch by inch it crept down the animal's gullet.

Ray Legge telephoned me early in the morning. "Will you come over and look at one of the young pumas? It's an odd case. There's one piece of string hanging out of the mouth and another from the anus."

When I arrived at Belle Vue the position had not changed. Sure enough, the animal had about three inches of string dangling from one end and a slightly smaller length trailing from the other. Ray and I agreed that both bits of string looked very much alike and might well be one and the same piece. The puma was not bothering to lick at the fragment hanging from his lips and appeared perfectly healthy. The possibility that we were looking at two ends of a single piece had ominous undertones. Endless opportunities for trouble in the bowel were offered by such a foreign body. I would have to anaesthetize the animal.

Ray had designed a new cat house with special squeeze compartments where I could get to grips safely with my patients, but it was not easy to entice the animal into the restraining device to give it a shot of anaesthetic. I made a mental note to order one of the new darting pistols that I had just heard were being produced in the United States. At last the puma was immobilized and I gave my anaes-thetic. In ten minutes he was sleeping peacefully and we pulled him out into the passageway of the cat house so that I could examine him.

Kneeling down and concentrating on the puma, I made the cardinal error of forgetting about my rear when in a confined space flanked by caged animals. As I bent to give a gentle pull to the string hanging from the puma's jaws, a nearby leopard whipped its forepaw through the bars, dug a hooked claw deeply into my right ankle, anchoring itself behind my Achilles tendon, and tried to haul me into its cage. In agony I tumbled round and literally unpicked the tough hook of nail from my bleeding leg. Thank goodness Matt isn't here, was all I could think, I've fumbled it again.

Pausing to stick some of the penicillin cream normally used up cows' udders into my wound and bind it with gauze, I returned my attentions to the puma. Tugging the string at either end did not budge it a millimetre. I decided that it might not be wise to pull really hard; I was not sure why, but I felt that if the string did not slip conveniently out the force might do untold damage to the animal's insides. Besides, I still could not be certain that the two portions were not separate. "I'll have to open him up," I told Ray. "I'll go into the abdomen first to find out how far the string extends and then maybe open the intestines."

We carried the unconscious big cat on a wheelbarrow over to the dispensary and the operation was soon under way. I inspected the loops of bowel. Sure enough, I could feel the firm thread of string running right through the animal's alimentary canal.

"My hands are sterile—will you try pulling the string at the back end, Ray?" I asked. The zoo director pulled lightly at the puma's rear beyond the draped operation sheets, while I watched the effect on the exposed bowel loops. When Ray pulled, the intestines began to concertina together as if he were drawing the cord on a pair of unoccupied pyjamas. I told him to stop pulling at once. Any more of that and the string would begin to cut into the delicate folded lining

251

of the bowel tube. Thank God I had not tried brute force in extracting the string—it would have sliced open the intestines at a couple of dozen points. There was only one way. At six places between the duodenum and rectum I had to pierce the intestine wall, fish in for the string, cut it and then sew up the wall with waterproof stitching. At every second incision I pulled out the freed section of string after cutting it.

An hour later it was completed. The puma had six patches in his food canal and I had all the string. With his abdomen sewn up and pumped full of antibiotics to prevent peritonitis, the still-sleeping puma was wheeled back to his night house.

"Marvellous job," said Ray, patting me on the back, "really worthwhile." Pity old Kelly wasn't there, I thought. Telling him tomorrow won't have the impact of the real thing.

Ten days later I took the stitches out of the recovered puma with Matt helping me to give the anaesthetic. "You ought to have seen it, Matt," I said proudly. "String from end to end like a bunch of black puddings. Good thing I operated."

Matt nodded and spat accurately at a drain. "Pumas," he said, "pumas. Sure, they're a drug on the market. Dime a dozen these days. Makes me wonder if they're worth spendin' money on."

Despite Matt's scepticism, my experience was beginning to extend beyond split toenails and lousy llamas. If there was the slightest chance of saving an animal's life Ray and I took it, and Matt was roped in to help as I fitted a custom-built wooden leg, complete with ingenious articulated foot, to a flamingo whose limb I had amputated because of gangrene; he held the bowl of water while I took casts of a newborn zebra foal's neck which had been bitten and broken by its father shortly after birth, and for which I designed a glass fibre support to keep the foal's head up while the bones healed. Times were gradually changing, and a major turning-point came the day I received through the post from America my gas-powered dart-gun. What was more the drug company, Parke, Davis, had sent me a supply of a promising new drug, phencyclidine, to try out on zoo animals. Concentrated enough to be used in the dart-gun syringes, and said to be fast-acting, it gave me a new optimism about my future as a zoo vet.

I took my new toys over to Belle Vue to show Ray, but he was not in his office so I drove through the grounds to the animal kitchen. Walking into the room where the diets are made up, I found Matt standing at the sink shaving. The foamy lather from his face was dropping onto a tray of frozen sprats that were being thawed out for the penguins.

"Dear me, Mr. Kelly," I said sternly, "what are you doing? It's hardly the right thing to do one's ablutions all over the animal food. The practice will have to stop at once."

The stocky Irishman glared at me like an apoplectic Father Christmas, blew a few soapy bubbles but said nothing. He began rinsing the sprats. I went out, leaving the crestfallen Matt with half his beard still on. I grinned to myself when I was out of sight. A belated comeback, I thought; one point to me.

Now that I had a dart-gun and the new drug, I was all set to break for ever with the old days of impotent guesswork from the other side of the bars or the opposite bank of the moat. The use of tranquillizers in the food of zoo animals had not proved to be very reliable—most of the drugs then available were designed for humans and did not necessarily work on wild beasts. Anyway, the animals could not be guaranteed to take the pills ground up and mixed with their food, and if they did the stuff often got lost among the vast quantities of digesting material churning around in their stomachs and either produced no signs of sleepiness or did so hours later when we were long gone and in bed. The doses of human tranquillizers also had to be multiplied many times when administered to exotic animals, even small ones, and the thousands of pills that would be required for a biggy like an elephant made the whole business farcical. Ray Legge and I had also tried jabbing injections of dope into awkward animals like giraffe with syringes attached to the end of long poles, but it never really worked. We just broke a lot of needles and even more poles.

The first animals on which I tried my gun and phencyclidine were some wolves that Ray wanted to move from one lot of quarters to another within the zoo. Nervously I loaded a dozen darts and then, one after the other, fired them at the prowling animals. Plop, plop, plop. I learned how easy it was to hit shoulder, thigh or neck muscle. Within ten minutes all the wolves were asleep—we had never seen anything like it. The whole transfer was completed within half an hour. I went on to lions and then bears. Never a hitch, never a fatality. The drug was ideal on monkeys, chimps, gorillas. It kept the animals unconscious for about an hour and then wore off gradually over the next day or so. Phencyclidine appeared to be the universal bringer of dreams I had been seeking.

Then I hit the first snags. I lost my first elephant, Mary, after a long operation to remove a tooth with a root abscess; the prolonged period of recovery from phencyclidine in such a large creature resulted in fatal congestion of the lungs. I experimented on zebras needing emergency suturing of wounds. The phencyclidine put the animals down but the nightmares they seemed to experience, and the hours of frantic crashing about as the chemical faded slowly from their systems, were painful to witness. After one awful night spent with Matt Kelly in a straw-smothered loose box, soothing and struggling to hold down a lathered, wild-eyed zebra stallion that was coming round from phencyclidine anaesthesia, I vowed never to use the drug again on equines. Fortunately, two newer drugs, xylazine and etorphine, would soon appear and prove the answer to doping zebra.

Although phencyclidine was first-class in bears, the polar bear was more sensitive to it than its cousins were and needed a much smaller dose to knock it out. It was my success in anaesthetizing polar bears at Belle Vue which led to my first piece of circus work. Billy Smart's Circus was at Prestwick in Scotland and had a male polar bear with the irritating condition common in these deceptive and highly dangerous creatures, ulceration between the toes. Polar bears have lots of fur on their feet to insulate them against the cold of ice and snow, but in captivity it often becomes matted between their toes into hard little balls. The balls act as foreign bodies and rub uncomfortably at the soft flesh on either side of them. Gradually ulcers are formed which attract fungus and other types of infection, and the accumulated hair balls must be cut out. The Smarts and I had met at the circus held every Christmas at Belle Vue, and they asked me to go up to Prestwick to dope the bear and clean up his feet.

I felt wildly elated as I drove back down from Scotland after darting in the phencyclidine and then taking my scissors and soothing ointments to the massive paws of the slumbering white giant. Zoo work is one thing; impressing the hard-bitten animal men of the circus world, who tend to have firm prejudices about veterinary matters, is another thing altogether. The Smarts had seemed very impressed with my fast, no-nonsense anaesthesia.

The gun and the new drugs could be the key to bringing veterinary help to circus animals as well, then, but the next patient on which I used it was back at Belle Vue. One morning Matt Kelly telephoned in a terrible flap; Ray Legge was away on holiday and he was acting zoo director. He sounded desperate yet resigned. "Get down as soon as ye can, Doctor. It's an oryx cow. She's just calved and all her insoides are hangin' out. It looks very bad."

Listening to Matt's brief description I could guess what

had happened, but I did not waste time telling him about it over the telephone. I told him to keep the animal quiet, to cover the "insoides" with a clean, moist sheet to keep them from becoming damaged or dirty, and to wait for me. Then I jumped into my car and set off for Manchester.

Matt's face was long and sombre as I walked into the oryx shed. I had never seen him looking so downcast. He did not bother to greet me but just announced bleakly, "She's had it. No question. Oi've never seen such a mess in all me years as a zoo keeper."

The Beisa oryx was lying on her side on a pile of straw, her hind quarters draped in white sheeting stained with large fuzzy shadows of red. Under the sheet a bloody pink balloon of flesh, studded with purple cherry-like objects and as big as the animal's head and neck, lay on the straw. It was attached by a narrow neck to the vulva. As I had guessed, the oryx had calved and discharged the afterbirth; then the whole of the womb, with the ovaries attached, had turned inside out and fallen through the pelvis into the fresh air. The oryx's entire womb and associated structures had prolapsed and were lying on the ground for all to see.

"Just look at her," continued Matt. "She's had it, oi can tell ye that. No animal can survoive havin' all its insoides turned out. Fancy drugs and such can't help her!" He clicked his teeth agitatedly.

Uterine prolapse is fairly common in sheep and cattle and occasionally occurs spectacularly in sows. It is rarely seen in wild animals. This was the first time Matt or I had come across it in the zoo, but unlike him I knew what it was and had wrestled with many similar cases in farm animals. I decided to keep that to myself for the moment. "Get some warm water and plenty of towels," I instructed. Matt went out sighing.

As I went towards the oryx's head to examine her, she threatened me with her wicked straight horns which I had seen driven with accuracy through two-inch wood planking.

256

I would have to dope her before tackling her hind end, although I could not be sure what the effect of phencyclidine would be on her four-stomach digestion. Matt watched while I also injected 10 cc of local anaesthetic to paralyse her spinal cord and stop her straining by reflex action when I began to work. Next I thoroughly washed the exposed lining of the womb and its "cherries", which were the attachment points of the calf's placenta, and picked off bits of straw and grime. "Now then, Matt," I said when it was clean, "I want you to put a towelling sling under the womb and hold it clear of the ground to stop it getting dirty again."

He took a towel, looped it under the flabby mess of raw flesh and lifted it off the straw. I coated the womb liberally with a sulphonamide antiseptic cream. Now for the tough bit. As the womb had fallen inside out, I had to replace it gently but firmly by rolling it inwards from the centre as if it were a plastic bag or woollen sock that was inside out. Womb walls are thick and spongy but easily punctured by too rough fingers, so I had to be extremely careful to use only the balls of my fingertips. Bit by bit the womb began to fold inwards. I kept lubricating it with obstetric cream. The size of the exposed womb began to decrease as I worked away with both arms groping in the oryx's pelvic canal.

Matt said nothing as he strained to hold the towelling up, and I knelt below him, concentrating, with my tongue stuck between my lips. At last, with a satisfying sucking noise, the last bit of the womb disappeared inside the vulva. I pushed it well forward inside the animal. Luckily I have a long arm with a smallish hand, ideal for this sort of obstetrical problem.

"Get me a milk bottle, Matt," I said finally.

The head keeper broke his silence. "A milk bottle? What for?"

"Get it please, and quick!" I replied sternly.

Matt dropped the towel and disappeared again. He came back with a milk bottle which, while he watched curiously, I disinfected with iodine soap. Then to his amazement I plunged my arm back inside the oryx's womb with the bottle held firmly by the neck. Using its blunt bottom as an extension to my arm, I made sure that the part of the womb beyond the reach of my fingers was folded back into its proper position. If I did not do that, the thing would be out again in no time. Withdrawing the milk bottle and still not explaining its function, or what indeed the whole business had been about, I finished off by putting a few clips into the vulva as a precaution. I would remove them after thirty-six hours. Done. The animal's colour, pulse and respiration were good.

I scrubbed my hands and arms and then turned to Matt. "She'll be right as a clock by tonight," I said. "It was just a prolapsed uterus."

Matt stared at the clean and tidy hind end of the oryx and cleared his throat. "Incredible," he said at last. "Incredible. The foinest bit of work oi've ever seen in all me years. Oi take me hat off, Dr. Taylor."

That was some reward, coming from Matt. Better still, just as I had predicted, by evening the oryx was indeed as good as new, and I tried hard not to gloat as Matt and I stood watching her suckle her lusty calf.

The disease problems of primates, apes and monkeys, had always fascinated me, so I was stung by a remark by Ray Legge that medical doctors were by tradition more equipped to deal with such animals than veterinarians. I decided to embark on a study course in an attempt to prove him wrong and in the process to gain a Fellowship of the Royal College of Veterinary Surgeons. After a year and a half's hard work, sandwiching the studies in where I could between my day-to-day clinical work and attending postgraduate courses at the medical school in Manchester, I got my Fellowship, the first ever given where zoo animals were named as the speciality. Not only did my practice with great apes in particular now have a firm base, but through the study I had

had to do at home for the Fellowship Shelagh was becoming increasingly involved with some of my simian patients.

Soon after I gained my Fellowship, Jane, a charming female orang-utan at Belle Vue, was pregnant for the first time. Then, with about two months still to go before her time was due, she suddenly had a miscarriage. A premature scrap of an orang infant was born dead one night.

The effect on Jane was remarkable and profound. All the other female orangs had live, healthy babies. She sat alone in a corner hugging the shrivelled corpse of her baby, trying in vain to make it suckle and whimpering in distress. I am not a sentimentalist prone to seeing the whole range of human emotions in animals, but when I first saw Jane after the miscarriage, I felt tears in my eyes. She was heartbroken. Try as we might we could not get her to give up the baby's body. I began to consider darting her with a sedative in order to remove it before it putrefied further. The distraught female would not touch food and she began to lose weight alarmingly.

I took Shelagh with me to the zoo when I finally decided to knock Jane out and take the infant cadaver. We went into the isolation room where Jane sat pitifully in a large cage. Shelagh looked at the orang and the orang looked at her. I saw her eyes fill. Matt and I stood silently.

"Before you try darting," said Shelagh suddenly, "I want to go in with her."

My wife was asking to go in with a full-grown orang that was undoubtedly in a disturbed and unpredictable mood.

"I mean it," she said. "Open the door please, Mr. Kelly."

Matt started to speak but I interrupted him. "OK," I said. "Open it, Matt."

Matt undid the lock and cautiously swung open the barred door. Shelagh climbed into the cage and on hands and knees crawled straight over to Jane. When she reached the orang, she at once began talking to the animal in soothing low tones. "What's the matter, love?" she murmured. "I know all about it. Come on, put an arm round me." On and on she talked, with the orang looking straight into her face. Shelagh sat down beside Jane and gave her a cuddle that was full of love and understanding. To our delight and astonishment, Jane snuggled into her and put her broad lips to Shelagh's mouth. Shelagh stroked Jane's hair and kept up the flow of sympathetic talk. Then, just like that, Jane gave Shelagh the dead orang. Shelagh took it, cradled it, talked admiringly about it, then slowly slipped it into one of her pockets. Jane did not make one gesture of protest.

"Pass me some food," Shelagh said to us. We handed in some bananas and grapes. Shelagh took them, broke them into portions and presented them to the orang's mouth. Jane took them one by one.

"I'd like to give her a stimulant, Shelagh," I said quietly. "I'll come in too."

"No, you won't," she replied. "Fill your syringe, tell me where to put it and I'll do it—won't I, Jane dear?"

"But Mrs. Taylor," Matt remonstrated, "she'll boite. Oi think we'd . . ."

Shelagh was having none of it. Reluctantly I made up a syringe and passed it in to my wife. "In the thigh muscle," I instructed. Cooing to her friend, with one arm still hugging her, Shelagh slipped the needle into Jane's leg. She did not budge a millimetre.

After a while, Shelagh left the cage and gave us the little corpse. Jane was no longer whimpering. She looked more tranquil as she watched my wife close the door. "I'll be in again tomorrow," said Shelagh briskly to Matt and me. She had taken over.

And that is how it was. Every day Shelagh went in with Jane, feeding her by hand, talking to her just like women do to their girl friends, particularly when they have suffered some misfortune, and giving her lots of loving cuddles. Jane responded. She began to cuddle Shelagh in return and stopped losing weight. Gradually she started to feed herself again. In three weeks she appeared completely normal.

I am certain that the injections that Shelagh gave sitting cheek by jowl with a great ape that could have broken every bone in her body did not play much part in Jane's recovery. As Shelagh said, "There are some things in zoo work that just can't be left to men."

Seven

I had landed the practice with a thumping big bad debt, and Norman Whittle was not amused. After chasing about for several weeks treating a touring circus's arthritic elephant with injections of gold salts, I found the circus had done the dirty on me. Its owner claimed that the animal rightfully belonged to such and such a clown, who in turn maintained that I had originally been called in by one of a family of acrobats while the circus was in Rochdale. The company was a small one, everyone seemed to be interrelated and the clowns doubled or even trebled as ice-cream sellers, bareback riders or jugglers. Trying to get my fee out of anyone was futile and embarrassing. If I called during a performance everyone was dashing round concealed under greasepaint and tomato-sized rubber noses, and at other times the trailers were silent as the grave when I knocked miserably on the doors for my cash. Strange, when the elephant had been creaking painfully about on puffy, tense joints, I had been able to find the staff in a trice in order to make my examinations. But gradually the circus moved farther and farther away from Rochdale and debt-collecting forays became impossible.

The bad debt led to a bitter exchange with Norman of the sort that made me long to make the great leap and to throw in my lot with wild-animal medicine lock, stock and barrel.

"Apart from the time you've spent gallivanting all over England away from the practice," Norman said in his undemonstrative, clipped manner as we stood over the unconscious body of a tortoiseshell cat on which we were doing a hysterectomy, "we're over a hundred quid out of pocket. This circus farce can't go on. Anyway you can't trust travelling folk, fly-by-nights, gipsies. I warned you time and again. And even if they had paid, look at all the time and effort and driving. Compare that to work like this." He waved a needle holder at the supine she-cat. "Thirty shillings, nearly all profit and done in five minutes!"

Looked at from a purely financial point of view, it was true; one vet we both knew frequently said that his ideal practice would consist of doing nothing but sterilizing she-cats, six in the morning and six in the afternoon. But that was not my view of veterinary work. Could they not see that taking the pulse of an elephant, feeling the thick artery deep under the dry, crinkly skin, was a reward in itself? Cash cannot be equated with seeing a cub in its foetal membranes emerge like a vacuum-packed pigeon, especially if you have helped it out. Even more especially if, as you peel the membranes from it, it writhes and natters the first feeble protest of its independent life. No, I felt as strongly then as I do now that it was a rare privilege to be allowed to try to heal wild living organisms. Can a stockbroker or banker know anything of the happiness which I have had when seeing a leg walk that I, somehow, have helped tack together?

I had talked before in this vein to Norman, but decided it would be pointless to start again this time. I think he thought I would grow out of it, so he was exasperated by my enthusiastic acceptance of our next circus call. It was from an outfit completely unknown to us at Great Yarmouth, two hundred miles or more away across country on the coast of the wind-washed fens of Norfolk. Again the problem was an elephant, an elephant suspected of foot-and-mouth disease.

"You can't go off down there," said my partner angrily. "This zoo and circus work is getting too much. No, we just can't have it."

An elephant with suspected foot-and-mouth? Nothing could stop me. "I'm off," I said, and slipped out of the door before he could say another word.

It was a long drive that took nearly six hours. By now I was receiving calls to exotic animals from all over Britain as the knowledge that I had a special interest in such creatures spread by word of mouth from one owner to another. My mileage was increasing rapidly, and on long journeys I was troubled by being out of contact with my surgery and the rest of the world for most of the day. Anything could be happening while I was doing nothing but acting as taxi driver to myself. To remedy this I had recently done something which was to prove the key to roving zoo practice: I had installed in the car a radio telephone operating on a private network that extended virtually all over the country. My call sign was the zippy "Jet eight-seven" and I got a great kick from receiving messages on the road like the first one that came over the air from Belle Vue: "Calling Jet eight-seven, Jet eight-seven. Mr. Kelly reports pigmy hippo born. All well. Repeat, all well. Over."

I had plenty to ponder as I crossed the flat marshes of East Anglia. There were the problems with Norman and my role in the practice: I owed Norman a lot for introducing me to zoo work, and I could understand his frustration at being left to cope on his own so much, but I knew that my first duty was to the animals I was trying to help. Then foot-and-mouth disease. I had never seen a real live case. As for such a thing in elephants, I had heard of a few suspect cases where large ulcers had formed at the back of the mouth, but that was all I knew apart from the fact that no foot-and-mouth disease was being reported in Britain at that time. There must be some likelier explanation.

At last I rolled into Great Yarmouth, a place exactly like dozens of other holiday towns dotted round the English coast, redolent with the faded fashion of Victorian and Regency days when Majorca and the Costa Brava were as far away

264

as the moon. The circus was inside the Hippodrome Theatre, and I soon found the elephant lines. Near three adult female Indian elephants an old lugubrious-faced German, who turned out to be the elephant trainer, a midget in a Charlie Chaplin outfit, a policeman and another man in a black rubber coat and gumboots were arguing. The midget seemed particularly agitated.

I went over. "I'm Dr. Taylor to see the elephant."

The man in the rubber coat put out a hand. "Tompkins," he said, "Ministry of Agriculture vet. Came out to see what this report of F-and-M was all about."

"And they won't pay me my half-crown," squeaked the midget, tapping me on the knee. "I want my half-crown."

"I am Herr Hopfer," said the German. "Please, Doktor, come zis way. Gerda iss very ill." He looked as if he was about to burst into tears.

"My half-crown! It's the rule! My half-crown!" The midget was fairly hopping about by this time and was waving his miniature bent walking-stick at the policeman.

The latter cleared his throat and sighed. He had obviously been saying something similar for the past half-hour. "I 'ave told you once, Mr. Lemon, and I 'ave told you twice. I know nothin' about no 'alf-crown. You'll 'ave to go down to the station and see my sergeant about that."

"What's this all about?" I asked Tompkins.

"Oh, it's all because he, Mr. Lemon, reported the suspect case of F-and-M. Apparently there's something in the law that says if any private citizen suspects a notifiable disease in anybody's animal, whether he knows what he's looking at or not, he can claim two-and-sixpence from the police."

"Is that right?" I queried.

"Can't say I know anything about it, but the little fellow's mad as hell on getting his cash. Claims to know all about it."

"Done my duty, done my duty! Where's my half-crown?" The midget started buzzing again.

"Now look 'ere, Mr. Lemon," said the policeman.

"Just give me the money," yelled Mr. Lemon.

Tompkins and I looked silently at one another and simultaneously put our hands in our pockets. We produced one-and-threepence each and pushed the coins at the midget. "Now can we please have some hush while we look at the bloody elephant!" I said tetchily.

Mr. Lemon waddled off, and later I learned that he was quite right; he was indeed entitled to the reward whatever the diagnosis turned out to be.

Gerda the elephant was standing miserably in a pool of water which streamed slowly from her lower lip to the cobbled floor. The water was her own saliva. I must look inside her mouth at once, but Matt Kelly had warned me of the danger of sticking one's hand blindly into an elephant's mouth: "If the craytchure moves her lower jaw, ye've a pulverized hand."

"Get her to open up, Herr Hopfer," I said. It is one thing all elephant trainers can do with their animals.

"Gerda, auf, auf!" he shouted.

Gerda slowly raised her trunk and opened her soft pink mouth. Tompkins shone his torch in and we both peered into the narrow space between the teeth. Not a blister or an ulcer in sight.

"I don't think elephants can get F-and-M," said Tompkins. "Better check her feet, though, just in case."

He walked cautiously round the elephant, looking at her neatly filed and oiled toenails. Nothing that looked like ulcers there. Tompkins was shining his light on the left rear foot when Gerda felt the urge to pass water. Unwisely, the ministry vet was not wearing the Government-issue black sou'wester that is supposed to be part of the uniform for investigations into notifiable disease. He took the cataract square on top of his head. It went down the inside of his coat and ran out below.

"I 'ave 'eard that yoorine is very good for the complexion," observed the policeman, as deadpan as if he were making an arrest.

"I'm off," spluttered Tompkins. "Negative F-and-M here. End of the affair as far as the Ministry's concerned. Get on with it, Taylor." Spitting, he squelched away.

"Now, Herr Hopfer," I said, "tell me the full story."

"Zis morning I find her streaming from ze mouss like zis. She vill not eat, not even drink. Maybe she hass a bad tooss."

Toothache was indeed a possibility. One of the commonest ailments in elephants is an infected or badly positioned molar. I got Hopfer to make Gerda open her mouth again and shone my torch carefully on each tooth with one hand while pressing down the slippery ball of her tongue with the other. One slip and I could lose a finger or three. All the teeth seemed normal. I felt Gerda's glands, ran my hands down over the outside of her throat, took her temperature and drew a blood sample. Everything was OK. But Gerda was miserable and would not eat or drink, and her saliva ran and ran. There was no evidence that her throat was inflamed, her swallowing muscles were not paralysed, there was no logical reason why she should be producing excessive quantities of saliva. I was left with one ominous probability.

"Bring me some bananas and a bucket of water," I said to Hopfer. I wanted to watch her reaction to food very carefully for myself. Treating elephants was not much different from treating cattle, I was finding, as long as you knew how to handle them and how to love them.

When the elephant trainer returned, I presented Gerda with a peeled banana. She took it with her trunk tip, popped it in her mouth and swallowed readily. Then slowly, slowly, the pulped banana came back and dripped in sticky blobs from the corners of her lips. I put the bucket of water in front of her. Immediately she sucked up a trunkful and squirted it into her mouth. She swallowed. For a moment nothing happened and then the water gushed back out onto the floor.

"What did you feed the elephants last thing yesterday, Herr Hopfer?"

"Chopped carrots and apples."

"Chopped?"

"Ja, chopped."

I was certain now that one of the apples had evaded the chopper's cleaver and was jammed somewhere in the gullet. And I could predict that it would be in one of three places: where the gullet enters the chest, where it passes over the heart or where it pierces the diaphragm. Wherever it was, Gerda was in big trouble.

In cattle, similar jammed objects often pass naturally if the animal is left alone for twenty-four hours. That was my first feeble line of attack. I booked in at a nearby hotel and made sure that the hungry and thirsty elephant at least had plenty of water to suck up. Maybe a trickle would get past the apple, I thought optimistically as I added nourishing glucose to the water. The next day, Gerda was much worse. She was sunken-eyed, weak and obviously dehydrated. How to move the apple? If I pushed it somehow, I could rupture the oesophagus. Operating was out of the question; no machine could keep the six-ton monster's lungs inflated with oxygen when the chest cavity was opened. Drugs designed to relax the muscles of the gullet had no effect.

By the third day the poor elephant was so weak that she could almost be pushed off balance by one man. Her eyes were red and her breath was foul. The apple was still firmly lodged and the river of saliva flowed on. Gerda was now desperately thirsty. Stripped down to my underpants, I started a series of hourly enemas, trying to pump water and glucose as far as possible into her lower bowel with a plastic tube and an old stirrup pump borrowed from the Hippodrome's fire-fighting equipment. It was slow, dirty work.

"Ooh!" said the waitress in my hotel when she learnt that I was working at the circus. "What a super job. Lovely animals and able to have a holiday by the seaside at the same time!"

She should have been there all night, pumping ten gallons of sugary water up an elephant's backside and getting nine gallons sprayed back over her, I thought, as the waitress flounced off for my pot of tea and kippered herrings. Still, it had been worth it. A gallon had stayed up, a gallon that might just keep Gerda going till something turned up.

On the fifth day I had to make a crucial decision. The elephant was deteriorating rapidly. The only thing left was to push a probe down her throat. This meant anaesthesia. By now Gerda was unwilling to lie down for fear of being unable to rise. Left much longer, she would not tolerate doping, for lack of sleep had now been added to starvation and thirst and debility.

I walked along the shingly beach and thought long and hard. I considered phoning Norman but, remembering the coolness between us, decided against it. The seagulls chivvied me in the cold, grey sky with incomprehensible advice. For a moment I envied the fishermen sitting muffled on the end of the pier, sucking contented pipes and off home soon to baked beans and TV. Then I decided. I would dope Gerda lightly, pass a probang, a long leather tube with a bulbous brass end, down her gullet and take her life in my inexperienced hands.

Later that day I gave the elephant a massive dose of acetylpromazine, a strong sedative rather than a true anaesthetic. After half an hour she slowly sank to the ground and lay, still drooling, on her side. Herr Hopfer pulled the upper jaw and the diminutive Mr. Lemon, who like most midgets was immensely strong for his size, tugged on the lower. Greasing the probang with cod-liver oil, I pushed it carefully to the back of Gerda's throat. When a couple of feet of tube had disappeared, I stopped and went to the end of the probang outside the elephant and put it to my ear. I could feel no puff of air as Gerda breathed, so at least I was not going the wrong way, down the windpipe. I pushed the probang on slowly. Suddenly it stopped; it would go no farther. I marked the tube and withdrew it so that by measuring it over the outside of the elephant's body I could tell exactly how far down the obstruction lay. The mark on the tube told me that the apple was jammed at the point where the oesophagus passes the great heart. I must push it on. I re-introduced the probang and arrived once more at the obstruction. The moment had arrived. The next strong shove could stop the heart. It could burst the gullet and send the apple into the chest cavity. Or it could succeed. I gritted my teeth and steadily increased pressure on the probang. All at once it began to move freely once more. Something had given. I was sweating and my lip was bleeding where I had bitten it. Had the apple moved on or was it now bobbing around on the lungs with a ragged, gaping hole in the gullet beside it? Through my stethoscope I could hear no ugly noises from the lungs. Hardly daring to breathe, I slowly withdrew the probang. After what seemed an hour, its gleaming brass end flopped out of Gerda's mouth. It was coated in clear slime and shreds of banana pulp but not one drop of blood. I had done it!

Gerda was drowsy for many hours as the sedative wore off. The waiting was intolerable. I went to the cinema but came out after five minutes. I did not feel like eating or drinking. I ran along the beach. I played the one-armed bandits on the pier. Every half-hour I was back at the Hippodrome. At last, at nine o'clock that night, Gerda regained enough energy to rise groggily to her feet.

"Don't do a thing, Herr Hopfer!" I shouted. "I'll do this."

I took a bucket of hay tea, an infusion of hot water and new meadow hay, and placed it in front of Gerda. Her trunk flapped weakly. I grabbed it and stuck it into the golden liquid. The bucket half emptied. Gerda's slow and unsteady trunk curled towards her mouth and injected its contents. I saw the gullet muscles contract. A wave passed down her throat. She had swallowed. We waited, frozen like statues. The hay tea did not come back. Gerda's trunk was already back in the bucket, draining it dry.

"A banana, a banana!" I shouted excitedly.

The German ran for a bunch of fruit and handed it to me. I stuffed one straight into the elephant's jaws without peeling it. Squelch! It was gone. Nothing drooled back. The ropes of saliva no longer hung from Gerda's bottom lip. Her sunken red eye was on the remainder of the bunch of bananas. A perfect lady, and anyway still appallingly weak, she reached delicately for them. We were on our way.

That night I stayed up with Gerda again, making sure that she was not overloaded too suddenly with food or water, but gradually building up her much-needed intake. By daybreak she was visibly much stronger and the signs of dehydration were disappearing fast. I went back to my hotel when Herr Hopfer woke and relieved me.

"Ooh!" said the waitress as I slumped into my chair at the breakfast table. "Been out on the town, eh? Naughty boy! Told you you'd have a smashin' time at Great Yarmouth. Must be all play, your job."

"Yes," I said wearily. "Bring me an extra pair of kippers, will you? I'm celebrating."

On my return from Great Yarmouth Norman tackled me again about my travels round the country in pursuit of exotic patients. "Anyway," he said, "can you really square your conscience with being involved in zoo and circus animal work? Aren't you just part of the shady business of exploiting wild creatures?"

It is a question people often ask me and from time to time, as I lie in bed, I ask it myself, just to make sure that the answer I give is still the same one, the one I believe in.

I believe in zoos, marinelands, safari parks. To come into close contact with the creatures of the earth—to see, to smell and, if you are lucky enough, to touch the beasts—is a

271

vital part of human experience. Just as cinema cannot catch the atmosphere of the live stage, films of elephants or lions or buffaloes cannot give that spark of magic which flesh-and-blood presence provides. To be snuffled over by the damp tip of an elephant's trunk, to have one's hair lifted by the curling rasp of a giraffe's tongue—out of such experiences spring real feeling and love for fellow animals. There is nothing more rewarding than escorting a group of blind people round a zoo. They truly appreciate, in every sense of the word, camels, puma cubs, snakes, ostriches and the rest of the species to which I feel it is safe to introduce them.

It is pie in the sky to talk of us all going to see the wild animals in their natural habitats. The habitats are shrinking fast, not least because of tourism. The cruel impact of man on animals' natural homes will inevitably lead to more and more birds, mammals, fish and insects becoming extinct in the wild. Wilful greed and careless pollution are taking a terrible toll, and zoos and marinelands have a real part to play in helping at least some creatures to avoid the fate of the dodo, the Steller's sea cow and the quagga. No, zoos are essential for all the kids in New York, London, Rome and a thousand other cities who will never in a million years get the chance to go on a jet-set safari to the Serengeti.

As for me, my job is to represent the animals' interests, to see their point of view. There are disgraceful black spots, disgusting examples of cruelty, neglect and naked exploitation, in animal trapping, zoos, circuses and laboratories in all parts of the world. But by working from the inside, by encouraging breeding here and improving diets there, by trying to heal the sick animals, educating their ignorant owners and proving to them that cruelty and neglect are counter-productive purely in terms of cash, I know things are slowly but steadily getting better. I am proud to be part of it.

When I explained how I felt to Norman, he grunted and said that was all very well, but how was he expected to run a two-man practice when one of the partners was never there? I wondered what he would say if he knew that I had just received my first call abroad, to go over to Holland the following weekend to inspect and then accompany six young African elephants to England. Since it was Norman's duty weekend anyway, I thought it would be more prudent just to go, and to tell him about it when I got back.

I made the tedious journey by truck and ferry. After the truck had burnt its brakes out and hours had been wasted finding a replacement, I eventually got my charges onto the Rotterdam–Hull overnight boat. I sat alone during the crossing, guarding the elephants and feeding them from time to time with hay, bananas and apples. It was further invaluable experience in animal handling and transportation.

One of my jobs was to keep curious passengers and crew from interfering with the elephants. All went well until the middle of the night when, tired out by the day's exertions, I was unable to keep my eyelids open any longer. Fighting against it, I finally fell asleep propped up in a sitting position against one of the elephant crates.

Three hours later I woke to find that some misguided animal lover had fed my entire stock of apples and bananas to the ever-willing beasts. So much fruit in so short a time could cause six elephantine cases of colic before we docked, and I prepared for the worst. Luckily colic did not develop, but the surfeit of fruit certainly made its presence felt. After half a day spent ministering to a handful of elephants with acute diarrhoea, I knew a little of what it must have been like to be a bell-carrying leper in the Middle Ages, and when I got home Shelagh made me strip down to my underclothes outside the back door.

A few weeks later I was back in Holland, to capture Mr. van den Baars's onagers, and soon after that I took a much longer trip. Its purpose was not to treat any one case but to learn more about one great group of wild mammals of which

I still had no experience. These creatures, taking their name from the Greek word for sea monster, second in intelligence only to man himself and descended from insignificant pig-like foragers that rooted around marshy land millions of years ago, were the cetaceans: whales, dolphins and porpoises. In the mid-sixties dolphins became the most fashionable and popular of zoo animals in America. Then Flipper and his relatives came to Europe, and I decided that it was time for me to start learning something about the care and medicine of these beautiful but mysterious beasts. I suspected that marinelands and dolphinaria were going to mushroom in Britain and on the Continent, and that dolphin doctoring was going to become an established branch of the veterinary art.

Today we know more about the dolphin than about any other animal except man and the dog, yet little more than a dozen years ago virtually nothing was known and still less published about cetacean disease. It was uniquely challenging, for this was not a case of trying out horse techniques in zebras or cattle medicine in buffaloes. Cetaceans do not abide by the rules. They have reconquered the watery places of the earth by adapting to a marine existence all the benefits of being a mammal, and combining that with ingenuity in doing things that mammals out at sea would not be expected to do. For that they have to be different: different in body structure, function and behaviour. The Atlantic bottle-nosed dolphin is an air-breathing, warm-blooded animal with three stomachs like a cow's, kidneys like a camel's, a brain as big as a man's, the swimming skills of a shark and the sonar equipment of a bat. It can dive deep and ascend fast without fear of decompression illnesses, endure long periods without oxygen but ignore levels of carbon dioxide that would black out other beasts, and drink nothing but sea water, the brine which drives thirsty casta-ways mad, and it has a bundle of other feats of mystery and imagination at its command.

Only the handful of veterinarians working full time with

marine mammals in the United States had the knowledge I would need if I was to treat cetaceans effectively. Leaving the long-suffering Norman in sole charge of the practice once again, and digging deep into my personal savings, I went first to Point Mugu in California, where the U.S. Navy Undersea Warfare Division had a small but high-powered veterinary team led by Dr. Sam Ridgway. Among their research pools and complex of laboratories set on the shore of the Pacific, I embarked on a crash course of sea-going veterinary medicine. Apart from the very different surroundings, it was rather like my first months at Belle Vue under the thumb of Matt Kelly. I learned that dolphins can contract influenza, mumps, polio and gastric ulcers, that their anatomical and physiological adaptations make them the safest creatures in the world to pass a stomach tube on but the most tricky to anaesthetize, and that they require each day three hundred times more Vitamin B_1 than a human of the same weight. An apparently simple thing but most vital of all, I was given my first opportunity to take blood samples from the animals. The smooth, shining skin of a dolphin betrays almost no evidence of where blood vessels might run. You can fish the beast out of the water and apply tourniquets to the flippers or the tail, but still the unco-operative veins and arteries refuse to reveal themselves. They lie beneath a tight, inflexible layer of blubber, each artery completely surrounded by a cluster of veins. Find the areas where the blubber is thinned and you find a cluster of blood vessels, the vets at Point Mugu told me. Easier said than done. Slight skin discoloration, a depression here and there, the glint of a shallow groove if the moistened tail is held to reflect the light; by such things I would be guided. Then a short needle could be placed in a vessel and a sample of venous, arterial or frequently a mixture of the two bloods taken.

My first essay in blood sampling was right on target. I struck oil. "It doesn't matter much," said Dr. Sam in his relaxed Texan drawl, "if your needle takes blood from vein or artery or a bit of both if you're doing routine analysis and such, except of course oxygen levels, but don't forget the layout in these critters if you ever want to do an intravenous injection. It's easy as hell to get some of the drug into an artery, with it lying so close to the veins. So watch out, David."

I saw the point. A drug inadvertently injected into an artery instead of a vein will damage the delicate arterial lining, stopping the circulation to tissues supplied by the artery beyond the injection site and causing them to die. At least in land mammals the tough-walled, pulsating arteries are usually easily located and are rarely close to the veins in places where the veterinarian roams in search of injection sites. Already these mermen were leading me, as they were said to lead ancient Greek seafarers, into a new life.

Eight

From Point Mugu I visited other marine-mammal vets and all the major marinelands in the United States before turning my attention to the dolphin-catching side of the business. Just as a zoo vet must understand the housing, handling and transport of his charges if he is to deal competently with their health problems, so it seemed to me best in this aquatic arena to try to find a water-borne equivalent to head keeper Matt Kelly from whom I could learn the nitty-gritty of the non-veterinary side of dolphins. I found him one March day in Fort Myers, Florida. He made his living catching dolphins in the Gulf of Mexico, his name was Gene Hamilton and with him I had some of the most exciting days of my life.

Like Alice I decided to begin at the beginning and asked Gene if he would take me out with him. A tall, lantern-jawed individual with a taciturn but kindly nature, he agreed, provided that I did exactly what I was told. His catching boat, with low sides and a cutaway stern for pulling animals on deck, could touch sixty miles an hour skimming over the shallow Florida waters, and it could turn on a sixpence at almost full speed. It was no place for novices who got in the way when the hunt was on.

The first thing I learned about catching is that wind is one's prime enemy and patience the greatest virtue. Even a slight breeze, which was welcomed by the yachtsmen and sweating sunbathers of Fort Myers, was enough to put a chop on the water that extended to the horizon. Under such conditions every triangular wavelet could be a dolphin's dorsal fin. The ocean seemed filled with dolphins or, looking

277

at it another way, totally devoid of them. After an overnight storm, the water would be opaque, full of stirred-up sand, and the spotter plane which worked with us as our airborne pointer could not see the groups of dolphins hunting fish shoals under water. So if there was wind or had been wind, and that was most of the time, we sat cutting fish on the rickety old jetty where Gene moored up and put a fortune into the pockets of Mr. Schlitz, brewing beer far away in Milwaukee.

When we did have a calm and glassy sea we would be off early, sometimes before sun-up, to the shallows where the waking dolphins might be collecting a breakfast of mullet, blue runner or butterfish. As the sun climbs out of the grey water we hear the crackle of our spotter plane's radio. In the first good light of the day he has located a group of twelve dolphins feeding quietly ten miles to our north. The pilot, experienced at estimating size and age from a height of several hundred feet, tells us how many animals of the right length, not too young and not too old, not pregnant and not suckling babies, are there for the taking—if we have luck.

We make for the area while Gene's two assistants, bronzed teenagers in frayed jeans shorts, check the catching gear. This is a mile of lightweight, fourteen-foot-deep net which has been carefully folded into zigzag layers and sleeved onto a long bamboo pole which projects over the stern. The top edge of the net is attached to a series of floats and the end nearest the water carries a small sea anchor. The sea anchor is watched carefully. If it were to fall into the ocean before the appointed moment, one mile of net would be unfolded in seconds and it would take an hour or more to retrieve it, sort it out and reposition it along the bamboo pole. While we sail for the catching zone I stand at the wheel talking to Gene, taking lungfuls of cold, morning sea air and munching my share of a bizarre but delicious breakfast of fresh clams, fried frogs' legs and doughnuts,

278

washed down even at that hour with cans of foaming Schlitz.

Before long we hear the buzz of the spotter aircraft some-where overhead, and the pilot tells us the latest position of our quarry. Cutting the engine speed down to avoid alarm-ing the feeding dolphins, Gene takes the boat towards the school of animals while the spotter keeps up a continual commentary. Suddenly I catch the first thrilling glimpse of a low, dark-grey dorsal fin breaking the water surface for a second as its owner takes in a gulp of air. Then we see another and another. Gene at this point relies almost completely on the aircraft. The pilot, seeing the dolphins' reaction to our approach, for their sensitive ears would have picked up our engine noise miles away, gives instructions that put us in a favourable position for our sweep. To us at almost water level the directions do not seem to make sense, but the pilot is looking down on the chessboard from on high and has a perfect view of all the players in the game. With luck, the dolphins will assume we are just another of the many pleasure boats in Florida's teeming waters. Nevertheless, some of the cowboys who sail such craft are known to in-dulge in the "sport" of using dolphins for rifle practice. It has made many old bulls wary of any sort of vessel, and the bullet scars that some of them bear are the reason why.

Today all goes according to plan for once, and the spotter plane tells us we are in an ideal position, with the dolphins quietly browsing a hundred yards to our right at two o'clock. He then leaves the scene, and the hunt from now on is con-ducted solely by Gene. His first action is to tell me, "Sit squarely down on the deck, grab hold of something firm and hold on!" Then he opens the throttle to the full, and the boat leaps forward with a deafening roar and with a punch that leaves the thrill of a ride on Belle Vue's roller coaster in the novice class.

Over the sparkling skin of the water we charge, the boat heeling over as Gene cuts a trench of frenzied foam that arcs across the path of the leading dolphin. The g-forces play musical chairs with my innards and I cling on for dear life, certain that at any moment I will be catapulted through the air like a human cannonball to join the dolphins. The boat stays flat out and the arc continues into a full circle. Gene takes us completely round the school of dolphins and keeps the wheel locked over for a second circuit. Peeping tensely over the gunwales, I can see the animals bobbing and blowing puffs of rainbow-shot vapour in the centre of a broad ring of white water. Gene's aim is to confuse the dolphins by encircling them with a continuous wall of sound from the powerful engines. We have encountered one or two wiser, pluckier leaders of schools (not always bulls, sometimes redoubtable matriarchs) who have made a high-speed beeline run for it, leading their weaker brethren straight through the noise wall and away safely into quiet water, but today the animals are hesitating and milling in the water, uncertain of the best plan of action. Gene observes their indecisive movements, tightens his circular run still further and then roars to his boys, "Shoot!"

At his command one of the boys throws the sea anchor overboard. Gene continues to carve out yet another circle, and all the while the mile of net is being dragged off the bamboo pole like an express train. Round we go, leaving the net floats bobbing in a great curve in our wake until, having completed the full 360 degrees, we come back again to the sea anchor and first float. Gene kills the engines and peers anxiously towards the now fully cast ring of netting, one mile in circumference. There has been no last-minute dash by his quarry, he has not misjudged the water depth, and the nets are deep enough to stop escapers diving underneath; in the centre of the circle a cluster of dark-grey dorsal fins swirl about.

At this stage in the proceedings I was able to stand up again and start to be useful. The first thing was to scan the line of net floats. Evenly spaced, they should all be visible on the water surface. If one or two were submerged it might well mean that the net at that point was being dragged down by some heavy object—like a dolphin enmeshed several feet below and in imminent danger of drowning. "In y'go, Dr. Taylor," Gene would say if we saw such warning signs, and with goggles and a short snorkel tube I would drop over the side into the cool, dark water and make for the spot where the floats had disappeared. Once there I would make an awkward duck dive and pull myself down to where a grey shape might be struggling to free itself from the net. As I glided down I would sometimes hear through the water the alarmed, high-pitched communication squeak of the trapped dolphin. If the animal was not too severely entangled I might free it by hand; otherwise Gene's treasured net had to be cut with a diver's knife.

Trapped dolphins were not the only cause of the net floats sinking. My first experience of other accidental catches came one sunny afternoon off Key Largo when Gene dropped his nets in a perfect "set" round six or seven immature adult dolphins. The line of floats dipped at two points and, while one of Gene's boys dived to investigate one, I went down to look at the other. Kicking myself under, I followed the net down to where the expected grey form thrashed furiously twelve feet under the surface. Through the fuzzy shadows I could tell that the beast was caught by its head in a hole in the net. It should not be too difficult to pull it back by hand and release it so that it could surface for a welcome gulp of air. Coming closer, I saw to my horror that I was within inches of a seven-foot shark that was lashing its tail to and fro and gnashing its rows of razor-like teeth. I identified it as a black-tipped shark, a species strongly suspected of attacking humans. Should I release it? What would Gene do? Would it attack me if I freed it? Looking at it held in the net by its pectoral fins, I decided to risk a few cuts with my knife before going up again for air. Surely it would be too relieved at its near squeak to try tangling with me. I reached for the knife in my belt and then I saw the second black-tipped shark. Bigger than its companion, it was weaving figures of eight two yards to my left and below me. That made my mind up. In a flurry of bubbles I kicked for the surface and pulled myself thankfully up onto the boat.

"Don't ever fool around with those guys," Gene said when I had told him my story. "If he ain't dead when we pull the nets in, I'll kill him. Hate those guys. Sometimes get a hammerhead or two in with the dolphins messin' up the nets. Ain't no good for anythin' 'cept bait."

"What are blacktips like around here?" I asked.

"Cain't trust 'em," he replied. "Know a dolphin catcher up near Steinhatchee lost a couple o' pounds o' thigh muscle from a blacktip. The doctors who stitched him up knew it was a blacktip by the pattern o' the tooth marks."

That was not the last time I went down to entangled sharks, but whenever I found one I came up fast and left it for Gene to deal with later. I often watched one or another of Gene's boys make similar hurried exits from the water while he laughed and shouted, "Sharks down there? Well, get on your Jesus shoes and walk on the water, fella!"

After clearing the nets of trapped animals, Gene would supervise the slow and meticulous pulling in. The area of the circle was decreased gradually to stop the dolphins panicking and entangling themselves en masse. Little by little the group of captured animals was brought closer to the boat until finally, with one or two men in the water to help, they could be hauled up onto the stern decking. Unsuitable animals were released while those that were to be kept were placed on foam mattresses amidships. There, while the other men pulled in all the net, I had my first experience in handling one hundred per cent wild, dripping wet, fresh dolphins. The older animals usually lay resignedly, chirping plaintively to one another but not objecting to my touching their bodies. I got, and still get, a sheer physical

282

thrill from contact with the flesh of animals that a few minutes before had been masters of a virtually limitless three-dimensional world where man is a feeble, groping amateur.

When the net was finally aboard and Gene started the engines ready for a fast cruise back to the holding pens at Fort Myers, another unwanted kind of captive often caused us problems and pain as we tended the dolphins. These were stingrays. This flat relative of the shark, which flies through the water like some marine bat and carries a poisonous flick knife at the base of its whip-like tail, abounds in Florida waters. Very often a number of these fish, even a hundred or more and some weighing up to twelve pounds, would be pulled in along with the dolphin haul. We would throw them back into the sea after picking them out of the net, but some of the slippery, plate-like creatures would fall onto the deck and flip about, unsheathing their poisonous spines and making it perilous underfoot. Occasionally we were inundated with the stingrays, and dead ones would lie all over the boat as we made for home, but even up to many days after its death the poison spines of the fish remain highly active. Once we had the net in, I put on rubber boots to cut the risk of being stung, but the spine of a big ray could easily go through the rubber covering my leg and would go through jeans with no trouble. Gene did not make it any easier for himself by working at all times barefooted, relying on his nimbleness and quick reactions to keep out of the way of the spines that would click up into the armed, offensive position in the twinkling of an eye if a ray was touched or even if it just felt ornery.

It was Gene who gave me one of my most important lessons about the extraordinary ways of the dolphin. It was a bitter but salutary experience; at the end of it a dolphin was dead and I had killed it.

We had caught a young dolphin which was on the point of weaning. It had been captured along with its mother, and both were destined for a famous marineland in California. The youngster struggled and fought when brought aboard and, most significantly, stopped breathing.

"Right now," commanded Gene, "listen good. Young critters like this one will commit suicide by holdin' their breath if you don't watch carefully. Once they're out of the water you gotta time their breathin'. If they go for a maximum, a maximum of two minutes without breathin', we put 'em over the side in a turn or two of net as a sling and let 'em be in the water again. Then they breathe."

"And what then?" I asked.

"Then we pull 'em on board again after a short while and try 'em some more. If they do it again, we dunk 'em again and so on. Usually by the time we get back to Fort Myers and put 'em in the holdin' pens they're OK." Gene wagged a leathery, sun-blackened finger at me. "Now your job, Dr. Taylor, while I get us home lickety-split, is to do nuthin' but watch that little feller and your wrist watch. If he goes more'n two minutes, give a holler and we'll stop and dunk him."

We set off and I sat close to the agitated baby, timing its respiration and pouring sea water over it from time to time to keep the skin from cracking and the body temperature from rising too high. Two minutes went by without the little blowhole opening to suck and blow.

"Whoa!" I yelled, and Gene slowed the engines and came back to help me sling the dolphin and immerse it in the sea. Hanging over the side I watched the youngster breathe normally once it felt the ocean around it. Gene told me that he never had this trouble with bigger specimens.

After two or three minutes we pulled junior back aboard and continued on our way. He took one good breath when he was settled on his pad again, and I noted the time. Two minutes passed with no further breathing. I stopped the boat a second time and we repeated the ducking. Once more the young animal went back to a normal respiration rate of four per minute. Back in the boat again he took a breath and Gene returned to the wheel.

I stared at my watch, following the movement of the second hand, and reflected silently as I squatted by my charge. The breeze streamed through my hair and the sun scorched my naked back. Suicide, Gene had said. Could any animal commit suicide? The mystery of the mass self-drowning of lemmings was a different matter. Could an individual animal just stop breathing and die? Some canonized Catholic virgin was supposed to have taken her life in this way, but normally in mammals the brain simply forces its owner to breathe when the body senses a deficiency of oxygen and an increase of carbon dioxide in the blood. Will power, design, psychological state do not come into it, and shock is a separate thing that produces collapse of the circulation and unconsciousness before death. This little dolphin, though obviously agitated, was conscious and alert and, as far as I could tell from its colour and pulse, its circulation was good.

The seconds ticked by. One minute fifty. I sat on. I knew dolphins' brains ignored high levels of carbon dioxide in the blood when they were diving, but they needed oxygen, demanded it, in the end. That is why eventually they have to surface for air. That is why they drown if trapped in nets. So some involuntary mechanism must make this dolphin breathe and soon.

One minute fifty-nine. I wondered why Gene had said "Two minutes." Surely this was just a good estimate—no, more likely it was a dolphin catcher's unscientific bit of mythology. I watched the second hand pass the two-minute mark and decided to let it carry on without calling Gene yet again. As the watch ticked out the third minute, I knew that orthodox, reliable physiology would prove Gene wrong. It was the unbreakable rules of oxygen deficiency versus the crude rule of thumb of the dolphin catcher.

Four minutes. Still no breath taken by the dolphin. I

began to sweat slightly and bite the tip of my tongue. Gene was busy navigating through the shoals. He probably did not know whether two minutes or twelve had gone by. Four and a half minutes. I felt my heart pounding but still trusted the laws of physiology which are common to all mammals from tiny vole to giant elephant. An arrogant voice still whispered, "Oxygen demand must prevail." Four minutes forty-five. The baby dolphin became as still as a plastic model and the pulse faded. My idiot resolve broke and I yelled to Gene, "He's stopped breathing!" The boat came to a stop again and Gene came back to help me lower the dolphin into the water, but it was obvious that this poor creature would never breathe again. It was limp. The eyes were glazing. I had murdered it.

In deep misery I told Gene what I had done. He grimaced but said nothing. Then, as he knelt by the gunwale to release the corpse from the net and let it fall away into the gloomy depths where the sharks patrolled, his knee touched a sting-ray that had been dead for some time. The erect spine pierced his leg and the barbed point delivered its poison into the vein. White and sweating with pain, he had to endure the worse agony of me withdrawing the spine against the direction of the barbs. Using one of the rubber tubes of my stethoscope as a tourniquet, I bandaged the wound, but within minutes the pain worsened and Gene became very ill. The tough dolphin man stood the wracking agony without uttering one sound, and I made him comfortable on a foam pad while one of his boys took us the rest of the way in. Gene was in bed for nearly a week after that. Dolphin catching was off and all I had to do was to sit on the old jetty, throwing bits of stick into the water and staring miserably out over the dark green expanses of the holding pools, where a big female dolphin dipped and rose without her young son by her sleek side.

When the newly caught dolphins destined for Europe

were fully acclimatized and feeding well in the holding pools, they were judged fit to make the long journey over the Atlantic. I had much to learn about this important aspect of dolphin management, too, and the best way to learn was to go with the animals from start to finish, from the sunny coast of Florida to New York and then on to London, Scarborough, Cleethorpes, Nice, Hamburg, Antwerp or Stockholm. Everyone thinks that accompanying dolphins by air from Florida to Europe must be an ideal way of earning one's living. It is not. It is hard, boring, wet, smelly work and it can last for two or three days, particularly if, as happened this time, the first leg of the journey from Miami International to JFK New York is delayed and a missed connection means a twenty-four-hour lie-over in the Big Apple. You cannot take a pair of dolphins along to the nearest Holiday Inn and stick them in your bathroom. If they stay in a cold and windy warehouse in mid-January, you stay too—night and day.

First comes the road journey to Miami with the animals smothered in vaseline or lanolin which gets on your clothes and makes everything tacky. At the airport are the loading and paperwork formalities. I was to find that experienced dolphin handlers avoid excess weight charges by emptying all the water from the crates and removing the recirculating spray pumps and their twelve-volt batteries just before checking in at the freight warehouse. The animal and crate are then weighed and the weight entered on the papers. Now everything can be loaded. On the way to the aircraft, the handler nips quickly round the corner, turns on a tap, runs tens of gallons of water into the crate and replaces the spray equipment and batteries. The dolphins then go onto the plane with the whole load weighing several hundred pounds more than the amount accounted for on the waybill. The alternative, I was told, is to carry water at a cost of five dollars a gallon for the trip. Another source of free water is the washroom on board the cargo planes. The trouble is that if this is overdone the crew of the aircraft complain later that they found no water on board for their needs during the flight and there might be inquiries made.

Batteries for the pumps have a nasty habit of failing at some crucial point along the way. If you are prepared to go completely without sleep in the uncomfortable cargo hold, the constant squirting of water through a large rose spray helps to solve this difficulty. The equally tiresome alternative is to try to buy eight twelve-volt car batteries in the middle of the night somewhere near Kennedy Airport. At that time of day, if you can find a handy garage that is open, the disbelieving guy on duty is likely to demand a fistful of dollars and to regard an American Express card with the enthusiasm he reserves for four-dollar bills.

The endless flight to Europe in what resembles the inside of a giant cigar tube has none of the amusements enjoyed by travellers on passenger flights. Damp and grease go through to your skin. There is the perpetual chore of unclogging the holes in the spray system which become choked with circulated dolphin droppings, and on bumpy flights the shifting positions of the dolphins in their crates means constant vigilance and a handy supply of cotton-wool pads in case of wounds, eye damage or bedsores. Meanwhile the crew sit forward in their snug cockpit and once in a while pass back a liverwurst sandwich or a beaker of Seven Up as you shiver in your duffle coat and try to find a comfortable squatting position for a minute or two on the treacherous ball-bearings which stud the floor of the cargo hold.

Probably the worst part of the whole journey will be the arrival at London Heathrow. It is not uncommon for a dolphin to wait in the bonded warehouse there for a couple of hours while the customs men take their time about sorting through the mass of paperwork. Rarely will they agree to let the long-suffering beast get on its way while you stay behind to sign all the necessary documents and answer any questions. It is not as if they ever inspect the animals thoroughly for diamonds or contraband hooch, even though it would be quite possible to slip small packages into a dolphin's stomach and the animal would tolerate them for months. No, however much suffering it causes the animals, the customs men work by the book and the dolphins must do likewise.

My first experience of the Heathrow customs was when I went there to receive a giant Pacific octopus from Seattle that arrived, all fifty angry red pounds of him, neatly packed in water, ice and oxygen. This finest of all octopuses is extremely difficult to transport because it tends to pollute the water in which it travels and eventually poisons itself with nitrates produced by its own excrement. Anxious to resuscitate my giant octopus and to give it the chauffeur-driven limousine treatment at express speed all the way to the Yorkshire zoo that had bought it, I had gone out of my way to co-operate with customs.

"There's nothing in my book of duty rates concerning giant octopus," said the official sternly as the minutes ticked by, "but I can't let it go without classifying it. I've got to fill in the right tariff."

"It's a mollusc," I insisted, "like oysters, snails and so on."

The official glowered at the massive, scarlet, tentacled creature in its plastic bag and insulated box. "You mean it's edible?" he queried.

"Well, no, but to make it easier you can classify it as an oyster if you like."

"Oysters are on my list, but he doesn't look anything like an oyster, or a snail."

"Don't you eat little squid, calamares, in Spain or Italy ever?" I asked. The octopus was getting madder and redder and passing more droppings. I had to get it out of there and away with new water and oxygen.

"Nope," said the customs man, "don't like nasty foreign food. Squid? Yuk!"

"Please, please," I said, "take my word for it. It's the same

289

family as oysters. Look that lot up in your tariff book and charge me at the same rate."

At last commonsense prevailed. My octopus was entered on the import documents as "One unusually large shell-less whelk". The customs man had had the last word, and what did it matter to me if he considered this scarlet kraken a variety of the humble whelk which is so good with vinegar, salt and pepper? At least I had got away.

As a direct result of this experience, when I returned with the Florida dolphins I did my first and only bit of animal smuggling. I was bringing back an unusual present for Belle Vue's aquarium in the shape of a bunch of horseshoe crabs, primitive, helmet-shaped creatures that abound in the canals and round the shores of Florida. I put a dozen adults, each ten inches across, in the water beneath a dolphin slung in its crate. Coming to count the single "fish", the customs officer noticed the spiky, rod-like tails of the large crabs projecting above the water surface as the creatures shuffled about below.

"Whassat?" asked the official.

"Horseshoe crabs," I replied.

"Crabs? What for?"

Oh dear, I thought, not again. I bet my bottom dollar that this unique descendant of the trilobites, a group whose other representatives became extinct two hundred million years ago, would not be in the tariff book.

"Er, the crabs are for the dolphins. Animal food for en route," I lied.

"Oh, fine. Of course," said the customs man. "I suppose they've got to have a nibble on the way like us." The crabs and I had won through.

Arrived at their destination, the dolphins were lowered into a shallow pool, their first feel of salt water in days. Even then, my work was not done. Stiff and sore from the journey, the animals had difficulty balancing themselves in the water. This went on for a further eight hours, but until they were able to swim freely and safely, I had to go in with them. Though dog tired, I would walk them round and round their pool, guiding them by holding onto their dorsal fins. No, dolphin transporting is not much fun.

One of the dolphins I brought back from the Gulf of Mexico was destined for the London Dolphinarium on Oxford Street, a place where dolphins, sea lions, penguins and beautiful girls put on non-stop shows in a converted theatre. There were marvellous sound and lighting effects, and professional actors presented the shows. Behind the scenes, beneath Soho Square, there were holding pools and facilities where I crammed in among leggy chorus girls and kept the dolphin stars up to scratch under intensely artificial conditions. It was a good training ground for me in working against the odds in show business, preparing for the days when I would go to Paris to examine dolphins in the glass pool at the famous Moulin Rouge, the only dolphinarium where the management has ever informed me that "When 'e 'as finished, ze veterinarian can take a shower weez ze girls eef 'e wishes, like ze French vet used to do."

Unfortunately, although brilliantly conceived, the London Dolphinarium was built in the shopping area of the West End where passers-by were more likely to seek coffee shops than wander into Flipper shows in their breaks between bouts of buying and window gazing. The Dolphinarium was eventually forced to close, but before it did I had driven down from the north at least once a week to sort out one problem or another with the animal and occasionally with the human performers. When the dolphins started roughing up some of the girl "aquamaids" swimming with them in the water, I was called in to help. The girls were getting bruised and alarmed by the dolphins' boisterous attentions, the shows suffered and some of the ladies talked of resigning. I found that the animals were detecting minute quantities of pheromones, sex chemicals, in the water during the days that the girls had their monthly periods. The attacks turned out in fact to be vigorous amorous advances, triggered off by the chemicals. Once the dolphin roués had been given shots of a drug normally used to turn the minds of human sex criminals to higher things, peace and good shows returned to the Dolphinarium.

One day, Clyde, the dolphin at the London Dolphinarium whom I had accompanied across the Atlantic, fell severely ill with liver inflammation. I struggled with the case, sleeping for a couple of nights beside the pool on a makeshift bed of an upturned rubber dinghy, and gradually Clyde began to pull round. He would need a massive dose of vitamin B complex by intravenous injection, so he was taken from the water and laid carefully on a thick mat of plastic foam. With two men holding the dolphin firmly, I slowly pressed a new, fine needle into the tail. A dark gout of blood welled up. Vein. I improved the flow by edging down a fraction more and stared intently at the blood. It was blackish, surely all of it de-oxygenated blood from a vein. Then I noticed the finest hair-thin wisp of pillar-box red. I recalled Dr. Sam's "Watch out, David" at Point Mugu. Probably the needle was drawing from veins and from the central artery. I pulled the needle back a whisker. Now all seemed blackish blood again. I must be in a vein and a vein alone. Trying not to alter the needle's position, I carefully connected the loaded syringe, sucked back to check all was well and then gently depressed the plunger. The vitamin B went into Clyde's circulation, he was returned to the pool apparently unperturbed and continued to make a fine recovery over the next forty-eight hours. We were all delighted.

Then, three days after the intravenous shot, I received a worrying phone call. A strange mark had appeared on Clyde's tail, a pale streak that was long and showed smaller branches, rather like a fern. Clyde was showing signs of pain and irritation in the area, an area as important to the motive power of the dolphin as a propeller is to an ocean liner. I went to look. Sure enough, the fern-like mark was distinct but only on one half of the tail, the half where I had given my shot, and it began at exactly the point where I had introduced my needle. For the first time in my life I had given at least part of an injection by mistake into an artery. Glumly I knew that the vitamin B, an irritant chemical, had gone whipping along the artery and into its tributaries. Thrombosis had occurred, the tissues supplied by the artery beyond my injection had died and I could expect them to drop off. It was a classic case of iatrogenic gangrene or, in honest layman's terminology, a real screw-up by the vet. There was little I could do. Dead tissue is dead tissue. I could encourage it to slough off, prevent secondary infection and wait. The nub of the question was how much tissue did that artery supply and so how much had died? If half the tail dropped off eventually, how would Clyde swim? I lay awake during those nightmare hours between two o'clock and five o'clock in the morning when only ill humours are abroad and sweated as I imagined the prospects.

As the days passed the pale, fern-like area became an ugly yellow colour, expanded and began to soften. At last after a week it was clear that I could see all the dead area; it had stopped expanding and the rotting tissue was beginning to peel away. A broad band ran down the centre of one tail fluke, but to my relief it seemed very unlikely that half the tail was going to fall off since the rest of the fluke looked healthy and was apparently well furnished with blood. What had seemed to be the main vessel supplying the tail fluke must have been backed up by other, smaller arteries which were not its tributaries and had been undamaged. Dolphins were obviously designed marvellously in yet another respect, to keep erring veterinarians from screwing up their engines.

After many anxious days, Clyde's tail eventually cast off all the dead tissue, leaving a deep wide trench which had gone right down to the fibrous core of the fluke. Still, the tail worked. Clyde jumped, somersaulted and spun. My job was to get this gaping hole filled as quickly as possible. Twice a day I arranged for it to be coated with a healing cream and then thickly plastered with Grandmother's water-resistant denture fixative. After a month Clyde had completely healed and I could sleep dreamlessly again, but a long, fronded snow-white scar remains to this day to remind me whenever I see him that "mainlining" a dolphin is one of the most hazardous of procedures.

Nine

After the exciting days at Point Mugu and on Gene's boat off the coast of Florida, I began to consider seriously what had always been just a dream: setting up a practice to treat nothing but exotic species. It would be some time yet, though, before my zoo experience and contacts would be wide enough to take such a big step into the unknown, and until then it was back to cows and sheep on moorland farms and cats and dogs in the Rochdale surgery. For exotic animal work I would continue to rely mainly on surgery cases and on Belle Vue Zoo.

It was from there that Ray Legge telephoned me one autumn evening. I hardly had time to pick up the phone and put the receiver to my ear before his unusually strident voice rapped out the message: "I've got a bear on fire! Get here sharp as you can!" Before I could ask any details, there was a click. He had rung off.

When Ray's abrupt call came in I was just putting the final touches to my favourite dish of hare, Lièvre à la Royale, an exquisite casserole containing cream, cognac and pine kernels. From the dressing of the shot wild hare after it had hung a week, something Shelagh insisted I do alone in the farthest corner of the garden, through the marinading in wine and herbs and the blending of the chopped liver and heart with the brandy, a relaxing and enjoyable culinary exercise with which I insisted Shelagh should not interfere, the whole process took twenty-four hours. Now at last, with its accompanying wafers of glazed carrots and rosemary-sprinkled potatoes, it was almost ready for the table. But the burning bear banished all thoughts of dinner.

"Don't worry, love," said Shelagh, as I whipped off my blue-and-white-striped cooking apron and picked up my emergency bag, "it'll warm up tomorrow." She pushed a couple of apples into my duffle coat pocket.

As I wound my way laboriously through the evening traffic towards the zoo I puzzled over Ray's call. He had sounded worried all right, but more than that I had the impression that he was mightily angry. I had never seen Ray, the epitome of the well-mannered English gentleman, blazing with rage the way he had sounded on the phone. A burning bear? It sounded like vandals. We have more than our fair share of those in a city zoo. Yes, vandals must have done something particularly obnoxious to raise his wrath. A burning bear sounded just that.

When I arrived in the zoo grounds my headlights illuminated a cluster of men standing near the bear pit. One of the group was in a state of great agitation, almost literally jumping up and down and stamping round in small circles. It was Ray Legge. The other figures I recognized as members of the Board of Directors. I stopped the car and walked over to join them.

"And if it happens once more, just once more, I'll walk out of this place and, by God, I'll . . ." Ray was white with anger. The Board members were listening silently; some looked crestfallen, others embarrassed. "Just look at that animal, will you?" Ray was in full spate. "You can't have it both ways, you won't have it both ways! It's my animals or your Battle of Waterloo. Your damned Battle of Waterloo will have to go!"

In the bear pit a brown bear sat on a rock licking at a frizzled black patch as big as a saucer on its side. On the ground nearby lay a large burnt-out rocket, a firework with a stick at least four feet long. From its charred casing a plume of grey smoke curled lazily upwards. I understood.

Damned Battle of Waterloo! Every autumn Belle Vue presented for two or three weeks a lavish evening firework display. Combined with son et lumière and several dozen men in period costume, historic battles would be re-enacted in a deafening, dazzling pyrotechnic spectacular. Last year it had been General Wolfe storming the heights of Quebec. This year it was Waterloo. The problem was that the hour-long barrage of star shells, firecrackers and smoke bombs was all staged in an arena backing directly onto the bear pits where the collection of Himalayan, brown, sun, polar and sloth bears ate, slept, went about their quiet daily business and, most importantly, mated. They were literally only inches away from the crackling rockets and roaring catherine wheels.

Both Ray and I had been complaining bitterly about the effects on the animals of being compulsorily in the orchestra pit during every performance of the ear-splitting extravaganza. We were particularly concerned for the polar bears and their efforts to produce young: we were certain that each year our lovely adult female conceived and, if things had progressed as nature intended, she would have delivered one or maybe two little cubs in November or December. It never happened. On came the fireworks at the end of September, and within a few days the keeper cleaning out the dens would find a smear of blood or perhaps remains which proved conclusively that the bear had once again miscarried and devoured the half-grown embryo. It was heart-breaking, but now this!

Ray broke off his tirade and came over to me. "That bear felt like sleeping outside on the rocks tonight. The keeper couldn't get him into the sleeping quarters." If a bear feels like napping al fresco on a mild night, there is no easy way of changing his mind. "Then that bloody pantomime started up, a rocket went off course and landed in the pits." He was quivering with fury. "Do you know, when the keeper called me the bear was actually alight!

Fur in flames!" He spat out the words with slow, precise venom. "I've told them. That's the last straw. The fireworks must go because we can't move the bears."

I darted the bear with a tranquillizing syringe and climbed down a ladder into the pit. The burnt area of the skin had been largely insulated by the dense, sizzling hair but it was still a serious and painful injury. I plastered it liberally with a paste containing local anaesthetic, antibiotic and cortisone. It would heal all right. Climbing back out of the pit, I found Ray still expostulating and gesticulating with the directors.

To our amazement, his war dance did produce all that we could have hoped for. The stray rocket turned out in the end to be a twenty-four-carat blessing in disguise, for it was decided that the annual fireworks displays at Belle Vue should end. Ray and I were delighted. Now maybe we would get our first baby polar bear.

The key to successful breeding of this species in captivity appears to be ultra-quiet privacy for the female. We decided that from October onwards next year, Crystal, Belle Vue's female polar bear, would be placed in strict isolation in a secluded, dark den, with food placed silently from time to time in an adjoining compartment which she could reach through a small door. No mucking out, no regular inspections by flashlight—just leave her alone. Then, if all went well, we might hear the soft squeaks of the hidden cubs some time before Christmas and get our first glimpse of them in the following January when she decided to show them to us.

The next breeding season came round, and true to form the female polar bear conceived. We went ahead with our plan and treated her like a hermit. Just after Christmas the keeper heard faint mewing noises in her den. They continued for a day and then ceased. Some days later the bear moved into the feeding compartment and insisted on staying there, clawing at the door that led to the outside pits. We let her out and searched her den. Inside was the shrivelled body of a full-term cub, but without a drop of mother's milk in its tummy.

The following year the same thing happened, but this time she half ate the baby. Ray and I were despondent. "Well," I said, "next season we'll hand-rear the cub right from birth."

"How do you reckon to get the cub away before she eats it or at least does it some harm?"

"As soon as the keeper hears any squeaking or gets any hint at all that she's given birth, you (I'm bound to be at least half an hour away, maybe more, and that could be too long) you will knock her out with phencyclidine and grab the cub. Beginning in mid-October we'll have a dart already loaded with the right dose of phencyclidine standing permanently in a jar outside her den. And we'll start the little 'uns off on Carnation milk."

Ray nodded. All we had to do now was to wait an interminable ten or eleven months to see if our plan would work.

Ironically, in view of my hard-won connection with the zoo and the amount of time I spent there, Belle Vue could not help very much with my increasing interest in learning about marine mammals. The only ones in the zoo were three big old Californian sea lions that lived in the wooden Victorian pavilion, jealously guarded by their trainer, an elderly German lady called Mrs. Schmidt. Mrs. Schmidt had a lifetime's experience in working with sea lions. She worried and doted and fussed over the honking, snorting, four-hundred-pound monsters, rarely taking a day off and meticulously selecting and preparing all their food herself. No one, but no one, be he head keeper or zoo director, and certainly not that meddlesome harbinger of death, the veterinarian, got within spitting distance of her beloved Adolf, Heinz and Dieter. Mrs. Schmidt took no chances; she even took her baths in the sea-lion house, sitting in an old tub and bellowing shrill Teutonic oaths if anyone made to approach the door. It was tacitly accepted by everyone that the sea-lion house was Mrs. Schmidt's private preserve. Left alone in her sanctum sanctorum she caused nobody any trouble and asked for nothing but the regular delivery of fish. Even Matt Kelly was a little in awe of her.

There was no salt water in the sea-lion pool, no filtration or chlorination equipment. The sweet water was changed when it became foul. The fish for the animals was fresh from the Lancashire docks and thus did not undergo the deep-freezing that would kill any parasites it contained. As a result of all this, Adolf, Heinz and Dieter were constantly taking in worm eggs by mouth and from time to time would excrete the long, wriggly, clay-coloured adult parasites. This would send Mrs. Schmidt hurrying to the nearby chemist's for extract of santonin, the stuff that she had always used on sea lions, as had her father before her. Santonin extract generally resulted in a pleasing expulsion of a biggish bundle of worms, but in the process the animals would suffer a few hours of griping pain in the guts and would grind their teeth with a most despondent air.

Mrs. Schmidt was used to that. "Those verdammte worms!" she would explain. "They fight to their last gasp to keep a hold. See how they make my three lieblings unhappy while they thrash about and struggle to resist my santonin. Still, all will be well shortly. I always get those verdammte Würmer!" And she would nod contentedly.

Sure enough, the three sea lions would soon recover from the worming and would be rewarded with choice whole whiting—whiting which contained invisible worm eggs and sometimes even invisible baby worm larvae.

If Adolf had a cold, Mrs. Schmidt gave him Fenning's fever powders, cloves of garlic and spoonfuls of honey secreted inside the fish. When Dieter got a boil and would not eat, she smeared the throbbing lump with Germolene and kept him locked in his pen away from the pool in the hope that he would drink from a bowl of water into which she had mixed some mysterious "blood-purifying" salts. In all the years and years that she had been at Belle Vue she had never once taken veterinary advice. I rarely ventured inside her domain and then only to catch the sea lions' show with the paying public. It struck me that the big animals were slow and lethargic considering their high degree of training, but my knowledge of marine mammals was still limited and perhaps it was just their great weight.

There were times when Ray Legge knew that one or another of the sea lions was not up to the mark and he would diplomatically suggest that perhaps Dr. Taylor might be able to help—after all, he was being paid for his veterinary advice—but Mrs. Schmidt would simply retreat within her pavilion, bolt the door and prepare to withstand a siege. If Ray took a firmer line she would just as adamantly but politely refuse the offer, send her assistant to the chemist so that her lines could not be infiltrated while she herself was away, and even sleep at nights by the side of her charges just in case we tried a secret nocturnal examination of the beasts. "You can't be too careful" seemed to be her motto.

The worms in the sea lions came and went and new ones took their place. One day Mrs. Schmidt noticed an unusually large number of live worms lying on the pool bottom. Mein Gott! The three boys had picked up a bigger load of parasites than ever. She decided to take stern measures with the disgusting invaders. It looked as if a particularly numerous band of the pests was involved; ach so! A double dose of the santonin extract would deal with them. Adolf, Heinz and Dieter duly swallowed their medicine hidden inside a whole fish. Half an hour later it appeared to Mrs. Schmidt that the worms were fighting far more ferociously than normal. The sea lions were getting the expected gripes and colly-wobbles, but something she had never seen before was also happening. The animals were beginning to vomit violently, tremble uncontrollably and shake their heads in a bizarre, glassy-eyed fashion. Sudden powerful spasms shook their sleek, chubby bodies. They were in trouble. The worms were winning!

As the minutes passed and the sea lions showed no signs of recovering, Mrs. Schmidt made a momentous decision; she would ask Mr. Legge's advice. Ray went down to the sea-lion house as soon as she appeared white-faced in his office to tell him with much agitation what had happened. It was plain when he saw the distressed trio that something had gone horribly wrong with the worming, and he called me right away.

Adolf and Co. were in fact showing all the symptoms one could expect from an overdose of santonin. Santonin is a poison derived from the dried buds of a plant named wormwood by ancient apothecaries after they had observed its properties. The use of it in the old days relied on the poison bumping off the parasitic worms at a dose which was low enough not to do the same to the worms' host. It is a chemical that attacks the central nervous system, and the signs that the worms were putting up a heroic resistance, as Mrs. Schmidt interpreted them, were in fact the effects of the toxic substance on the sea lions themselves.

Now at last I was presented with my first marine mammal case at Belle Vue. It was a breakthrough, but I could hardly have chosen a more inauspicious debut than three un-restrainable sea-lion bulls with the signs of nerve poisoning produced by a chemical to which there was no antidote.

Although the vomiting and diarrhoea should evacuate any of the santonin that remained unabsorbed by the intestine, the dramatic convulsions continued. I decided to try a tran-quillizer, but it would have to be injected, and sea lions are one of the species on which it is risky to use the dart-gun because of the danger of dirt from the skin being carried into the animal's system by the dart.

Kelly had arrived on the scene and was shaking his broad head pessimistically as he looked at the agonized animals.

"Can you and Matt hold them somehow while I give them a shot?" I asked Ray. The sea lions were in a small pen containing a pool from which the water had been drained. They were conscious and obviously aware of our presence. It would be impossible to pin down such heavy creatures and, like most sea mammals, the sea lion is designed without any convenient grab handles.

"I'll get a chair," said Ray. "If you can get a needle into the back flipper muscle somehow, I'll try to distract the head end."

Mrs. Schmidt produced a chair, and the zoo director took up the classical lion tamer's pose with the four wooden legs pointing towards the jerking head of the agonized Heinz. We both knew how dirty sea-lion teeth are and what severe bites they can inflict on one another and on man; Mrs. Schmidt bore gnarled scars on her hands and arms. Protected, I hoped, by Ray and his chair, I splashed some disinfectant onto Heinz's skin and jabbed a new needle into his rump. He was too wracked with the convulsions to do anything more than turn his head slightly in my direction. The tranquillizer slipped into the muscle. Adolf and Dieter were treated in the same way, then we stood and waited while Mrs. Schmidt continued to marvel at the powerful rearguard action by the worms. Slowly the sea lions relaxed, the convulsions diminished and the vomiting ceased. After three quarters of an hour it looked as if the three sea lions were going to be all right. They were drowsy but undoubtedly out of danger.

"Now, Mrs. Schmidt," I said, feeling able to take advantage of the situation, "that's the last time that you will use santonin on *our* sea lions." She blinked and did not say a word. Matt stood by, looking like a sergeant-major quietly enjoying the dressing-down of one of his privates by the CO. "From now on," I continued, "we will use something new. It's very effective and not at all poisonous. I'll send you a bottle of piperazine tablets tomorrow."

Adolf, Heinz and Dieter did fully recover but in a few weeks began to show evidence of worm infestation again. Obediently, Mrs. Schmidt gave them the piperazine tablets. Delightedly she watched the worms expelled a few hours later, and much to her amazement not one single worm put up a struggle. The sea lions had no gripes, no diarrhoea, no grinding of teeth.

Mrs. Schmidt continued to feel, I think, that although I might be Lord of the Worms, the rest of my medical art was still suspect. At least I had penetrated the sea-lion house and was allowed to look at the animals whenever I wanted—unless their keeper was bathing. It was a major advance, but I still had the impression that the sea lions were slow and sluggish in their movements. They seemed to tire easily and they lay around idly; there was none of the zest I had seen in sea lions at other zoos. At the time little of importance had been published about sea-lion medicine, so the special nutritional problems that pinnipeds (seals, sea lions and walruses) and other marine mammals can develop in captivity had not yet been realized.

One day, as I watched Mrs. Schmidt prepare fish pieces for Adolf and his partners, it struck me that for every bucket of fish she filled with choice cuts for her "boys", she was filling another bucket with waste pieces to throw away. She was neatly filleting the fish, removing bones, heads, tails and all the internal organs. The sea lions got only one hundred per cent meat, first-quality steaks. In the wild, sea lions naturally eat the whole fish, bones, guts and all, as well as huge quantities of squid and cuttlefish. I discovered that for years the Belle Vue sea lions had received only the boneless middle cuts of herring, whiting and mackerel.

"What about supplements?" I asked. "Do you give minerals or vitamins?"

"No. Nor have I in all the years I've been keeping sea lions, Doctor," came the reply.

"Right, I'm going to give you some multivitamin syrup,"

I said. "Put a tablespoonful in their fish each day." She agreed. "And what's more," I added, "I want you to stop filleting the fish. You can remove the guts if you like, but I don't see how these animals can get enough calcium without the bones in their diet."

Mrs. Schmidt looked horrified but she promised to do what I asked. I sent down to her the first multivitamin syrup I laid my hands on in the dispensary, a lemon-flavoured concoction made up for human geriatric patients. Apart from the flavouring it contained nothing but a mixture of the vitamins A, B, C and D.

A few days later I was driving through the zoo grounds when I saw Mrs. Schmidt running towards my car waving her arms to attract my attention. Oh-oh, here's trouble, I said to myself as I wound down the window.

"Dr. Taylor, Dr. Taylor, you must come and see my boys," she said, puffing with the exertion. Apart from her flushed face I was surprised to see that she did not appear alarmed or angry. If anything she was in rather a pleasant mood. Good Lord, Mrs. Schmidt had actually smiled at me!

I went into the sea-lion house. There were Adolf, Heinz and Dieter playing in the pool and gambolling around on the stage. But how they were playing! The three ponderous fellows were no longer torpid or slow-moving. They were sliding, rolling, diving and leaping in the water like young otters.

"It's the vitamins, Doctor," crowed Mrs. Schmidt, "it's the vitamins. I've never seen them so alert and active. I thought they were in peak condition but look how wrong I was."

She was right: it was the vitamins, probably the vitamin B_1 in particular. It is a wonder that those animals survived at all when they were deprived of minerals and the all-important vitamin B_1. Years later we were to discover how essential these substances are to marine mammals fed on dead fish like herring and mackerel, which contain a potent enzyme that utterly destroys vitamin B; and how dangerous the lack of salt could be to specimens kept in fresh water.

The conquest of Mrs. Schmidt and her sea-lion house was complete, but I became increasingly nervous about driving near the pale blue wooden pavilion. She seemed to sense that I was in the grounds and would come flying out with a thousand questions about every minute thing that might or she imagined might be wrong with her boys. As for the lemon-flavoured liquid, she refused ever to change from it. When more suitable, more concentrated tablets with the same constituents were given to her, she swore that they did not work as well as the lemon syrup. And when the drug company making the product changed the flavouring from lemon to orange for some reason, she kicked up a mighty fuss in Ray Legge's office. "Dr. Taylor said I should use the lemon syrup and look what wonders it performed," she thundered. "I must have the *lemon* one!" When it was made absolutely clear that no more lemon was ever going to be produced and that Dr. Taylor had personally checked the credentials of the orange substitute, she gave in. I do not think Mrs. Schmidt ever treated another ailment in her sea lions again, and she made it her business to see that no one, but no one, except myself went anywhere near her precious boys.

Driving back to the surgery one day after I had been to the sea-lion house at Mrs. Schmidt's excited request to see the effect of my vitamins on her threesome, I stopped at some traffic lights. Casually looking at the other vehicles around me, I thought I recognized an individual sitting next to the driver of the car on my immediate right. Bigger and shaggier than when I had first encountered him when he was a baby, he was dressed in corduroy dungarees, purple chunky-knit woollen sweater and Sinatra hat. He was holding one side of an unfolded road map while his human chauffeur held the other and studied their whereabouts. If I was not mistaken it was Billy, a chimpanzee I had once treated for pinworms. He had been owned at the time by a rather overwhelming woman named Mrs. Lomax. I tapped on my window. Billy glanced superciliously in my direction and then, apparently unable to place my face as belonging to anyone important, and bored stiff by yet another of those oddballs who would insist on gesticulating, waving, winking and generally making asses of themselves every time he did nothing more remarkable than go out for a drive, he yawned histrionically and looked down at the map. I could not quite see Billy's companion at the wheel, and wondered whether it was Mr. Lomax and he was trying to make his way to see me.

I had not been in the surgery for five minutes before Billy and his friend were ushered in. It was indeed Mr. Lomax, a portly, pink-faced man with a high-pitched voice, an ever perspiring brow that required frequent mopping with a large blue-spotted handkerchief, and a tight grey suit the pockets of which bristled with pencils and ballpoints and the seat of which was so polished that I might have expected to see Billy's impish reflection glinting in it. Mr. Lomax wore socks that did not match.

"Dr. Taylor," he piped, "my wife sends her apologies. She couldn't come because she has a speaking engagement in Bradford. I've been sent—I mean, I've brought Billy with his problem."

"Problem? The worms again, you mean?"

Mr. Lomax shook his head vigorously. "Oh no. We, well, he's absolutely OK in that respect these days. What's worrying her, us, is the way his tummy's swelling."

I looked at the now mature ape sitting placidly on the floor holding the neatly folded road map in both hands. He was big, hairy, muscular and very much the macho male chimpanzee. True enough, he did look eight months pregnant. His purple piece of home knit was stretched over a distinct pot belly.

"Can you handle Billy?" I asked, noting the chimp's now well developed fang teeth, which he displayed from time to time as he gave me the apprehensive chimp grin.

"Not really, to be honest. Billy's a mummy's boy. But if you wouldn't mind looking at him on the floor, and if I keep giving him these Smarties"—hesitantly he produced a large bag of iced chocolate drops from a pocket—"you can probably examine him down there."

I certainly did not mind. Not for the first time I would sit on the floor with a patient to avoid starting a potentially disastrous rough-house by trying to get the beast onto the examination table. I am one Mahomet who, for the sake of a peaceful and productive examination, is prepared to go to any mountain anywhere.

"Apart from the swelling has Billy shown any sign of illness?" I inquired.

"He's a bit more peeky than usual, we think. He threw a milk bottle at the next-door neighbour's dog last week—knocked a tooth out and we had to pay the vet's bill—and he's not eating quite as well as usual. Gone off his fried liver and onions and his bedtime Ovaltine. He's still fairly lively though. He got into the bathroom when my sister-in-law was washing her hair, pinched her electric drier and dropped it down the loo. Blew all the fuses. Sister-in-law had to go to a Masonic dinner with a wig on. He's taking his fruit and vegetables fine, though. Droppings? Well, she —my wife—changes his nappies, you know. He did take his clothes off the other night when we were asleep. Nappies and all. Did his business on the piano. No, no sign of diarrhoea or anything. Very normal, I'd say—I know because I cleaned the piano myself."

I sat on the surgery floor near Billy, and Mr. Lomax bent down and started to feed Smarties into the mobile black lips with the frenzy of a slot-machine addict. Cautiously I stroked Billy's head and slyly let my hand caress downwards over one cheek. Billy seemed to like it. He stuck one index finger into my ear. I let it stay there; it was only marginally uncomfortable and seemed a reasonable quid pro quo. As my fingers lay on Billy's cheek I gently pulled down the lower eyelid. He seemed paler than normal. Pretending to flip idly at his lips, I pulled them out a little so that I could inspect the gums; they were not as freshly pink as I would have liked either. Billy kept his finger in my ear and with the other hand tried to push the corner of the road map into my mouth. I pursed my lips and quietly raised my hand to ease away his arm and to indicate that while I might tolerate an earful of finger, a mouthful of paper was out of the question. I also used the opportunity to take his pulse as I held his wrist. It was normal. So far so good. The examination was proceeding well and Billy was still unperturbed. Next I slipped my hand under his sweater. The chimp hooted a warning at me and pulled the finger from my ear, making ready to clout me if I showed any sign of trying to take his clothes off. I cooed at him and tickled his navel as I explored his abdomen beneath the sweater. Billy relaxed, but took a grip of the hem of his sweater just in case.

The swelling of the stomach was undoubtedly more than just obesity or slack abdominal muscles, conditions often seen in young, imperfectly fed great apes, particularly gorillas. A tense, round mass the size of a large grapefruit lay in the body cavity. It did not seem to be painful, and it was possible to move it slightly from place to place within the abdomen.

For ten minutes I carefully explored the contours of the mass and went through the possibilities in my mind. Abscess, cyst, tumour? Amoeba cavity, common in chimps? Tapeworm hydatids? Which organ was involved: liver, spleen, intestines? Or no organ—just an independent mass attached to the peritoneum? I debated whether to take a biopsy sample, but decided that it would only delay the major operation which I felt sure would be necessary. Better perhaps to operate and remove the mass and then confirm its true nature. That would avoid both the need for anaesthetizing twice and the possibility of the biopsy producing side effects like peritonitis; it would also save time if the lump was in any way malignant. On balance I thought that the mass was most likely a non-malignant cyst, lying fairly free in the abdomen or possibly embracing most of the spleen and containing pus produced by the same amoeba parasite that causes dysentery in man. Whatever it was, Billy was going to undergo major surgery.

Mr. Lomax had to have a chair to sit on when I stood up and told him what I had found. "It's not the thought of the operation that upsets me, Dr. Taylor," he squeaked, sponging his pink jowls with his handkerchief. "It's, well, it's the thought of telling her—my wife. She'll have a fit! She'll want to know how he got this trouble—she's sure there's no healthier chimp than Billy."

"I understand," I replied truthfully—I remembered her as a formidable, excitable woman—"but it would be unwise to pretend that there is anything else to be done in the circumstances. No operation and there may well be no Billy before long."

I saw them to the door and watched as they crossed the outer office, Billy carrying the road map in one hand and belabouring Mr. Lomax's backside with the Sinatra hat held in the other.

I had arranged for Billy to be brought to the surgery in four days' time, with an empty stomach and a spoonful of tranquillizing syrup administered in a cup of fruit juice just before setting out. Operation day arrived and promptly at ten o'clock Billy, accompanied now by Mrs. Lomax herself, was brought into my office. She was a stringy, pale, middle-aged lady, with a querulous voice and fidgety manner. To my dismay the chimp showed no signs of having taken any tranquillizer, and I did not fancy jabbing needles into him while he was fully conscious.

"He just would not drink the fruit juice with the drug in it," his owner confessed. "He seemed to know there was something added."

At my request, the normally modish chimp was undressed. He looked mean and hungry. Spotting a small packet of Nescafé powder and a sugar cube lying on my desk ready for my mid-morning brew of coffee, he swept both items into his mouth with one fast "lodger's reach", as Lancastrians call such swift light-fingeredness. After swallowing the goodies, he spat out the indigestible paper. Still mean and still hungry, he looked round the room for something else to eat. Ominously he began cracking his knuckles. Everything else was ready for the operation, but first I somehow had to get some injectable anaesthetic into Billy. He was obviously in no mood to be trifled with and there is no way to restrain a full-grown chimp who does not feel like letting folk prick him with needles. I would have to use the dart-gun and, for the first and only time in my career to date, I prepared to shoot a knock-out syringe at a free-ranging chimpanzee on the prowl in my own surgery waiting room. Loading the gas-pistol with a small syringe charged with a dose of phencyclidine, I explained what I planned to do. "Billy will have to be left on his own in the waiting room."

"No, never!" wailed Mrs. Lomax.

"Yes, definitely. There's no other way and I can't risk having humans about when I start firing darts in a confined space. No one can stay in with Billy. I'll open the door a crack, shoot at him, close the door and then, when he goes to sleep, we'll carry on in the normal way. By the way, Mrs. Lomax, I suggest that you go shopping for a couple of hours after he's knocked out." I did not want her hanging round the premises while I operated.

Vulnerable items like photo frames, potted plants and an electric fire were removed from the waiting room and Billy was slipped in there. Behind the closed door we listened. I had to be certain he was at the other side of the room before I did my bit of sniping. There was a bumping as Billy moved among some of the chairs; then I heard a shuffling noise. He was rifling through the magazines on the table by the far wall. This was my chance.

I opened the door a few inches, put my foot against the bottom of it and held firmly onto the door handle, ready to close it should Billy try joining us. With one eye at the crack I glimpsed a crouching Billy looking at me from a distance of three yards. I took aim with my gun hand and squeezed the trigger. Plop! From the angry screeching I knew that the dart had struck chimp flesh. Before I could close the door, Billy had snatched the missile out of his buttocks, where it had lodged and discharged its contents in a fraction of a second, and flung it accurately back at me. Not for the first time I nearly took a returned dart full in the face. Great apes often return my ammunition in this way, which is helpful of them I suppose, but I shudder to think what would happen if I was hit by one which had not fired its drug load. There is no antidote to a big dose of phencyclidine, and I can just see the headline in the *Rochdale Observer*: "Veterinarian put to sleep by chimpanzee." A different way to go.

The dart whipped through the still partly opened door and embedded itself firmly in the corridor wall. With a crash I shut the door just before Billy hurled himself at the other side. Hollering with annoyance, he pounded the door and threatened to split the panelling. Then he wreaked his fury on our chairs. There were tearing and shredding noises, too, as copies of *The Field* and *Illustrated London News* were turned into ticker tape. Gradually the echoes of bedlam subsided and all was still. Six minutes had passed since the darting. Billy should now be chasing lady chimpanzees in a sunlit happy valley, for we know that small doses of phencyclidine in humans tend to produce fanciful erotic dreams. I opened the door. Sure enough, Billy lay sprawled and sleeping on a heap of chairs and pieces of chair.

With Mrs. Lomax sent fretfully packing, the chimpanzee was carried into the operating room and I deepened his anaesthesia with oxygen and halothane gas. Scrubbed and gowned, and with the patient shaved and painted a startling antiseptic red over his bulging belly, I took a scalpel and unzipped his abdomen from top to bottom. Spreading the operation wound open with a set of ratcheted retractors, I felt inside for the round lump. Bit by bit I pulled it close to the opening where I could see it. It was not part of any organ, but an independent, tense sphere containing some sort of thickish fluid and stuck at dozens of points to the loops of intestine. It was going to take a long time to free all those attachments. Beneath it might lie large blood vessels that I could not see; there might be weaknesses in the wall of the thing which would rupture as I separated it. I began cautiously and laboriously to break the adhesions with the handle of my scalpel, as using the sharp blade might pierce the sphere and release the contents, with appalling consequences. After half an hour I had still freed only a small part of the mass. On I went, stopping from time to time to check Billy's pulse, colour and breathing. He slept deeply. Two hours later I had freed all of the mass that I could see. Now for the underneath bit.

As I tried swinging the sphere over so that I could approach the lower adhesions less blindly, I noticed something that made my stomach turn. A pink-brown creamy liquid was beginning to seep up between my fingers. I swabbed it away hurriedly and looked closely. More of the stuff welled up. I gently pressed the spherical mass. It was less tense than before. Somehow, somewhere below it had begun to leak. The unpleasant pink-brown cream was running over Billy's intestines.

Cursing silently, I pressed on rapidly with the complete removal of the lump, now a collapsed and flabby bladder. With that gone, I surveyed the terrible sight before me: an abdominal cavity which was awash with pus full of amoebae and nasty bacteria. No matter what, Billy was going to have quite a case of peritonitis. How could I remove most of the foul stuff? If I put a drain into his tummy, as is done in humans, he would only pluck out the rubber tube when he came to. But would the wound hold if I stitched it with much of that rubbish inside?

Then I recalled watching as part of my surgery course at university an operation on a human patient whose gastric ulcer had burst just after being bombarded with a meal of steak pie, chips and peas, covering his liver, spleen, stomach and all the other bits and pieces of organs inside him with gravy, peas and chewed-up bits of food. The surgeon had not made a big fuss about this dinner that had gone so sadly astray but had dealt with it in a thoroughly down-to-earth, commonsense sort of way: he had ordered up two or three sterilized stainless-steel buckets full of warm saline solution and simply swilled out his patient's innards by pouring in a couple of gallons and letting it wash out. Then he had done it again, just as if he was washing down his garden path after a spot of untidy gardening. The peas and all the rest of the meal were washed away and what small quantities of foreign matter and bacteria remained in the abdominal cavity following this practical bit of laundry were easily controlled by antibiotics. I decided to use the same method. Sending Edith for some bottles of sterile saline solution, I sucked out as much of the pus as I could with a special tube and vacuum pump. When the saline was ready I used it to wash the intestines and surrounding organs, rinsed them again and again, popped everything back into place and sprinkled antibiotic powder in nooks and crevices. The rest was simple: stitching up the various layers of peritoneum, muscle, fat and skin.

Billy gradually began to come round when he was taken off the gas, but because of the phencyclidine still active in his body he would not be fully back to normal until the following day. Mrs. Lomax did not object when I insisted that Billy

314

would have to go naked and unadorned until his operation wound healed; chimps' tissues heal rapidly when left dry and open to the oxygen in the air.

By the time Billy came to have his stitches out, he was his old fighting self once more. I did the job only when they had finally succeeded in slipping him some tranquillizer in a sweet plum, seven days after the date originally planned for the appointment. Billy had recovered excellently. There was no sign of peritonitis and he looked the picture of health. My examination of the pus from his lump had shown the presence of both amoebae and bacteria, as I had suspected, but these were dealt with by a course of fruit-flavoured drugs originally designed for children.

"By the way, Dr. Taylor," said Mrs. Lomax, when she brought Billy for his final check-up with her perspiring, pink-faced husband standing by, "this amoeba. Is there any chance that George here brought it home from the office?"

George mopped his forehead and looked appealingly at me, saying nothing.

"No chance, Mrs. Lomax," I replied firmly, "absolutely no chance."

George Lomax let out a sigh of happy relief. "Now, how much do we owe you, Dr. Taylor?" he asked.

Ten

It was a dark, wet night. The roads were empty and sheeted with rain as I drove home from a 3 a.m. call to an old cow whose calf had a head three sizes too big for her mother's pelvis. I had removed the big-headed infant by Caesarean and then, sticky, sweaty and covered with pieces of chaff, set off for a bath and what remained of the night's sleep. By nine o'clock that morning I would be at Belle Vue to begin a day's chiropody, trimming the overgrown hooves of every one of three dozen agile, unco-operative aoudads. Not my favourite occupation wrestling with those fellows, was my last thought as I fell asleep. Yes, today looked like being a hard one.

But I was learning that in zoo work it is impossible to plan ahead. As I sat bleary-eyed at breakfast, the telephone rang and the distant elfin voice of a frantic Tunisian animal importer delivered a message in a mixture of French and English over a line that crackled and howled like a banshee.

"Dr. Taylor, this is M. Taouche. Mr. Legge at Belle Vue told me where to contact you. *Please* come quick. I have twelve dying giraffes, ici en Tunisie!"

I stood looking through the persistent autumn drizzle at the cotton-mill chimneys impaling the low, early morning clouds hanging over the town, while M. Taouche told of the happenings on the farm near the town of Sbeitla, below the Atlas Mountains, where he had set up a quarantine station for African animals bound eventually for Europe. When his Arab keepers had risen that morning they had found that every one of the twelve magnificent Rothschild's giraffes on

316

the farm was lying prostrate on the ground with legs askew, necks arched back and bellies bloated so grotesquely that the skin seemed about to split.

My mind whirred as I listened. I had only a few seconds before I must come up with advice that could give twelve helpless patients, unseen and unexamined fifteen hundred miles away, a fighting chance. This was ludicrous! How could I ever consider seriously working a one-man practice that might extend over half the globe? Some medical doctors will not take on patients living at the other side of the same town, yet here was I listening to a man paying ten dollars a minute in long-distance charges to plead for help. Come on, lad, I said to myself, this is what independent full-time zoo work would be all about. Every day things like this would be happening; was this not what I had always wanted? There had never really been any choice, had there? Cats with coughs and ponies with pleurisy had been the qualifying heats; the main race for me was supposed to be just this sort of situation. My mind cleared. No time to mull over a considered review of possibilities, diagnoses and prognostications. I had to learn the art of making snap decisions about critical situations in Cathay or Katmandu and always be right—or at least never harmfully wrong.

M. Taouche had finished his account of all he knew about the giraffes. Clearly the animals were bloated by gas produced by something they had eaten fermenting in their warm, wet stomachs. The gas pressure must be released before any distended stomach ruptured or pressed on the heart and stopped it.

"OK," I said, "I'll fly out at once. Meanwhile do this: get your man to find the biggest, broadest hypodermic needles he can—from a clinic or a doctor somewhere—and tell him to stick one into the swollen belly of each animal at its highest point on the left-hand—repeat, *left*-hand—side."

"Mais oui," came the Tunisian's faint voice, "but would

it not be better for Abu al Ma'arri, my man, to release the pressure with a sharp knife?"

"No, repeat *no*! Do that and you will lose all the giraffes for sure!" I had seen too many cattle that had overgorged themselves on lush spring grass lanced in that way by farmers. Gas came out all right, but when the knife was withdrawn, the hole in the stomach moved away from the hole in the skin and the remaining gas forced stomach contents into the abdominal cavity. Peritonitis followed and none survived.

"One last thing," I continued. "If possible, see if your man can find some washing detergent."

The line hissed and crackled. "Washing detergent?"

"Yes. Tell him to give a teaspoonful of detergent powder— detergent, *not* soap—in water by mouth to each giraffe. He should be able to handle them if they're down and in such a bad way."

"But detergent powder in the stomach! It will froth, will it not? Like in my bath? Have I understood you correctly, Doctor? Detergent? Hein?"

"I repeat: detergent, d-e-t-e-r-g-e-n-t. Got it?"

The phone hissed more furiously than ever and the line went dead. I hurried to pack a bag while Shelagh dialled Air France. There was a plane to Paris from Manchester in ninety minutes, and in Paris I could pick up Tunisair. Shelagh followed me into the bedroom and stuck chunks of toast and grapefruit marmalade into my mouth while I used both hands to cram shirts, syringes, tins of emergency surgical equipment, drugs, dart-gun, toothpaste, mosquito cream, money belt, alarm clock and water-purifying tablets into a bulging grip. Also, never left behind, the dog-eared collected poems of John Betjeman.

"Ring Belle Vue, love, will you?" I said as I went out to the car. "The aoudads will have to wait for their chiropody. Oh, and ring Norman Whittle. I know he'll be a bit browned off but would he do my surgery and the RSPCA clinic and could he be on instead of off duty this weekend. Tell him I'm off to Tunis to see a bunch of bloated giraffes."

"Leaving me to do the dirty work," she replied, making a face. "Norman won't be pleased. This means the end of his sailing on Lake Windermere on Sunday, and you know how he feels about the way you keep rushing off."

"My profuse apologies to him," I answered. "Oh, I almost forgot—just in case detergent powder is hard to get on the Algerian border, be a good girl and nip and fetch me your packet of Daz."

At Tunis airport a rotund little man in a white suit and pink tie stood by the arrival gate sweating profusely and holding aloft a piece of cardboard with my name crayoned on it. Beside him a tall black man wearing a crocheted skull cap and grimy grey jibba was mopping the perspiration from his companion's brow with a large silk handkerchief.

M. Taouche threw his cardboard away as I walked up to him. "Thank heavens you've arrived," he squeaked, shaking me vigorously by the hand. "No, I've no further news from the south, except Abu al Ma'arri thinks that the giraffes' trouble might be because of some peaches he fed them last night. He says the fruit was over-ripe when it arrived. Pour moi, I believe he has been selling the good fruit to the villagers near the farm and keeping only the worst for my animals. It's important you go down there tout de suite."

"But aren't you coming too?"

"Sadly, no. I want to, I need to, but I have important work here in Tunis. Anyway, I am sure that I personally could be of little assistance. Nasser here will drive you, and Abu and the other men will do anything you ask." He fidgeted with his tie with fingers like cocktail sausages.

"Let's go then," I replied. "We may be too late already, you realize. Giraffes don't usually last long once they're down."

M. Taouche's forehead oozed fresh sweat globules and Nasser blotted them up as we walked out to the parking lot. Nasser jumped into a pick-up truck and Taouche pumped my hand again. "Au revoir, Doctor," he said. "In'ch Allah, all will go well down south." Nasser and I set off on the long drive to the village near Sbeitla.

The journey was interminable. We travelled south at first, passing through lemon groves and tobacco fields glowing red-gold in the afternoon sunshine, then turned west, away from the Gulf of Hammamet, into a smoky twilight, rattling over mile after long mile of scrub and steppe. Every few hundred yards we would be brought to a juddering crawl by jay-walking flocks of sheep or goats, by donkey carts slewed across the road while their owners loaded bales of esparto grass, or by smoke-belching trucks weaving dangerously down the wrong side of the road. Darkness came suddenly, an indigo sky with a half moon dodging between tufts of cloud, and the truck started to climb up into the hills. It was too cold and too bumpy to sleep, and I could see little beyond the few square feet of grey dust picked out by the headlights. Nasser, having been disappointed to hear that no, I was not a relative of Elizabeth Taylor, had long since lapsed into silence. The only words to pass between us were an occasional "Imshi, imshi!" from me, a tentative stab at the Arabic equivalent of "Faster, faster!" It brought no perceptible increase in speed.

The low houses and narrow streets of Sbeitla showed no sign of light or life. We climbed on through winding valleys where the wind blew coarse dust into the open-sided pick-up and my eyes became sore with squinting. At last, ten hours after leaving Tunis, Nasser hauled the wheel over and we lurched off the road and ran down a rutted track. The head-lights picked out a group of white buildings set on three sides round a yard—the quarantine farm. Nasser skidded to a halt and shouted something in Arabic, and Abu al Ma'arri with his three companions came out of a doorway carrying kerosene lanterns. All wore jibbas and skull caps except for Abu, who sported a tattered old French army greatcoat. He had two black teeth remaining in an ever-smiling mouth, and a snow-white scar like forked lightning zigzagged across the cornea of each eye. Like one of my chimpanzee patients at Rhenen Zoo in Holland, he had six fingers on each hand. He introduced the others, Hussein, Abdul and another Abdul.

"Venons, where are the giraffes?" I said, anxious to get started.

Abu's happy face glinted in the soft glow of the oil lamps. His melon-slice smile broadened as he said in halting French, "Five are dead, Doctor. But seven live. I pricked them as you instructed." He led the way through the darkness to a rough wooden stockade behind one of the crumbling cement-block buildings.

The feeble light of the lanterns showed me a horrific scene. All on their sides, with limbs and necks in a higgledy-piggledy heap of unnatural and agonized positions, the giraffes sprawled like a collapsed log-pile. At first it was impossible to tell the dead from the living. All had swollen bellies.

I climbed over the fence and picked my way warily between the horizontal legs, but the flickering lantern made it difficult to avoid contact with the limbs. Accidentally I brushed against a hind leg. That animal was still alive. It gave a weak kick that had none of the pile-driver force that can disembowel a predator snapping incautiously at a giraffe's heels on the African plains, but it was enough to sweep both my legs from under me. On my knees I crouched and hunched my shoulders. There were five or six iron-hard hooves within inches of my head. Touch one of those again and I could be brained. With the delicate care of a man in a minefield I rose to my feet and continued my rounds of this charnel house-cum-hospital ward. Yes, there were seven animals still breathing. The mounts of small hypodermic needles sprouted from the belly walls of some of them.

Despite my instructions to place them on the left side only—the point at which the stomach lies closest to the skin in giraffes—some needles gleamed in the lantern light on the animals' right sides. They were in the intestine and useless for releasing gas in the stomach.

The surviving animals bore their agonies with the mute fortitude typical of the dignity of my sort of patient. People often say giraffes have no voice. That is not strictly true; I have sometimes heard them give a short chirping cry. These poor creatures were utterly silent.

"Bring another lantern in and watch the feet," I shouted to Abu.

At last he understood and picked his way over to me. As he held both lanterns high, I picked one giraffe and, with a quick stab, stuck a special device for tapping off gas through the skin into the stomach. There was a flatulent puff of foul-smelling vapour from the instrument, the giraffe's belly subsided a little and then, to my dismay, a noisome khaki foam began to pour out. As I had feared, the gas in the stomachs was not in one giant bubble; it had produced a vast, fine froth that the animal could not burp. This was where the detergent came in. It would break up the foam in the animals' stomachs in the same way that a drop of detergent bubble-bath liquid will instantly destroy a soap foam.

"Did you give them detergent?" I asked the Arab.

"Detergent?" He looked puzzled.

"Poudre, poudre à laver—dans la bouche!" I struggled wretchedly with the words. Abu smiled broadly and shook his head.

I went round all the living animals and released what gas I could. All contained foam. Thank God for Shelagh's Daz, I thought, and prayed that, shocked and far gone as the giraffes were, I might be able to save at least some with my wife's washing powder. I mixed a little with water in a wine bottle. To Hussein and Abdul number one I said

slowly, "Hold the head of the giraffe. I give this drink."
I gesticulated and they understood. "Manchester United,"
said Hussein, for no apparent reason. From Greenland to
Indonesia, wherever I work, I always meet at least one person whose English extends to soccer terms, usually
"Manchester United", the most famous soccer team in the
zoological world. The man who catches the first yeti and
brings it to me for a check-up will say, if nothing else,
"Manchester United".

One by one I drenched the giraffes with the detergent
mixture. Now to tackle the intoxicating effects of the food-
stuffs fermenting in the giraffes' stomachs. I shot high-potency
vitamin B directly into the bloodstream, the treatment
applied to humans who became hospital patients after
swigging a bottle of whisky in an hour or so. A heavily
pregnant female was one of those still alive. Cautiously I
made an internal examination and felt the calf kick in his
comfortable water bed. It was amazing that it, or indeed
any of the giraffes, was still putting up a fight.

I could do no more that night. Abu al Ma'arri led the
way to my quarters. "Please, Doctor, I hope you will be
comfortable here." He showed me into a small room which
had no door and was bare except for a straw-filled mattress
on the floor, two carefully folded blankets and a picture of
President Bourguiba on the wall. The other occupant of the
room was a gecko, with a body like a smouldering crusty
heap of jewels. He scuttled behind President Bourguiba as
Nasser brought me a bowl of greasy water in which to wash
and a jam jar full of strong sweet tea. In the light of a
lantern I washed, dried myself on my shirt, drank the tea
and arranged myself uncomfortably under the blankets.
From the Arabs' room came laughter and murmurs of ad-
miration as Abu demonstrated his prowess at catching rats
with his bare hands and his ability to pop live scorpions
into his mouth, roll them about with his tongue and slowly
extrude them sting first, unharmed and unruffled, onto the

palm of his hand. Despite the noise, the cold and the blankets' reek of goat and garlic and sweat, I was soon in a deep sleep.

The next morning I was up early. One more of my patients had died during the night; the remaining six were no longer lying on their sides but sitting up on their briskets. The bellies of five, including the pregnant female, were no longer resonant like drums when I tapped them but the sixth was still very blown out. While the men dragged out the cadavers of the six dead giraffes, I went round again in the grey light before dawn giving more vitamin B and circulatory stimulants as well. By sun-up most of the animals were looking distinctly better and I started paying attention to the "bedsores" on the recumbent creatures. The still-distended sixth animal I drenched again in the hope of avoiding more drastic surgery.

Giving the drench some time to act, I looked round the dilapidated farm. Dirt was everywhere, and a long sloping dung heap ran right up to the round stone well at which Nasser and the others drew water by means of a bucket on a rope. There was a smell of manure and burnt wood. As I sat with my back against a wall, letting the sun warm my face, I heard a screeching noise from one corner of the yard. The Arabs were gathered round what looked like a dog kennel, watching intently and chattering as Hussein bent over the kennel with a stick in his hand. Abu was laughing happily and clapping his six-fingered hands. The screech came again. I could not identify it. Pig? No. Cat? Whatever it was, it did something to the hairs at the back of my neck. I stood up and walked over to the knot of men. They looked round as I arrived and parted to give me room to see.

Hussein stood in front of a wooden box with a door made of stout iron bars. Proudly he re-introduced his stick between the bars and jabbed fiercely at the interior. There was another awful screech, a scrabbling noise and a thumping and a banging from inside the box. I bent down and looked inside. The most tragic animal face that I have ever seen confronted me. The box contained a hyena. Almost as big as the container itself and with no room to turn round, there stood a full-grown striped hyena, trembling, panting, open-jawed, with every visible tooth freshly broken, one eye wide with frenzy, the other a bloody mass. His neck and forelegs were a mass of cuts and sores, his ears were torn and bleeding. By my side, Hussein thrust the stick into the box and ground it into the cheek of the hyena. It turned its head as far as it could, but no matter how it tried it could not retreat from the cruel point. "Tottenham Hotspur," crowed Hussein.

I felt my head drain of blood and my face prickle with cold anger. I straightened up and opened my mouth. I wanted to shout something, anything. Not a sound came out. The Arabs looked at me and grinned pleasantly.

"Bad dog," said Abu, leading me to the back of the hyena's prison. There were more bars there. The animal's hind-quarters showed the same loathsome lacerations as his head.

Hussein came round with his stick. "Kick off," he said, and pointed to the hyena's hock joints. I saw what he felt so proud about; the poor beast had been hamstrung. The Achilles tendons on both legs had been severed by a sharp instrument.

I stood with my back to the bars so that Hussein could not introduce his stick again. My voice returned trembling. "What do you bloody well think you're doing?" I wished I knew the worst Arabic or even French obscenities.

"Bad dog," said Abu again, his smile growing. "He kills chickens. Dirty. Smells. No good."

"Not bad dog," I said, wishing I could vomit the words. "Why do you wound him? Pourquoi blesser?"

All the Arabs laughed gently. Abu's two black teeth were bared as he explained politely, "But Doctor, to teach him. To teach him. A good idea for a bad dog, n'est-ce pas?"

Hussein, blocked from his victim by my legs, went round to the front of the box again. I roared, dashed after him and grabbed the stick from his hands. "No you don't!" I shouted, and broke the stick over my knee. "Rien va plus!" I picked up the halves of stick and broke them again and again until I found it impossible to destroy the small bits further with my fingers. The Arabs watched. Abu smiled. Hussein glared sullenly, then kicked viciously at the hyena's box and walked away. The others followed. I crouched in front of the terrified animal and looked deep into his one eye. He must have been a maverick, trapped when he left a pack in the hills to come foraging on the farm. There was nothing I could do for him. Both ends of the box were secured by rusty padlocks and even if I could have got to him, severed Achilles tendons are a major injury in man and domestic animals, not to mention wild creatures.

An hour later the giraffes were continuing to improve except for the one whose stomach was still swollen. I decided to operate and literally unload the offending food. It was my first major operation on a giraffe, a notoriously difficult species to anaesthetize safely even today in the best of animal parks, but I injected it with a stiff dose of tranquillizer, then numbed a large T-shaped area over the left abdominal wall with local anaesthetic. Abu and the others drifted over to watch as I disinfected the skin and cut through to the stomach. It was full of stinking fruit and vegetables, and the overpowering smell of alcoholic peaches confirmed the cause of the distended bellies. With my bare hand and arm I reached deep into the digesting broth, cupped my palm and ladled out handful after handful of the stuff, making sure as I cast it aside that some would accidentally splatter my audience's jibbas. Then I placed a small quantity of penicillin into the remaining stomach contents to knock out over-enthusiastic fermenting bacteria and stitched up. But as I threaded my needle, positioned the layers of muscle and skin with my forceps and swept the persistent flies from the operation site I could think of only one thing: the hyena.

That night I sat alone on the floor of my room to eat my supper of mutton stew and pitta bread. The giraffes were almost forgotten as I agonized over the plight of the hyena. If I broke the padlocks off the kennel, the poor beast could not get anywhere. I knew the Arabs were giving him food and water occasionally; he was likely to stay alive for their cruel amusement for weeks. Then the answer came to me.

By eleven o'clock the Arabs had gone to bed. The farm was quiet except for the occasional bleat of a goat and the restless murmurings of drowsing pigeons. After an hour or so I lit my lantern, took what I needed from my bag and tiptoed out into the yard. No one stirred. Holding the lantern high to avoid slipping into the dung heap, I quietly approached the hyena's box. I could hear him breathing tensely in the darkness and could imagine his pulse beginning to race and his shoulder hairs bristling as he sensed my approach. I pulled the syringe and injection bottle from my pocket, filled the syringe and blew out the lantern. Going round to the back of the box, I put a hand gently through the bars and felt a quivering ham muscle. The hyena growled lightly. Quickly I jabbed the hypodermic into his ham and pressed the plunger. He gave a short screech and I pulled away the empty syringe. I looked round; no one had been roused by the sound of the "bad dog."

I crept swiftly back to my room without relighting my lantern, so I did not see the dung heap until I walked into it. I did not mind, for as I sat on my mattress decontaminating my shoes with cotton wool, I knew that the hyena would by now have passed painlessly into oblivion. Rarely in zoo work do I have to destroy an animal; even with modern humane methods it is unpleasant work, bringing death to a living creature. But giving a shot of lethal T61 to the hyena that dark North African night was one of the most fulfilling things I have ever done as a veterinarian.

Next day the giraffes were improving still, and the one on

which I had operated was catching the others up fast. I gave more injections, and by the second afternoon I was delighted to see that all bar one, the pregnant female, were on their feet. They were groggy and only picked at the hay I had told the men to give them, but at least they were up. "When a giraffe goes down," Matt Kelly used to tell me, "he never ever gets up." The pregnant female was running with milk and making determined but unsuccessful attempts to rise. With any luck I could get away in a couple of days.

The third morning, going round the back of the farm buildings in the direction of the unpleasant hole in the rocks that was our toilet, I nearly walked straight into a tethered group of six camels, each with a large bundle of esparto grass on its back. The nearest spat balefully in my direction. Beyond them, Abu al Ma'arri and the others were talking intently to four other men, dressed like themselves in jibbas and skull caps. As I approached, the strangers began talking furiously in Arabic, addressing their remarks to Abu and looking suspiciously at me.

"Salaam aleikum," I said.

Only Abu answered, his smile flickering uncertainly. "Aleikum salaam, Doctor. You come for breakfast? Nasser will make tea presently and bring it to you."

The camel men stood silently staring at me. I certainly was not going to obey the call of nature with this lot watching.

"Merci," I replied. "After that we must begin darting the giraffes." The animals were no longer safe to inject by hand, except the pregnant female, and I would administer the necessary drugs by dart-gun.

I walked back to the yard, wondering uneasily what the Arabs and their new cronies had been nattering about. Twenty minutes later Nasser appeared with the tea. I drank it while I loaded my 10cc darts with chemicals, then went to look at the animals. The zebras were eating a new consignment of food the lorry had brought in yesterday, the rhinos

328

were still sleeping and the giraffes looked in fine fettle. None of the puncture holes in their bellies seemed to be going the wrong way and the operation wound on the one animal was healing neatly. I was as pleased as Punch. The mother-to-be was sitting up alertly and chewing her cud. Maybe today she would be up.

Suddenly there was a horrible strident scream. My first thought was, what the hell are they torturing now? But this sounded like a human and it came from behind the buildings, where the camels were. I ran out of the yard and round the corner. All the Arabs, Abu's band and the strangers, were gathered round the head of a standing camel. Two men were hanging tightly onto its leather bridle as it bucked and gurgled. Nearby Abu whirled round and round, hopping on one foot like a dervish. It was he who had screamed, I saw, for with his good left hand he clutched the wrist of his right, a pulped and bloody mass from which two of the six fingers dangled down, attached only by shreds of skin. As I watched in amazement the camel suddenly reared up, arched its neck and, with a bubbling roar, spat out from its mouth a flat oblong object about the same size and shape as a tobacco pouch. One of the camel men swiftly snatched it up and dropped it down the neck of his jibba, but not before I had time to see that it was made of oilskin and was neatly tied with cord. Every one of the men, except Abu, who continued his distressed dance, had his eyes fixed on me. Suddenly I realized what was in the pouch and how Abu had come to have his fingers ground between the powerful molars of a camel. Fear took a firm hold of my stomach and gouged deep. I had just glimpsed a rare, hidden, evil thing, the bungling of one link in a long and filthy chain that stretched from the poppy fields of Asia to the junkies of Times Square and Piccadilly Circus.

Abu's greatcoat was now soaking with blood. The men made no move towards him. They just stood looking at me. Pointing at Abu, I said, "Doctor. Médecin très nécessaire!"

Abu stopped gyrating and looked at me. He was not smiling. "Non," he said firmly. "I will come to your room presently for attention."

"But . . ." I began.

"I cannot go to the doctor," interrupted the injured man.

Hussein stepped forward and I froze to my marrow as he slowly pointed at me and then, with the same finger, drew a line across his throat. "Offside," he said. "Penalty kick."

Dizzy with fright, I went back to my room and took from my instrument box the largest scalpel I had. Wrapping a wad of cotton wool round the cutting end, I stuck it securely down my sock under cover of my right trouser leg. It was sheer fright, not melodramatic imagination, that spurred me on as I rammed a wicked-looking rhinoceros needle on the end of a 10cc flying syringe down the barrel of the dart-pistol. Its sharp point poked from the muzzle. Locking the breech, I cocked the pistol at full gas pressure. Then I sat on my mattress and laid the puny weapon within easy reach. I reflected that one of the lesser, but to me saddest, miseries in the whole squalid affair was that it was yet another example of the satanic ingenuity with which Man is prepared to destroy innocent fellow creatures in furthering his own ends. Those grumpy, imperious, fascinating camels tethered outside were unwitting couriers of vice. Once safely across the border into Algeria, they would be slaughtered and the precious cargo retrieved from their stomachs. I almost wished there might be some crooked veterinarian in the pay of the traffickers who, by an operation similar to the one I had performed on the giraffe, could recover the oilskin packages less wastefully.

Abu broke into these bizarre daydreams by appearing at the door of my room. I leapt to my feet, dart-gun in hand, but his face was haggard and he silently held out his bitten fingers.

"You need a hospital or doctor, you know," I told him.

He shook his head vigorously. "No. You can do it. Have

330

you not treated one camel bitten by another?" He stared hard at me. "Do it and forget it. It is nothing." Then, deliberately spacing his words, "It—is—nothing. Please remember that."

The menace behind Abu's words hung in the air as I cleaned up the stumps of the pair of fingers. I was preparing what little I had in the way of dressings when there was a shout from outside. Abdul number two came dashing in and jabbered excitedly in Arabic. Abu said, "The giraffe with calf—she has got up but has crashed down again."

Leaving Abu, I pushed through the knot of camel men who must have been watching the door of my room and dashed round to the giraffe stockade. There against the wooden fence lay the female, her legs still and her neck hideously twisted. She was not breathing and her eyes had the languorous gaze into infinity that I knew too well. She was dead. In falling she had broken her neck on the top rail of the fence. Stunned, I stood for a split second and then shouted to Nasser, who had come running, "Quick, a knife. *Vite!*"

Like a magician, from under his jibba he produced a sharp stiletto. I took it, jumped over the fence and, running over to the dead giraffe, for the first time in my life performed the original Caesarean operation. With a long, raking slash the womb was revealed, bulging between still flickering muscle sheets. I grabbed its glistening outer surface, steadied it, then cut again quickly and carefully. I thrust my hand in and felt a warm, slippery forelimb. With no time or need for elegance, I held the leg tightly and gave a great heave. The ungainly, tangled body of a baby giraffe rose into the sunlight through the lengthening split in the womb. I plopped it down onto the earth and stood gasping with the effort. The little form twitched. I knelt down and felt the heart. It was beating!

With a wild shout I picked up its hind legs and stood it on its nose to clear its mouth and nostrils. I slapped its chest, there was a sneeze, and an eyelid fringed with the most glamorously long lashes outside Hollywood fluttered. I called Nasser to help me pick up the heavy creature once again and we shook it with all our might. Down again. Up again. More slapping of the chest and then suddenly, wonderfully, the little calf was breathing stickily but strongly. Caesar himself had been born, it was said, in just this manner, an orphan from the womb. This little fellow was going to live, and I christened him Julius on the spot. He wriggled and sat up. His large round dark eyes looked at me, and I wondered whether, like ducks, baby giraffes are imprinted and emotionally bound to the first living creature they see.

The whimsy that Julius might be inclined to call me "Momma" vanished as I heard voices behind me. Looking round I saw the camel men talking to Hussein and Nasser. They seemed angry, and one of them pointed briefly in my direction. In the excitement of Julius's arrival I had forgotten other, darker things. With what I hoped was a disarmingly cheerful wave, I called out, "The baby is hungry. I must take him to my room and feed him," and began to half carry, half drag the struggling giraffe in the direction of the yard. My heart bounded as Julius and I staggered round the corner. The yard was empty and there was Nasser's pick-up truck parked by the dung heap—with the keys in. Without ceremony I hauled the baby across the uneven ground and pushed him like a sack of potatoes over the tailgate of the open vehicle. Furtively looking round to check that there was still no one about, I took off my jacket, wrapped it round Julius's legs and firmly tied the sleeves together.

Then, with adrenalin flooding through my veins, I ran into my room, grabbed the dart-gun and my grip and dashed back to the truck, dropping bottles of medicine, artery forceps and other bits of equipment on the way. I did not turn back for them, but as I was about to leap into the driving seat my eye caught the metal pot of mutton stew for the midday meal simmering on a wood fire outside the Arabs' room. As if by instinct I reached into the grip and fumbled for my small tin of Altan, a powerful horse and zebra purgative that looks like cayenne pepper and has very little taste. Still I was alone in the yard. A moment later, Abu al Ma'arri and his friends had enough Altan in their meal to produce dramatic effects in four draught horses, and I hoped they would pass a distressing and cathartic twenty-four hours.

"Compliments of one hyena, you bastards," I shouted as I threw away the empty tin and ran yet again to the truck where Julius lay uncomplaining and wide-eyed. Safely aboard, I turned on the ignition and pressed the starter button. The engine fired and I let out the clutch with a bang. With wheels spinning in a shower of grit, dust and manure we shot forward and charged out of the yard and up the rutted track. Ten minutes later, with a little giraffe sucking gently on my right ear, I roared through the main street of Sbeitla. With only one stop for fuel, Julius and I went flat out for Tunis.

Half a day later, weary and covered in dust, I was in the office of Herr Mueller, the surprised curator of Tunis Zoo. Julius needed expert rearing and with luck I would be on the next plane for Paris. "Take good care of him," I said before I left. "He's my boy!"

I just had time to call on M. Taouche in his lemon-blossom-scented garden and to tell my story to my client. When I came to the bit about Abu al Ma'arri and how he went back to having ten fingers like the rest of us, M. Taouche closed his eyes and chewed energetically on his cheroot. Whether he was involved with the sinister affair I could only guess. He said nothing except to thank me and to promise me a bonus along with my fee when I rendered my account. That account was never paid: three weeks later M. Taouche died of a heart attack.

Eleven

Christianity, unlike some of the world's other great religions, has no particular theology of animals. After establishing that the Deity constructed whales and other marine creatures on the fifth day and turned his attention to terrestrial fauna on the sixth, it has fussed and feuded pretty exclusively over one often rather unattractive and unreliable species of naked ape. True, Thomas Aquinas split scholarly hairs over the nature of the brutish soul, and Francis would have been on the Assisi branch committee of the RSPCA if there had been such a thing in the twelfth century; but Protestant bishops can be run to earth in the huntin', shootin', fishin' fraternity, devout Orthodox peasants of the Mediterranean trap small songbirds by the million, Latin Catholics leave Mass to attend the ritual torture of black bulls on a Sunday afternoon. I find it odd. The more I have studied, looked at and handled animals, seen their intrinsic beauty, the perfection with which they spin their strands in the web of life, the more I have tilted towards a unified theology of all living creatures, the scorpion and the maggot just as much as the tiger or the whale. Dead, beneath my autopsy knife, they reveal not just themselves but also what I am: part of the all-purposeful, all-beautiful, endless wheel of growth and change, of death and regeneration. Nothing is chaos. Look close, with seeing eyes, and even a blob of pus is a wondrous, active, ordered microcosm.

The Church of England often exhibits a rather dotty concern for animals, however, which I experienced soon after my return from Tunisia when a vicar friend of mine in a country parish across the Pennines in Yorkshire invited me to read the lesson at a special church service for pets. The occasion was graced by the presence of a bishop, who preached a sermon full of round plummy aphorisms about sparrows and their welfare-state existence, Daniel's way with big cats and how much happier we all would be if we lived like armadilloes, although for the life of me I could not make out what it was about these nocturnal miniature tanks that so impressed the gaitered cleric as epitomizing the Christian ideal. To illustrate his point he produced a small, curled-up representative of the species from beneath his purple cassock. It had been borrowed from a nearby zoo, and its dramatic appearance had an electrifying effect on the chancel full of nodding choirboys.

Unfortunately His Lordship mishandled the armour-plated ball and dropped it, whereupon it rolled down the pulpit steps, galvanizing the choirboys still more. A full complement leapt unceremoniously from their seats in both front rows and scrabbled to retrieve the creature, which made off towards the organ. The armadillo won by a short head, nipped behind the forest of pipes and was not seen again until halfway through Evensong a week later.

The young congregation would never have guessed from the bishop's admonition, "In being kind to beasts we are honouring the work of God's hands," that the reverend gentleman hunted two days a week and was the proud possessor of a well-used pair of Purdey shotguns. There were children with dogs and cats, budgies and rabbits. Some clustered outside the porch with their ponies. Doting parents, sly-eyed schoolboys with grass snakes in jars and toads in their pockets, girls clutching goldfish bowls, all sat side by side in the pews of the seventeenth-century stone church. There was one lad with a monkey, a chunky, muscle-bound pig-tailed macaque. It continually raised its eyebrows towards the preacher in the typical mildly challenging grimace of macaques, which made it seem like a sceptical, possibly agnostic listener. Its owner kept a firm grip on the leash with which it was restrained.

Blessing animals is, I suppose, a cut above doing the same thing to motor bikes or lawn mowers. Services for pets at least provide the small boys who attend such gatherings with the hope that something might turn up. On this occasion it already had, and the absconding armadillo brought back memories of forfeiting my place on the annual choir outing to Blackpool: a white mouse released under the long blue cassock of a middle-aged lady chorister at St. Edmund's Church had resulted in the unusual spectacle of the lady vaulting clean over the choir stall in the middle of the reading of the banns and streaking off into the vestry.

". . . and so I leave you with these words. Kindness, patience, goodwill to all creatures, not least the wonderful creatures that bring us so much joy. In the name of the Father" etc, etc. The bishop came to the end of his address. A final hymn was sung and everyone trooped outside. The bishop was going to move among the crowd assembled in the churchyard and bless the beasts—human and otherwise.

In the churchyard it was warm and sunny. My part in the proceedings was over. I stood watching the milling crowd and saying good-bye to the vicar before making my way back over the hills to Rochdale. The bishop was in a jolly, expansive mood as he wandered through the chattering throng, his right hand raised in benediction. He cooed to the budgies thrust up towards his face, tugged the ears of some of the dogs and had his picture taken as he sat perilously on a donkey. All at once the boy who had brought the macaque barged through the crowd waving a leather leash, at the end of which there was no sign of a monkey. The press of jostling humans and animals parted like the Red Sea before Moses as a squat brown figure bounded between them. The pig-tailed macaque shot down the church path, through the ancient lych-gate and straight through the partly open window of a sparkling new Bentley parked directly outside.

336

He was pursued by his owner, closely followed by all the small boys present, and behind came the rest of us.

Inside the car the monkey was having a fine time. He quickly pulled open the door of the glove compartment and spilled out all the contents. A tin of pipe tobacco lying on the front seat was thrown out of the window, and the plastic cover of the interior light was prized off and bitten in two.

"Harry!" shouted the monkey's owner. "Stop that and come here!" He opened the car door a fraction.

Harry bared his wicked-looking canine teeth, grimaced as histrionically as any villain of Japanese theatre, and savagely bit the right hand of his owner as it moved towards him. Bleeding profusely and in obvious pain, the gallant lad advanced his other hand. Harry grabbed it, pulled it up to his jaws and lacerated the palm with a slash of his fangs. The poor boy fell back and the door was slammed to. The vicar led the casualty away.

By now the bishop had pushed through the crowd. "I say," he said, his genial expression fading fast, "that's my car, you know." He looked through the window at the macaque, which by now was flying round the interior like an angry bluebottle in a jam jar. "We really ought to get the chappie out of there." No one volunteered.

Then Harry spotted the dashboard, a surface bristling with interesting knobs and levers, glinting bits of chrome, plastic and glass. Just beneath the dashboard was an inviting twist of coloured wire which the inquiring mind of the would-be engineer could not ignore. As he reached down and pulled it there was a satisfying click, and the panel covering the tangle of assorted gadgetry behind the dashboard fell away.

"We must get that monkey out of my car," said the bishop, pale but calm.

The jungle of gleaming electronics now exposed fascinated Harry. With one powerful leathery hand he grasped a bunch of wires and plugs and pulled. They came away and bits of metal and plastic tinkled onto the floor. The electric clock stopped.

Harry looked at the bishop, raised his eyebrows sceptically and pressed the horn button. As its wires had just been disconnected it did not work. Harry pulled and the horn button broke off. He threw it out of the window.

"Please, sir, you haven't blessed Chirpy yet," said a little girl, worming her way through to the bishop's side and straining upwards with a fistful of budgerigar.

"Hrumph," said His Lordship.

Meanwhile I was marvelling at the speed with which a small monkey was dismantling a solidly built vehicle. If a gang of Harrys could be trained to work as fast assembling the various pieces of metalwork that now lay around the inside of the car, the labour problems of the automobile industry would be a thing of the past.

"Somebody do something! This bloody monkey is tearing my car apart!"

"Please, sir, you haven't done Chirpy," persisted the little girl, her budgerigar by now almost suffocated in her grip.

"Next year, next year!" shouted the bishop, purple-faced now as well as purple-robed. He patted the child so hard on the head that I expected to see her reel away cross-eyed.

I must confess I had thoroughly enjoyed the unique experience. The inside of the car was now in utter ruin. Harry was sitting in the back seat, looking round for anything he might have missed. Stirring myself, I decided I must do something. Pig-tailed macaques are one of the toughest and most dangerous species of monkey, and to tackle one single-handed in the close confines of a car would be foolhardy. I had no dart-gun with me, but I did have some anaesthetic in my car and plenty of syringes. I sent the vicar's wife to fetch a banana while I inspected the partly opened car window. The gap had been big enough for Harry to get in, so he could get out as well if he wished, and I could not wind the window up without opening the door. I sent a choirboy into the church for one of the thick hassocks, or kneeling pads. "Now," I said when he returned, "get up on the roof of the car just above the window, and when I give you the word jam the hassock hard down over the side."

Enthusiastically the boy scrambled up the gleaming paintwork. The bishop leaned against the lych-gate groaning, a hand across his eyes.

I held a piece of banana through the window. Harry sniffed at it, passed it as undoctored and ate it. It tasted good. I proffered another piece, holding it just outside the window gap. Harry slowly put his hand out to take it. "Jam it down!" I yelled to the boy on the roof as I seized Harry's hand and pulled with all my strength. Harry screamed and struggled vigorously but the boy with the hassock had narrowed the gap enough to stop me pulling an agitated twenty-five pounds of steely muscle and teeth completely out of the car. In half a second I had plunged the hypodermic into Harry's arm and whammed down the plunger. I released my grip and Harry retreated onto the rear window ledge, hollering furiously. In two minutes he began to drool, his eyes became dreamy and he emptied his bowels over the bishop's top hat. In another two minutes it was all over; Harry fell into a drowsing heap on the back seat and I opened the door to pull him out. We had been lucky— he would never be taken in that way again.

There was no hope of getting the bishop's car to start. It had to be towed to the next town for major repairs. I offered to drop His Lordship at the station on my way home.

"Many thanks, Doctor," he said as I stopped outside the ticket office. "Wouldn't have your job for the world. Damned brutes!"

If the Right Reverend gentleman's last two words are literally true, Old Nick is going to have a hell of a time dealing with Harry one of these days.

Despite my experience with the bishop and his Bentley, in the normal run of things I do not have to cross swords with the Established Church. With other faiths things can be different. There are many Moslem Pakistani folk living in the north of England, and at certain religious festivals they slaughter lambs. The rules lay down that the sacrifices must on no account be eaten by human beings, but it is perfectly acceptable for the lambs to be fed to wild beasts. At these times vans containing beautifully dressed and wholesome carcasses arrive at zoos and Pakistani gentlemen request that the meat be fed to the big cats. Solemnly the lamb is unloaded into the meat store and the van driver goes away, happy in the knowledge that the tenets of the faith have been upheld. Later, nominally Christian zoo keepers can be seen assembling in the zoo kitchen, armed with meat saws and cleavers and ready to decide who gets what for their family's Sunday joints.

The Moslem calendar was pinned up in the office of one head keeper whose animals I treated, with red lines marking the weeks when the staff could be sure to dine daily on mutton. Even the youngest assistant keeper of the Pets' Corner could tell you when Ramadan ended, although I doubt if he even knew what month Easter was in. Beside the head keeper's calendar were pinned two other pieces of paper. One listed the staff in order of precedence for the share-out:

Zoo director:	Loin, 2 shoulders, 2 legs, breast
Veterinarian:	2 shoulders, 2 legs, also likes kidneys, breast
Head keeper:	2 shoulders, 1 leg, liver, breast
Asst head keeper:	1 leg, kidneys
Head bird keeper:	4 cutlets
Reptile keeper:	1 cutlet, head

and so on down to:

Trainee keeper:	liver.

340

The other piece of paper was most important. When the lamb came, it came in abundance, and the head keeper was hard put to it to see that his staff's taste for the meat did not become jaded. It read:

Suggestions for all staff:

Mondays:	Lamb Argenteuil
Tuesdays:	Carré d'agneau Dordonnaise
Wednesdays:	Lamb Kashmir
Thursdays:	Kebabs
Fridays:	Navarin of lamb
Saturdays:	Lamb and vegetable casserole
Sundays:	Epigrammes d'agneau

N.B. Recipes for the above can be had from Nellie in the cash office.

Nellie kept a pile of duplicated instructions, for which useful service she received a choice roasting shoulder from the head keeper every Saturday during the sacrificing season.

Came the sad day when one of the Pakistani meat donors forgot his gloves and returned to the zoo stores shortly after making a delivery. Inside he found a dozen amateur butchers merrily dividing the spoils according to the list of precedence under the eagle eye of the head keeper. The scene that ensued, with the Pakistani snatching up a chopper and advancing hysterically on the red-faced sacrilegists, could have been the start of a holy war. Luckily the zoo director made an opportune appearance (coming to collect the ingredients for his favourite crown roast with cranberry stuffing) and the matter was temporarily shelved.

Some days later a polite Pakistani called at my home and introduced himself as the imam of the community whose sacrifice had been profaned by the zoo. Wild beasts were not particularly common in the north of England, at least not ones big enough to devour whole sheep carcasses, so the zoos were an essential means of disposal. Dumping on the municipal rubbish tip or incineration were out of the question. Could I advise him professionally?

Much as I had enjoyed my illicit share of meat, I was ethically bound to give him the best possible advice. "When you have sacrificed the lambs," I said, "splash some non-poisonous green vegetable dye over the carcasses. That will not harm lions and tigers but will render the meat un-appetizing to humans."

The imam thought for a moment. "Yes, I can recommend that to my people. Such colouring will not defile the sacrifice."

It was settled. Supplies of sacrificed lambs to the zoo resumed. The big cats enjoyed the new arrangements and the threat of a jehad erupting in the zoo grounds receded. But the head keeper and his staff had the very devil of a job cutting any uncoloured meat out of the carcasses, and I noticed that the precedence list in his office had been altered. Now the very bottom entry on the list read:

Veterinarian: 1 kidney (if any left over).

The zoo which narrowly escaped being decimated by a holy war was one of several in the north of England which I was by now visiting regularly. Belle Vue was still my major zoo client, however, as it had been throughout the five years since I took over the care of its animals from Norman Whittle, and there Matt Kelly had noticed something odd about the way Simba, a four-month-old lion cub, was moving.

Simba led a happy, carefree life with his parents and brothers and sisters until one day, for no obvious reason, his father suddenly bit him on the back. The wound did not look bad, just a pair of small puncture holes in the skin, but the cub started to become wobbly on his hind legs. When Matt called me in I found from an X-ray of Simba's back that he was becoming steadily paralysed; one of the adult lion's teeth had penetrated down to his backbone and a spinal abscess had developed.

I anaesthetized Simba and took him back to Rochdale in my car and there explored the area deep in the lumbar region of his spine, where the dirty tooth had set up a nasty pocket of diseased, pus-filled bone. With a scalpel and a special spoon-shaped gouge I removed the infected bone and put a small rubber drain tube into the wound. Stitched up, Simba looked like an inflatable toy lion with a red rubber valve projecting out of the middle of his back, ready for someone to attach a bicycle pump. Now for a long period of post-operative nursing; Simba was partially paralysed and incontinent, symptoms which would not go overnight. I needed somewhere to hospitalize him where I could keep a personal eye on him, and it was Shelagh who came up with the answer.

Our home in Rochdale, a Jacobean stone farmhouse on the edge of the moor, had one acre of walled market garden attached. Shelagh decided to build a lion hospital there. To the passer-by, and eventually to the tax-man, who considered the lion hospital a poor cover story to use in industrial Lancashire when we were claiming the building expenses, it looks like a wooden garden shed. It later became the home of Henry, my favourite and most intelligent goat, who no doubt considered it a perfect goat shed. It was erected, however, Henry and the tax man notwithstanding, as a bona fide, custom-built lion hospital. There Simba would be nursed back to health and to full use of his limbs and bladder.

This was the sort of thing Shelagh loved. While I attended to the medical side, giving the daily injections and checking the reflexes, Shelagh was Simba's nurse, physiotherapist, cook, companion and latrine attendant all rolled into one. Every two hours she meticulously bathed the protesting cub in baby soap and water so that his hind parts would not become sore because of his incontinence, dried him on one of a specially commandeered bunch of my bath towels and smeared the vulnerable areas with silicone ointment. Nourished on an appetizing steak tartare mixture that had me drooling at the mouth, and encouraged to use his legs outside on the grass when it was fine, Simba gradually mended.

In these days when lion cubs are cheaper than ten a penny, when the boxes they are carried in cost more than themselves and they are worth a hundred times more as a dead skin than they could possibly be alive, it is sad to reflect that the very success of breeding and safely rearing lion cubs in zoos and safari parks over recent years has made some lion owners regard these big cats as characterless and as expendable as sausages out of a machine. I know they are lazy fellows but, like every other animal, the more you know them the more fascinating their ways and workings are seen to be. That was something Shelagh and I quickly learnt from Simba.

After a summer of Shelagh's physiotherapy, and to the relief of the farm cats who could not pursue voles in the market garden without finding themselves the quarry of a gleefully growling creature with sandy hair and enormous paws, it was time for the fully recovered lion to go back to the zoo. First I took him to make his and my debut on television. We were going to be interviewed about the cub's paralysis and subsequent recovery.

It became obvious when I led him into the studios on a dog lead that Simba, by now grown to an impressive size, was by no means filled with awe at passing the portals of the Temple of the Holy Box. An extra in full costume and make-up as a Roman senator came fussing down a corridor towards us. Busy primping himself in a small hand mirror, he had not noticed the lion ambling along by my side. His sandalled feet came level with us and Simba decided it was time for a bit of provocative rough-housing. As the senator passed, the lion clubbed with sheathed claws at the back of his knees, buckling them and bringing him crashing to the floor in a flurry of toga and velveteen jockey briefs. Apologizing, I helped the unharmed but fluttering actor to his feet. Then he saw Simba sitting blandly on his haunches

344

waiting for me to resume our exploration.

"Ooh, my God, darling, what's that?" he exclaimed, clutching me with both hands like a scrawny vulture. "Have props brought a real lion in for the *Julius Caesar?*" He scurried off, theatrically casting the loose end of his toga over his shoulder.

We found the studio where the interviewer was waiting for us. Simba did not like the lights nor the way the sound man seemed to tease him with the boom microphone, swinging it to and fro above his head. It was just out of reach; perhaps, Simba thought, it was some sort of game. He decided to find out. With a great leap upwards he managed to get one set of claws on the microphone before the sound man could whisk it away. The wire-gauze casing of the microphone crashed to the floor. Simba looked up with watery eyes; not a bad game, this.

When I eventually settled in my seat with the lion at my side, Simba had a call of nature. Waddling away from me into the middle of the floor, he squatted and relieved his bowels. Within moments the studio reeked with the heavy and unforgettable odour of lion droppings. I retrieved the animal and asked for a shovel and bucket. "Don't worry yourself," they told me, "it will be dealt with." Minutes went by and it wasn't. The smell got stronger. Two men came into the studio, walked over to the pile of droppings, talked for a couple of minutes over it and then went out. The droppings continued to sit noisomely in the middle of the studio floor. People wandered around with contorted features and handkerchiefs over their noses, regarding the monument to Simba's healthy colonic function from a respectful distance. I asked again for something with which to clear up the mess. No one seemed inclined to listen.

"Now come on," I said loudly, beginning to lose my patience, "all I need is a shovel and I'll do the cleaning up in a trice."

An elegantly dressed girl assistant hurried over to me.

"Please, Dr. Taylor, please," she said earnestly, taking my arm, "don't get involved. It's the unions."

"Unions—what unions?" I asked incredulously.

"Well, the question is, which union in the building should be responsible for cleaning up the, er, stuff?"

"But it can be done in less time than it takes to tell. What unions are involved?"

"There's the union that the television centre's normal cleaning staff belong to and there's the quite separate union for the people inside the studio here, the scene shifters and so on."

"And you mean they can't agree who clears up the, er, stuff?"

"No."

"Both unions want the privilege of shovelling that lot?"

"Well, not exactly. You see this type of, well, dirt is extraordinary according to the rule book. It's not only who does the cleaning, but how much extra pay will the chosen ones get."

More folk were now inspecting the mound of excrement which was the centre of the dispute and walking in circles round it, conversing intently. It might have been a suspected bomb. Another girl assistant came in with an air-freshener aerosol and filled the room with the stench of cheap rose perfume. Mixed with the existing odour of lion it made a still more repulsive blend.

"Well, what's going on now?" I growled in disgust.

"They're having a meeting in the corridor outside. Then it will be decided."

Time went by. The girl drifted off. "Oh, look here," I said to the assembled company, without addressing anyone in particular, "if it will ease matters, couldn't I as a paid-up member of the Lion Shitshifters Brotherhood get you off the hook by removing the stuff with a piece of newspaper?"

346

"'Fraid not, old boy. You're not a member of the right union," replied a voice.

Another ten minutes went by, with Simba's troublemaking offering lying centre stage, before a man came into the studio and announced that the matter had been settled. In just under ten seconds two fellows with dustpans and brushes had the studio floor clear and sparkling.

"Which union won?" I asked the girl assistant.

"The scene shifters. They argued that the, er, stuff should be regarded as a prop, not as ordinary dirt. Eventually that was accepted. The lion, er, stuff was a prop so they shifted it. As it was a prop extraordinaire and could be classed as dirty work in the rule book, they got a bonus."

I wished Shelagh had had a union from which to claim a bonus for all the lion, er, stuff that she had removed from Simba's convalescent home in the market garden at Rochdale.

There is of course a special satisfaction in helping zoo babies such as Simba, so I was delighted when Katja, one of the Belle Vue chimpanzees, presented Robert the thumb-remover with a daughter. Christened Topaz, this sister for Lee, in whose bed the remains of my pink shirt were still to be seen, had something of her brother's adventurous nature and an apparent interest in race relations! The quarters for the orang-utans and chimpanzees are side by side at Belle Vue, although they are separated by a solid brick wall so the two groups are unable to see one another. At the front of the centrally heated indoor compartments are widely spaced and decorative iron grilles, and outside these there is armoured glass sheeting dividing the animals from the humans and keeping airborne human bugs and viruses at bay. Between the grilles and the glass is a narrow passageway that runs without interruption the length of the house.

Normally baby chimpanzees do not venture far from their mothers, and although we realized that they were small enough to squeeze through the grille at the cage front, we had never known one do so—until Topaz came along. She would run happily in and out of the cage, playing some game such as chasing her shadow and passing between the metal bars with ease. Katja, her mother, did not seem to mind, and the little animal always returned after a few moments' expedition into what for her was the outside world. But one day, as Shelagh and I were standing with Len outside the plate glass watching young Topaz play, she suddenly did something new, something that made us all gasp as we instantly appreciated the possibly serious consequences.

Leaving the chimp cage she moved along the passageway to the left until she found herself for the first time in her life standing outside the living room of the orang-utans. She was fascinated. There through the grille was the great Harold, patriarch and sage of his group, sitting in the middle of the domestic circle with Jane and his other wives tending the orang babies, doing a bit of grooming of their lord and master and sorting through the day's ration of fruit and vegetables which Len had carefully mixed with their wood-wool bedding to set them a sort of treasure hunt to pass the time. The three of us stood in growing apprehension as little Topaz stared goggle-eyed at the covey of chestnut-coloured men of the woods, as their name means in Malay.

Of the three types of great ape, gorilla, chimpanzee and orang-utan, orangs have always been my favourite. They are a peaceable, gentle and tolerant species, and I have become much closer to them than to the saturnine gorillas or mercurial chimps. Nevertheless they can be swiftly vicious and immensely strong if provoked, as when Len had lost a toe and half a shoe to a liverish Harold. It was impossible to predict what might happen to a little foreigner like Topaz who suddenly came upon the scene. Harold and the family had already noticed the visitor waiting without. It was too late for us to do anything like rushing round to the back of the house. We might as well stay where we were, keep our fingers crossed and hope that the young chimp would quickly wander back to Katja before she was set upon as an intruder.

Having gazed at the family group from outside the bars, Topaz apparently found it most inviting, for without more ado she popped through the grille and shuffled up to the mighty Harold with her lips drawn back and her teeth showing in the grin that indicates friendship among chimpanzees. Now for it, I thought. If Harold or one of the females was in a bad mood, little Topaz might be pulled limb from limb before our eyes.

In fact, quite the reverse happened. The baby chimp was accepted into the orang family circle as if she was one of their young daughters who had just come home from school. She took her place at the feet of Harold, who looked down his nose at her and stuck out one index finger, apparently for her to play with. He never moved another muscle. The baby orangs came and sat next to her and solicitously arranged the wood-wool bedding round her bottom to make her more comfortable. Jane half peeled a banana and thrust it into Topaz's face. It was a wonderful spectacle. Here was Uncle Harold playing perfect host and benefactor to his favourite niece from next door; you would not have guessed that he had never before clapped eyes on her. Topaz enjoyed it immensely, and before long was sitting on Uncle Harold's capacious pot belly and gleefully wrapping his long tresses of red hair about her. Harold indulged her like a sultan with one of his numerous offspring.

Shelagh and I stayed watching the touching sight for half an hour. Then we saw Katja come to the grille of the adjoining cage and start chattering anxiously. She could almost have been calling to her infant, "Come on back home now, Topaz. You really can't presume on too much of Uncle Harold's time. Be a good girl and say thank you politely. There will always be another day."

Topaz slid off Harold's belly, put a finger to the lips of

the female orangs in a gesture of closeness and went back the way she had come. Katja gathered her up in her arms, far less hairy than those of Uncle Harold, and took her back to father Robert, who does not possess Harold's belly either. Were they saying to her, "Well, tell us all about the folk next door, and did you have a good time?"

So began a delightful association. When Robert and Katja were busy or had had enough of the ever-active chimp, Topaz would slope off and spend a few hours with the neighbours. On at least one occasion she was seen to take Uncle Harold a present of a carrot.

The visiting only stopped when Topaz grew too large to slip between the bars of the grille, but by that time she had other things outside to interest her. Ray Legge liked to take her on his rounds through the zoo and would sometimes let her sit with him in his office when he did his paperwork. She revelled in new places and new faces, and was particularly interested in a group of Arabian camels that had come into quarantine at Belle Vue some months before. They were a sorry sight when they arrived. Every one was thoroughly infested with the microscopic little mite that causes sarcoptic mange, a very common skin disease of camels that is related to human scabies. We began an intensive programme to try to rid the grumpy animals of the troublesome complaint. We sprayed them and dipped them and anointed the bleeding areas each day with soothing creams and ointments, but the mites had burrowed deep into the skin and were protected from chemicals by all the thickening and scaliness they had produced. In the end I decided to bring on the big guns of organo-phosphorus insecticides, helping them to penetrate the layers over the mites by scrubbing off the scales with specially bought yard brushes and hot water.

Topaz accompanied Ray on his many visits to supervise the keepers brushing and scrubbing the insecticides into the camels, and she became familiar with their routine of filling buckets with hot water, adding the chemicals and then applying them vigorously to the bodies and legs of the diseased dromedaries. One day after this had been going on for several weeks an assistant keeper in the great ape house rang Ray's office in a panic. He admitted his fault right away —he had left the door to Topaz's cage open while cleaning it—and now he had to report that the young chimp had disappeared somewhere into the zoo grounds. It was not that she was in any way a dangerous or unpredictable animal, she posed no threat to any child or little old lady that she might meet on her travels, but what might happen if she naïvely paid a visit to the lion compound or the polar bear pit? She might not be as lucky there as she had been with Uncle Harold.

A full search was started, and keepers combed every section of the zoo from aquarium to elephant house. Eventually Topaz was found. It was the keeper of the camels who sent for Ray to come and collect the fugitive, and quite a sight greeted the zoo director when he went into the camel house. Topaz had obviously been fascinated by all this business of treating the camels, and after escaping from her cage she had gone to their house to help us out with the anti-mange treatment. There she stood, in the middle of a group of camels that towered above her, but which had so far apparently tolerated her presence and had not begun covering her with ejected stomach contents, their normal sign of disapproval. The little ape had decided to give them a good scrubbing down—if the humans were making such heavy weather of it, she would see what a sharp young chimpanzee with muscles and application could do. She had pulled a fire bucket full of water into the thick of the forest of camels' legs and had armed herself with one of the keepers' sweeping brushes.

As Ray and the camel keeper watched, Topaz dipped the brush into the fire bucket and then, constantly displaying the wry grimace of appeasement and keeping up a fussy chatter, which was presumably her way of exhorting the camels to stand still, she scrubbed away at the limbs and the undersurfaces of the bellies all around her. She continued doing this after the humans arrived, pausing only occasionally to look over her shoulder at them as if to assure herself that her efforts to help were not going unnoticed by her superiors. It is hard, wet, repetitive work dressing camels and other hoofed stock for mange, so perhaps one day such chores might be carried out by trained groups of chimpanzee veterinary auxiliaries!

It was not quite the end of the affair when Topaz was safely restored to the great ape house. One week later she began to show signs of itchiness on her arms and chest, and I found that she had broken out in a very fine rash. At first I thought it was an allergic reaction to something she had eaten, but tests showed that she had contracted the mange parasite from the camels. Topaz had scabies. She was not very pleased when it was her turn to be thoroughly lathered and bathed in the special shampoo every few days but, as I told her, picking up such complaints is the sort of thing that a chimpanzee has got to learn to expect when she embarks on a career as a zoo vet.

Twelve

As if not to be outdone by his sister, Topaz's elder brother Lee was demanding a good deal of my attention at about this time. It was he, resourceful and innovative as ever, who proved to me that at least one hairy little ape, born without pockets and not in the usual run of things issued with a wallet, lunch box or handbag, could give some substance to the ribald fancy about where a monkey keeps his nuts.

I was driving through Belle Vue's grounds on my way home one day after a long session of anointing snakes with a cream to destroy skin parasites when Len, the ape keeper, waved me down. With Len you never knew. Not one to fuss over trifles, he would stroll up and quietly announce the advent of some dire emergency with inexhaustible sangfroid. Matt Kelly would buzz about, crimson-faced, teeth clicking and neck veins bulging like an apoplectic leprechaun, when a crisis broke among the animals, but Len in the same situation would make a Trappist reading his breviary seem like a hysteric. Being flagged down by Len, calm as you please, might mean that all the tigers had literally "gone over the wall" or that the elephant was in difficulty delivering quintuplets.

Winding the car window down, I asked, "What can I do for you, Len?"

"Lee, Dr. Taylor. He's bristling."

Hedgehogs bristle. Porcupines make a fine and flamboyant art of bristling. Dogs when they are in that sort of mood bristle. Chimpanzees do not. Apprehensive, irate or fighting mad, their shiny black hair stays as flat as a pancake.

"Bristling? What do you mean?"

"He's sprouting straw, sort of. His back end. His bottom." Len blinked and scratched his head. "Keeps putting pieces up, er, inside his rectum. Bits of twig too. I just don't know what's got into him. I'm frightened he might do himself some injury."

I got out of the car and walked over to the great ape house with the keeper. Robert leered at me as I went by, and the great Harold, supine in his sunlit seraglio as his womenfolk conducted his toilet, blew a friendly gobbet of saliva in my direction. Lee was sitting on a branch in his open-air quarters, throwing bits of banana skin at pigeons on the edge of the parapet above him. Lee is not a bird-lover and was not good-humouredly feeding the birdies. He was vainly trying to knock one down, a feat which he had achieved at least twice before, using more potent ground-to-air missiles in the form of half-apples.

"See what I mean?" said Len, pointing towards Lee's butt where it hung over the branch. "He's bristling."

Sure enough, Lee's nether portion was sprouting a fistful of stems, stalks and similar bits of vegetation. Pieces of straw and thin twig projected from the chimp's anus, making a stubby corona.

"Are you sure they aren't bits passing through his bowels?" I asked. "Undigested fibrous pieces that he's got jammed?"

"Oh, no. There's no question about it. Lee puts them in there like that. I've watched him at it for more than a week now. Doesn't seem to bother him, but I'm worried he might damage himself internally. Why does he do it, Doctor?"

Why indeed? Lee looked for all the world as if he was growing an embryonic tail. Had he been watching the pigeons so long that he had delusions of one day taking to the air? After fixing himself up with an airworthy straw tail, would he launch himself from the top of his tree one day, long arms flapping wildly, and pursue the pigeons in

354

their own element? A chimpanzee-versus-pigeon dogfight in the sky above the zoo would pull in the crowds on a summer afternoon. Sternly I put such whimsy aside and considered the possibilities. An itchy bottom? Worms?

"Has he been showing any sign of itchiness, Len? Scratching or rubbing himself?"

"No, I don't think so. He seems to select straw and twigs with some care and, well, just hide them there, as if it's a handy place to keep the collection."

My immediate suspicion was that Lee had pinworm itch and was using the straw to scratch the irritating area. "I'll leave you some worming syrup, Len," I said. "It's got a nice fruity flavour which chimps don't usually object to. Dose him with it. If he's got pinworms, that should do the trick. I'll look at him again in a week. With any luck he'll be bristle-free and unadorned by then."

One week later Lee was as healthy as could be. And he still had his tail. If anything it was somewhat denser and more luxuriant.

"He's still got a thatched bottom," said Len blandly. It was true; Lee's posterior had a hint of harvest festival about it, of dying country crafts like straw "dollies" and the ancient custom of well dressing in Derbyshire parishes once visited by the plague.

The other chimps in the house had not copied the fetish, so I decided to see if I could find out more by closer examination. Half an hour after I had slipped a stiff shot of tranquillizer into his mid-morning cup of hot chocolate, Lee was sprawled somnolently in the forked branches of his tree, his eyes glazed and his lower lip drooping. Len and I fished him out of his arbour and turned him upside down. Carefully I pulled the cache of straw stems and twigs out of his rectum, put them to one side and looked inside him with an auriscope, an instrument designed for looking down people's ears but which comes in handy for other more exotic orifices such as dolphins' blowholes and koala bears' pouches. The foreign bodies did not appear to have damaged the lining of the lower bowel, nor was there any sign of parasites or itchy inflammation.

I picked up some of the short straw pieces that Lee had collected and inspected them. Turning them over in my fingers, I discovered something that made my eyes widen. Even Len gave a low whistle of surprise. Lee had not been decorating himself, rooting for parasites or even trying to fly. If anything he had been taking a leaf out of the book of those luckless felons who, until the end of the nineteenth century, were condemned to serve their sentences on French prison ships. Living in the most abominable conditions among murderers, thieves and other desperate characters, they would safeguard their precious personal possessions—a knife blade perhaps, a flint, a needle or a few rolled scraps of paper—in the hollowed-out marrow of a bone. This *plan,* as it was called, was then hidden by being thrust deep into the recesses of the owner's lower colon.

Lee's pieces of straw and twig were his form of *plan* and the booty he was concealing, not from convicts but from a wily bunch of chimpanzee gastronomes, was sunflower seeds. Each day Len provided the apes with a few handfuls of dried sunflower seeds, rich in essential oils and other nutriments. These were especially fancied by the chimpanzees, who would root through their food the moment it arrived, trying to pick out and eat as many of the black and white seeds as they could find. The nimblest and deftest got most. Lee, quite amazingly, had taken matters much further and had provided a unique demonstration of the ability of these advanced primates to use tools.

The straws that lay in the palm of my hand had been split longitudinally. Neatly inserted into the hollow centre of each stem was a row of sunflower seeds. The twigs had not proved as handy. They too had been split at points and seeds pushed in towards the centre but, not being hollow, they had not made such excellent *plans* as the straws.

356

Altogether, Lee had a hoard of sixty-seven sunflower seeds in his little bundle. There was no question of their having got there accidentally; the chimp must have put them there after rations had been issued, no doubt gobbling down as many again at the same time. The ones in the straws and twigs were for a rainy day or at least for a beanfeast in the middle of the night when, with only the peacock's eerie cry breaking the quiet of the sleeping zoo, Lee could stealthily retrieve his haul and nibble happily away in the darkness.

Although Lee's squirrel-like ingenuity was of great scientific interest, it would eventually produce proctitis, an inflammation of the rectum. Reluctantly but firmly I told Len to change all Lee's bedding from straw to wood wool. Twigs, the bark of which contains chemicals important for normal bowel action, were not abandoned, but only ones of too large a diameter to make comfortable *plans* were provided.

Lee ceased to bristle. From watching his unchanged behaviour, his sparkling interest in everything that happens around him and his continued ack-ack barrage against overflying pigeons, one can see no sign that he was once thwarted in his bid to corner the market in sunflower seeds. But sometimes, as I stand and watch him watching me, I wonder. Maybe the gleam in his brown eyes means that Lee knows something that Len and I don't know: that chimpanzees have more than one ingenious way of hiding their treasures.

It was as well that we de-bristled Lee when we did, for a few days later Edith popped her head round my surgery door. "If you don't have any emergencies, you're invited to a party tomorrow," she informed me. "It's a party with a difference, at the Queens Hotel in Manchester. Some charity has organized a pets' luncheon."

"What's that?" I asked her. No one was going to get me

tucking into dog biscuits and tinned cat food. Anyway, whose "pet" was I supposed to be?

"Well, the idea apparently is for the diners to be an assorted group of tame animals who will 'bring along' their owners—show-business celebrities and well-known figures in the city. Belle Vue are sending Lee with Len to keep an eye on him. They would like you to go as well." I hesitated, remembering the fiasco of the pets' church service, but Edith went on, "The thing is, it's to raise money for animal charities, so I said you would go."

"OK, Edith," I said resignedly, "book me down tomorrow for a couple of hours' duty as gentleman-in-waiting to a high-living chimpanzee."

When Lee had been younger I had prohibited him and the other baby chimpanzees from going out to children's parties, fêtes and school visits because of the trouble I was having with the measles, colds and upset stomachs they were bringing back to the zoo. Now that Lee was older he was being allowed to attend the occasional function. He enjoyed getting out and about and was especially fond of going with Matt Kelly on some of his evening lecture dates. They invariably ended up after the lecture sharing a glass of beer in a nearby pub, and if Matt was feeling especially generous Lee might occasionally be treated to a glass of his favourite tipple, Advocaat.

Next day I drove to the hotel, one of Manchester's grandest, where already a seething throng of furry, feathery and scaly animals along with attendant personalities, city fathers and press photographers had begun to assemble. There was Lee, neatly dressed, not in the shirt he had stolen from me but in the red and white colours of Manchester United soccer team. He was holding the hand of an obedient and well-behaved Len. On a large dining table at one end of the room, feeding bowls and dishes and stainless steel trays had been prepared and filled with appropriate food for each of the animals according to a large seating plan which had been pinned up on the wall. There would be sunflower seeds for the parrots (I hoped Lee would not spot them first), fruit salad for the primates, meat and biscuits for the dogs and raw liver for the cats. There was a place but no actual food for each of the reptiles, as they were not thought likely to fancy lunch under such circumstances. By each plate or bowl was a container full of water. Although chairs had been provided for the dogs and the chimpanzees, there were also high stools for the smaller monkeys and perches for the birds. The idea was that the doting owners would stand behind their pets, watching as the Noah's Ark chomped away to the pop of flashbulbs and the whirr of cameras.

I located a gin and tonic and stood in a quiet corner, admiring the kaleidoscope of the animal kingdom before me. A movie actress with a pair of petite squirrel monkeys that she had borrowed from a photographer for the occasion stood sipping cocktails in speechless horror as the little creatures did unmentionable things on her mink stole, a portly alderman slopped martini down his waistcoat as the dalmatian on the other end of the leash he held lunged menacingly at a passing parrot, and a fruit bat brought along by a local disc jockey got itself frantically entangled in the hair of a waitress who was moving round the humans with a tray of canapés. The fruit bat had not been looking where it was going because it was fleeing the beady-eyed attention of a brace of hawks sitting unhooded on the gloved hands of a guest dressed up like Robin Hood. It was this incident which led to the trouble and to my becoming involved.

The waitress, terrorized by what she thought was a day-light attack by a vampire bat fancying a nibble at her scalp, dropped her silver tray and scattered the appetizing morsels all over the carpet. All hell broke loose, as dogs and monkeys, bush babies and macaws, all no doubt with empty stomachs in preparation for the famous luncheon, thought with one accord that this was it and scrambled, scurried or fluttered about the floor gathering up bits of smoked salmon on toast, stuffed olives, wedges of salami on pumpernickel and cubes of savoury cheese. There are inevitable consequences when a mean and hungry parrot descending on a tasty titbit of shrimp wrapped in cucumber finds himself eyeball to eyeball with a Yorkshire terrier, all tassels and bows and lacquered toenails and dying for a bite to eat, or when a pet goat, noted for always having her own way, is holding one end of a stick of celery while the other is grasped meaningfully by a muscle-bound Rhesus monkey in a sailor suit. The din was deafening: birds screeching and protesting, dogs barking, felines of various species spitting and hissing, monkeys howling and humans shouting and screaming.

Worse was to follow when, the canapés having been devoured, the animals began to look at one another with an eye to starting the main course. A swirling, screeching, colourful mêlée of fur and feather began to develop in and out of the legs of the distraught owners. Women wept as their dear Tiddles or immaculately groomed Fido disappeared gleefully into the scrum, glasses were knocked from hands by swooping birds and, worst of all, leads, chains, leashes and halters of every kind became tangled and intertwined round chairs, pinstripe trousers, high-heeled shoes and potted palms. Things worsened as a City Councillor was swept neatly off his feet, his ankles lassoed by strands of leather and chain link. Having been brought low, the worthy gentleman had to endure being crossed and recrossed by the paws and claws of the rioting beasts as they struggled to free themselves from the tangle.

To the noise and confusion another horror was now added. A man from a pet shop had come along with his twelve-foot python. At the outbreak of hostilities this non-venomous reptile had weighed up the situation, decided to adopt a neutral stance and, having extricated itself from the grip of its owner, made off across the floor to the relative quiet and peace to be found beneath some seating round the walls. Under the seating ran a line of central heating pipes, and around these the python wrapped itself, no doubt to observe the proceedings from the safety of a grandstand seat. The pet shop owner, pursuing his errant snake, got down on his hands and knees and started to extricate it from the piping. It is not an easy job with an animal of this size: just as you unwind and hold one part of the snake, another part is winding itself even more firmly into a tight hold. The owner tugged and tugged and the more he tugged the more the python resisted and increased its coils on the piping. Then, as his master's attempts to winkle him out became ever more desperate, the snake became somewhat alarmed. Like most other creatures, when snakes are alarmed they tend to lose control of their bowels, and very soon the dining room of this rather superior hotel was filled with the indescribable and unmistakable stench of upset python. Few of those present could have smelt such an odour before, but the glazing of their eyes and contortion of their facial muscles showed that none of them would ever forget the experience.

Meanwhile, the big dining table which had been specially laid out for the feeding of the animal guests was standing completely neglected. Its centrepiece was a large iced cake containing only sponge and sugar, which was thought to be acceptable to most of the birds and animals invited. Crowning the cake was a representation of the Manchester coat of arms in red and gold plastic. The public relations people had visualized the Lord Mayor cutting the cake and handing out slices to everyone from pekingese to parrot. Dining table and iced cake were deserted and forgotten as the skirmishes over the spilled canapés raged on. I was fully occupied trying to avoid getting bitten whilst acting as umpire and inter-posing portions of my anatomy between the contenders in the bouts around me. Len was clutching Lee's hand but the chimp, adopting a superior air as if such hooliganism was beneath him, waited calmly on the fringes of the battleground, stooping only to pluck the odd tail feather from a mynah bird or macaw if it came within reach. But his stomach was beginning to rumble as the canapé hunt reached its climax; still not a peanut nor a potato chip, not a cocktail onion nor a gherkin had passed his lips. Then he spotted the big iced cake. Invitingly unattended it stood, and the look of it appealed most powerfully to Lee's sweet tooth. Without attracting too much fuss, he slipped his hand from Len's and sidled over to the dining table.

Lee was actually up on the table sampling the icing with both hands before Len realized that his companion was no longer by his side. "Lee! Come off there this minute!" he shouted, pushing his way through the battlefield as fast as he could.

Lee may not have heard him above the hullabaloo, but he certainly gave no sign of obeying. He dug his hard black nails deep into the succulent sponge and scooped out a sweet mouthful.

Len's approach was hampered by an irate ferret clinging tenaciously onto his ankle. "Dr. Taylor, it's Lee! Grab him!" he roared, hopping on one leg and trying to unpick his dogged assailant.

I looked up, saw the looter at work on the table and decided to let my two canine opponents in one particularly bitter three-cornered match sort it out between themselves. There were still a lot of furious bodies between me and the chimpanzee.

Lee summed up the situation like lightning and realized that Len's expression was not only one of anguish at the needle-like teeth perforating his lower limb, but also meant the imminent confiscation of what was turning out to be a very tasty cake indeed. There was only one thing to be done. Picking up the whole cake on its wooden stand, Lee cleared off to look for a quiet spot where he could continue his lunch away from all these bothersome beasts. Out of the dining room, along the corridor, down the stairs went the small chimpanzee with the wounded-looking cake carried effortlessly on one shoulder. Looking back briefly, he saw us in full pursuit, accompanied by a very angry catering manager. Lee reached the lobby still without having spotted a suitable hideaway where he could hole up and do the cake justice. Visitors coming into the hotel stood dumbfounded as the little midget waiter, obviously some strange foreign immigrant on the hotel staff, scurried by with his short order. Some room service! A bellboy, arms outstretched, gallantly tried to halt the cake's progress. For his pains he was spat accurately in the eye as the chimp swerved by with all the skill of one of the international half-backs in the team whose colours he was wearing.

At last Lee found the ideal place, or so it seemed. An open door led into the gentlemen's washroom. Glancing back once again to check that his pursuers were not too close, chimpanzee and cake disappeared inside and closed the door. Cautiously I opened the door and went into the washroom, followed by Len and the catering manager. There was no sign of Lee, nor for that matter of anyone else. We were faced by a row of toilet cubicles, all with closed doors. Now we had a delicate problem. Behind which door was Lee? I decided to leave it up to the catering manager—at least he was a member of the hotel staff. Miserably this poor fellow went from cubicle to cubicle tapping on each door and inquiring in diffident tones, "Excuse me, we've lost a chimpanzee. Could you please answer so that we know he's not in there?" A succession of oaths and other sounds of indignation produced by obviously human occupants floated back over the top of the cubicles.

Eventually we came to a cubicle the door of which was firmly shut, but where the "engaged" sign was not showing at the lock. "Er, anyone in there?" called the catering manager. "Sorry to disturb you if there is."

No answer came. Lee had been run to earth, and when

Len shinned up the side of the cubicle and looked over the top, there was the chimpanzee sitting happily on the toilet seat with the cake in his lap and his legs wedged firmly against the door to keep it closed.

Len prepared to descend on Lee and what was left of his meal just as the chimpanzee was sucking icing from the little plastic coat of arms which he had removed from the cake and was using as a sort of spoon. When Lee saw that the game was nearly up he took one last frantic scoop of cake and packed it, together with the coat of arms, into his mouth. Down dropped Len, Lee made a futile jump to try to escape, the remains of the cake fell into the lavatory pan and it was all over. Carried out of the cubicle by determined hands, and with his cheeks bulging with cake, Lee gulped the final mouthful, forgetting in the heat of the moment that the little plastic coat of arms was also in his mouth. An instant later he was coughing and choking. Len had seen him take the piece of plastic and we immediately realized what had happened : it was jammed somewhere at the back of his throat.

"Quick, slap him hard on the back while I hold him upside down!" I shouted, hoisting Lee up by his ankles with both hands and letting his head dangle close to the floor.

Len slapped and slapped at the hairy black body and Lee coughed and groaned but no plastic coat of arms appeared. The chimpanzee was becoming markedly distressed; the mischievous escapade was turning into something much more grave. I laid the ape down on a chair in the washroom and sent Len to my car for my bag. Anxiously I looked into Lee's familiar face and saw that his gums and lips were already turning slightly blue. His breathing was hideously noisy and laboured. All his vital energy seemed suddenly drained out of him. He had neither the spirit nor the power to resist as I opened his jaws wide and probed over the back of his tongue with my fingers. I could feel nothing abnormal. Len came dashing back with my bag and I pulled out my stethoscope. Normally Lee objected to this instrument—he seemed as frightened by the rubber tubes as he was by a plastic or rubber toy snake—and given half a chance he would pick the head of the stethoscope off his skin and puncture the sound-receiving diaphragm with his teeth, but now there was no objection as I listened to his straining chest wall. What I heard confirmed that the chimp was just not getting enough air into his lungs. The plastic decoration for the cake was stuck somewhere in his airway.

Wedging one hand between his teeth, a hazardous position in a conscious ape were he not in such a critical state, with the other I pulled his lilac-tinged tongue as far forward as possible. Len shone my pencil torch down the throat for me. I could see Lee's tonsils and larynx very clearly. Across the opening to the windpipe was an arrow-shaped splinter of red plastic, a tiny piece of the coat of arms but enough where it was lodged to threaten to asphyxiate the chimpanzee at any moment.

Still using one hand as a mouth gag, I took a pair of long artery forceps from my bag and, with Len lighting the way, reached into the depths of Lee's throat with the metal jaws. The shard of red plastic fluttered with each in-and-out of the chimp's agonized breathing. Please God don't let it drop down the dark red hole into the trachea! I reached it and with a gasp of relief clamped the forceps firmly round it. Out it came. Lee began to breathe more easily but still far from normally. Most of the coat of arms was still missing. I looked down the throat again as Lee gurgled and his lilac-coloured parts began to regain a little of their healthier, salmon-pink tinge.

Where was the rest of the cursed cake decoration? It was surely too big to have actually gone down the windpipe. Then a terrible thought occurred to me. If Lee had split one piece off the plastic, perhaps he had crushed the remainder into a dozen smaller fragments, now sucked far beyond my reach into the bronchial tubes. Ice water ran down my spine as I imagined the consequences: chest surgery far beyond my experience in zoo animals. There was just one other place where the bigger part of the plastic might have lodged: above the soft palate. Suppose Lee had almost swallowed the coat of arms and then blown it up again by coughing when the splinter had broken off and wedged in his larynx. It could have been shot forward into the space at the back of the nose and above the roof of the mouth. Perhaps it was there, jammed between his adenoids. To look up and round the back of his soft palate I would need a mirror of the kind used by dental surgeons or something long and shiny which could be bent at the end.

"Please ask at the cocktail bar if they have any stainless steel plungers for mixing drinks," I said to the catering manager. One of those might do. If I could only see the smallest flash of red or gold for an instant I would know its whereabouts.

Lee was by this stage much improved, although still breathing noisily and with effort. Part of his airway was still obstructed: the thought of bits of plastic in the lung continued to haunt me. When the catering manager returned he was carrying a variety of plungers of differing lengths for my inspection. I selected one and then asked Len to hold the mouth open again while the catering manager was reluctantly pressed into doing something that catering managers do not normally do in smart hotels— putting a full nelson wrestler's hold on a now restless chimpanzee. With the chimp's breathing still embarrassed I was loath to give any form of anaesthetic which might depress his respiration still further.

Shining my light down the mouth, I passed the plunger between the tonsils and past the tip of the soft palate. The plunger's circular base was now in a position to reflect back up into the recesses behind the nostrils. Directing the beam of my torch onto the plunger, I moved the two instruments about, trying to bounce light off anything that might be hidden out of my sight. Suddenly I saw a hazy splash of red reflected in the stainless steel of the cocktail plunger. I wiggled the plunger and saw some more red and then a fuzzy flash of gold. It was there! The coat of arms was lodged above the soft palate.

As long as I could keep Lee breathing via the mouth, I should have time to get him to my surgery, where I could use special instruments to remove the plastic, but first I decided to try something that only works occasionally. Sitting the miserable little thief upright in his chair, I slapped him hard and abruptly on the forehead. His head flew back and he looked at me with an expression of surprise and reproach. Nothing happened. Again I slapped him hard between the eyes and the little head flew back onto the hairy shoulders. Lee gave a retch, coughed once and there was a tinkle as he spat a lump of red and gold plastic onto the washroom floor. When I matched it with the fragment that I had extracted with my forceps it fitted perfectly; the ornament was complete, not a scrap of plastic was missing.

Immediately Lee's breathing became normal and the strange noises disappeared. He was feeling more himself, for he back-kicked the catering manager in the solar plexus, winding him and forcing him to release his grip. Manchester's heraldic escutcheon had been saved, and Lee went home to Belle Vue somewhat chastened by his experience but with a stomach fuller than most of the other animals invited to the ill-fated luncheon. For some reason they have not held such an event since.

When I arrived home there was the delicious aroma of one of Shelagh's fish pies, the treat of the week made from cod, cheese and dry white wine. I rather fancied a large helping of that with mashed potatoes after the interrupted and rather insubstantial nibblings at the Queens Hotel.

"You'll never believe what happened with Lee today," I said cheerfully, slipping off my coat. "I'll tell you all about it while I'm getting some of that inside me."

"You won't, I'm afraid," Shelagh replied, darting into the cloakroom and unhooking her coat. "You're off back to Belle Vue. There's just been a call from Ray. He's got two polar bear cubs. And I'm coming with you!"

Good-bye, fish pie! Of course, it was December. I had known that Crystal, the female polar bear, was once again near her time. Ray must have heard the cubs squeaking and used the anaesthetic dart that we had had on stand-by as planned. And now it sounded as if he had successfully cub-napped a pair of twins!

If there was one of the frequent police radar traps on the Manchester road it would just be hard luck. I was going to get to Belle Vue in record time. If I was nabbed I would have a fine excuse, and if they did not swallow my story it would be worth a fine and an endorsement on my licence to get my hands on my first newborn, warm and squirming, snow-white polar cubs.

"What did Ray say?" I asked as I gunned the Citroën out of Rochdale.

"That things didn't look good at all," replied Shelagh.

My heart plummeted. I wish I had a jet helicopter, I thought. No doubt every household will have one by the year 2000, but here I am with twelve miles of road to cover and every vehicle in front of me seemingly being driven in the middle of the road, at a snail's pace, by an opium-eater.

Ray and the twin cubs were in the dispensary when we charged into the zoo. "I'm afraid it's too late," he said as we went through the door. His face was haggard with disappointment. Matt Kelly stood silently by. Two plump, grubby little bodies lay inert on the table. Newborn all right, but quite definitely not warm, squirming or snow-white.

"What happened?" I asked as I opened the miniature jaws and looked at the pallid gums.

"The keeper didn't notice anything until he heard her scratching away at her bedding. Then he thought he heard a faint squeak. I darted her straightaway and we went in.

We found she'd cleared all her straw away from one corner, down to the bare concrete, and had pushed the cubs there. They were probably born this morning. When I got to them they were cold, damp and not moving. Still attached to their placentas. She'd neglected them again."

Unstimulated by the tongue-licking and warmth that their mother should have provided, and left untended on the hard floor, the cubs had slipped into hypothermia. I picked one cub up in each hand and squeezed their chests firmly and rhythmically. I tried to feel an arterial pulse—nothing. They were floppy and chill and they had the familiar look of death about them.

"Get some hot water," I said. "From the tap will do. As hot as a good hot bath. Quick. In a bucket or anything."

Matt Kelly had the water ready in seconds. I plunged both cubs in, immersing their whole bodies except for their little muzzles. Underwater I continued squeezing and massaging their chests. "Shelagh, you do one while I do the other." I passed the manipulation of one of the babies over to her. "Pump rhythmically but don't dig your finger ends in too viciously," I instructed. I had seen lungs ruptured and heart muscles haemorrhaged many times where over-enthusiastic artificial respiration had been applied to tiny creatures.

Minutes went by and suddenly Shelagh yelled, "Mine's moving!"

I looked at its mouth; it was definitely much pinker. I told her to keep pumping and I struggled on with mine. "More hot water, Matt," I said. He topped the bucket up. Then I too felt it. My cub was moving slightly. It was not quite so floppy. There was a faint muscular tension growing in the furry lump within my clasping hands.

"Both out!" I said. "Stethoscope!" I listened to the two now warm little cubs. Dab-dab, dab-dab. I heard the faint soft heart sound in one. I turned to the other. Dab-dab,

dab-dab. "They're alive!" I shouted. "Back in the water, keep respirating!"

There was no doubt now, both cubs were wriggling their bodies under water. "Right, out again!" I said. "I'll take them both." I held both cubs by their back halves, one in each hand at arm's length. Then I whirled my arms round and round in fast, wide circles. I hoped the centrifugal force would throw out any mucus blocking the cubs' windpipes. Then it was back into the hot water. The cubs were struggling manfully now but there was not a squeak out of their little throats. "Out again! We'll try mouth-to-mouth."

Again Shelagh took one cub while I handled the other. Sticking the cubs' snouts into our mouths we blew gently but firmly. The minute chests expanded. We pulled out the snouts and let them expire our air. We waited. Moments passed. They were not breathing automatically. More mouth-to-mouth. And more. Puff in, squeeze out. The twins were developing the healthy feel of coiled wire springs in our hands. We stopped and waited again. The pink mouths opened a fraction, two stubby pink tongues tentatively probed the outside world and then, giving me an exhilarating "high" surely greater than any experienced by a main-lining junkie, they both voluntarily breathed strong and deep.

Shelagh cheered, Matt and Ray shouted in delight and I laughed and laughed. I picked up the cubs and turned them over onto their backs on my palms, a good test for vigour in the newborn. Cussedly they squirmed themselves round into the head-up, belly-down position which self-respecting little critters prefer. An excellent response, and as a bonus they voiced their protest at being so peremptorily upended and emitted their first, glorious squeaks of complaint. I had never seen Shelagh so thrilled.

Within minutes we began dripping a solution of pre-digested protein and glucose into the twins' mouths by way of a feeding bottle designed for premature human babies. The cubs were installed in an infra-red heated box, where they scrabbled and wriggled and grumbled lustily. I had no intention of going home until I had seen them do one more thing: start to suckle. The protein and glucose solution was ideal as a first-aid source of energy, but after that it was going to be all the way to weaning on tinned Carnation milk.

"Come on, Shelagh," said Ray when he had prepared the first milk feed, "you must have the first honour." He gave her the two little feeding bottles.

On tenterhooks we watched as she proffered the rubber teats to the two protesting cubs. Then there was silence. The twins had grabbed the teats hungrily and contentedly begun to draw in the milk.

It was now up to Ray and Matt to organize a two-hourly feeding schedule round the clock. It would be worth it. Bears grow very quickly and these little fellows were never to look back.

"Come on, Shelagh," I said after scrubbing up and going out to the car, "bugger the fish pie. Let's go and have a bottle of champagne at the pub."

Thirteen

The little old blind lady in Singapore's Lion City Hotel stamped her enthusiastic way up and down my back in bare feet, grinding her heels into every one of my ill-humoured vertebrae and accompanying each audible rending of my bones with a triumphant, high-pitched "Atcha!"

I was on my way back from Bangkok, the cesspool of unscrupulous animal dealing, where I had been to check a collection of beasts being offered for sale by Thai traders. Not only had the job meant Norman's wrath about yet another absence from the practice, it had been a depressing experience in itself. In noisome, unlit dungeons, I had run my hands over baby elephants as knobbly as blackberries with multiple skin abscesses and had gingerly pulled one live, tick-covered king cobra out of a stinking pile of forty of its long-dead fellows. I had seen giant bird-eating spiders that had died from thirst—they need liquid refreshment in hot countries just as much as the trappers who sell them for one cent and the dealers who buy them for retail at five dollars—and had discovered that even after death the reddish hair that covers their fearsome limbs can cause painful inflammation. I had also been knocked about while taking blood samples from a bunch of anaemic-looking water buffaloes. Slipping while drawing blood from the jugular of one animal, I had suddenly found myself with my nose in the mud and both hands protecting the back of my head as a dozen buffaloes milled round and over me.

Now, along with my bruises, I was in Singapore to spend a few days exploring this most kaleidoscopic of Asian islands and to recuperate from my "buffalo-ing". The ancient Chinese masseuse had done wonders in erasing the buffalo footprints, but she had beaten, drummed, kneaded and trodden copious quantities of oil of wintergreen into me. I could not scrub away the all-pervading mentholated smell, and for days after her ministrations I was as pungent as a bottle of smelling salts. When I was invited by Feng Lo, a rich Chinese importer of lapis lazuli, to visit his private menagerie of exotic animals, I arrived at his bungalow close to the famous Tiger Balm gardens with as much animal appeal as camphor has for moths.

The pride of Mr. Feng's collection were his four Hartmann's mountain zebras. Fine, plump animals in a shady corral in his back garden, they were as tame as donkeys, he told me; his nephew had actually sat on the stallion's back. The zebras trotted over pleasantly enough when Mr. Feng called them. They nibbled the sugar lumps he offered, then they looked at me and sniffed me over. A vapour rub in human form—ugh! Ears went back. The whites of their eyes flashed. Soft nostrils wrinkled and snorted. The three zebra mares spun petulantly away, but just to show how he felt the stallion lunged and bit me neatly and painfully right on the tip of my nose. Stung by spider hairs, trodden by water buffaloes, smelling like a throat lozenge and now this! Mr. Feng hopped from foot to foot in a frenzy of apologies, but as I clamped a padded handkerchief to my bleeding nose and watched the stallion fling up his tail and canter arrogantly away my attention was riveted. One of his testes was grossly abnormal, about five times the size of the other. I pointed it out to Mr. Feng.

"What could it be, Dr. Taylor?" he inquired, looking troubled.

"It could be a hernia or it could be a tumour. Whichever it is, an operation is called for without delay. If it's a growth it should be removed, and a scrotal hernia must be repaired before it strangulates a piece of intestine."

Mr. Feng scratched his head and sucked the bean-sized solitaire diamond on his right index finger. "But who can do it here in Singapore? The vets here know riding horses. But zebras?" He muttered quietly to himself in Chinese. Then he suddenly smiled and prodded me in the solar plexus. "Ha!" he said cheerfully, as if it was now perfectly clear to him. "No problem. You will do it, Doctor. What a good idea!"

"But I . . . " I began. Neither hernia nor tumour demanded instruments more complicated than those I always carry in my emergency pack, but the anaesthetic—that was the problem. I could buy barbiturates on the island, but they would be useless unless shot straight into a vein, hardly practical on a fighting, kicking zebra stallion. Chloral hydrate solution in the drinking water might work, but the stuff tastes so appallingly bitter that an animal will go for two or three days before, maddened with thirst, it drinks the knock-out drops; I had never used the method, feeling it to be slightly barbaric. I had phencyclidine, but no phencyclidine ever again in zebras for me after the dreadful night at Belle Vue when I had first tried it on the species. What I needed was etorphine or xylazine, both excellent drugs for zebras. There was not a drop of either in Singapore.

Then I remembered my motto, "Always say yes". In danger of extinction in its native mountains of Damaraland, South-West Africa, this precious creature was not likely to come my way very often. And it needed help. This maxim, of accepting opportunities positively in the knowledge that in almost every case there is time later to change one's mind if absolutely necessary, has paid off time and time again in my career. To be sure of being "in" is better than to risk being "out" through timidity or indecision. It stirs the blood, brings far fewer disasters than might be expected and should be heartily recommended to all except young ladies and, so they say, members of the armed forces. Quick affirmative decisions are like ice-cold champagne after a cloying meal, clearing the palate of the mind.

"Right, Mr. Feng," I said briskly, "I'll do it. I want your men to build a stout wooden crate for the zebra, the sort you might use to transport him. No holes in the sides, absolutely solid. But with no top on."

"It will be done by tomorrow," he replied. "Anything else you want?"

"Yes. A bottle of chloroform and the address of a good, quick tailor, the sort that runs up suits for tourists in twenty-four hours."

"Ah, yes." Mr. Feng looked faintly perplexed. "For you, of course. You want a suit?"

"No," I said, grinning, "for the zebra."

While Mr. Feng, clearly puzzled by my sudden attention to the zebra's sartorial welfare, set about organizing the crate building, a taxi took me to an address he had given me. It dropped me in the old Chinese quarter at the fringe of a large crowd watching the weaving dragons and warbling, white-faced maidens of a street opera. Gongs boomed, cymbals clashed, villainous landlords were revealed and demons machinated as I pushed my way through the rapt audience into the cool gloom of the tailor's little shop.

"I want you to make something unusual," I told the tailor, a young man with long vertical moustachioes and a Pink Floyd T-shirt. "By tomorrow, or better still tonight. For a zebra. Yes, zebra. Ze-bra. Z-e-b-r-a. Horse, black and white. Stripes." Pencil and paper were produced and I sketched what I needed.

Chloroform was a veteran method of anaesthesia and I had never used it in my life on a large animal. But I had watched horses knocked out by it while I was at university, and now I needed a mask of the sort I had seen being used there. A simple strap round the back of the animal's ears kept in place a canvas cylinder divided into two compartments; the horse's muzzle fitted into the upper one and the smaller lower one held a wad of cotton wool soaked in chloroform. A small hole between upper and lower compartments allowed air to be drawn through the cotton wool in the lower chamber into the upper chamber and so into the respiratory system of the animal.

"But I have no canvas," explained the tailor.

"Then use some of the firmest felt material you have, the sort you put inside collars and lapels of suits."

The tailor caught on quickly. It would be ready at five o'clock and would cost twenty . . . well, what about fifteen . . . OK but at eight you are getting it at cost price . . . well, agreed then at five dollars.

As I drove back to the Lion City Hotel to do repairs to my nose, I recalled with a shudder the last time I had seen a chloroform mask fitted to an equine. A final-year student, I had watched a hunter mare rear in the air at the first whiff of gas, snatch the halter rope from the groom and spin stiffly backwards through 180 degrees to crash with the back of her skull on the ground. Since then I had stuck purely to injectable anaesthetics. But chloroform was what I was going to have to use, and on a rare and unknown quantity. I wondered what Mr. Feng would have said if I had announced that I was literally starting to practise on his beloved zebra.

The mask was ready as promised at five o'clock and the tailor had made a very creditable job of it. It seemed strong enough, and had the silk square normally sewn inside jacket linings attached to the muzzle compartment: "Jerome Hua—Tailors of Singapore—By Appointment to Dukes and Kings since the Tenth Century and Mr. Rocky Marciano." "The World's One and Only Zebra Tailor" would have had even more panache, I thought.

Since the zebras lived completely outdoors with trees for shade and no kind of stable, I had decided to operate in the cool of the next day, just after dawn. Before turning in early, I strolled through the alleyways round Bugis Street taking in the aromas, colours and sounds that swirled in the soft evening air. Little boys scurried round with steaming buckets of rice. Hand-held firecrackers with a report like a hand grenade exploded showers of paper streamers over the shabby roofs. Pretty girls in cheongsams split limes by pulling them down taut thread and squeezed the juice over heaped half-moons of watermelon. At one stall a boy was passing sugar cane through an iron mangle and collecting the sweet, refreshing juice in jugs of ice. Stopping for a glass, I washed down a couple of painkillers to pacify my muscles, which were grumbling about water buffaloes once again.

As I stood drinking, I saw that the next stall specialized in cubes of some sort of meat, speared onto fine wooden skewers and coated with a spicy satay-nut sauce. The skinned little creatures from which the stallholder was cutting the meat were not immediately recognizable. Curious, I wandered over. Not rabbits or cats—knowledge of the subtle differences between those two carcasses once heads, feet and skins have been removed had come in useful when the Rochdale police were prosecuting a rogue of a market trader who went out at night nabbing stray toms for sale the next morning as "fresh meadow-trapped bunnies". Encouraged by my apparent interest, the stallholder pulled my sleeve and pointed to the back of his stall. Hanging there upside down, with its clawed feet lashed to a rickety cross-pole, was a live Malayan flying fox, or fruit bat.

"Him very fresh. You like me kill him? Roast quick. Taste very good fresh." The man smiled a solid gold smile and pulled my sleeve again. The furry brown creature's wings were bound tightly with thread that had cut into the flesh and was crusted with dried black blood. There were holes in the shining soft fabric of the wing membranes, like moth holes in cotton curtains.

"How much for him?" I asked.

"Six dollar. But I fry him good. You like." He grabbed a

meat cleaver. "Him very good with plenty soy."

"I'll have him," I said, taking off my shirt. "Wrap him in this."

The man looked flabbergasted. Then he dazzled me with the eighteen-carat palisade of dentures again. "Ah! You take home. You know how cook? You got good wife cook?"

"Yes," I replied, "I know how to deal with him." I paid my six dollars, snipped the thread and cord binding the animal and wrapped him carefully in my shirt with just the tip of his nose protruding.

"Good appetite, sir," bade the stallholder as I went off in search of a taxi.

Back at the Lion City I took the squeaking bundle to my room and carefully unwrapped him in the bathroom. The cords had cut deep and his wings were showing as much daylight when fully extended as a slice of Emmentaler cheese. It was tricky working single-handed; Malayan fruit-eating bats are up to a foot long and can nip severely if mishandled. Slowly I managed to clean up and treat his wounds, and for good measure I gave him a shot of long-acting penicillin. When I released him he managed to flutter up to the shower curtain and grab hold, upside down. From there he watched me with glinting, angry eyes. Out of the hotel I went again and from the street stalls which bustle merrily all night long I bought a selection of peaches, cherries, mangoes and bananas. I distributed the fruit along the bottom of the bath, used the bidet as a rather inefficient sort of upside-down shower and went to bed.

As usual before a major operation I lay in bed worrying about all the complications which might beset my treatment of the zebra the next day. Singapore nights are humid enough without the sweats such thoughts provoke. At least I found next morning that the flying fox had been down to eat some of the fruit and was now dozing comfortably, hanging from the edge of the lavatory cistern.

Sticking the "Do not disturb" card on my room door, I

went off as soon as the sky was light to begin operations at Mr. Feng's bungalow. Everything was well prepared. The stallion had been lured into the crate and was now securely fastened. Keeping a wary eye on the other three zebras and on their companions in the paddock, a pair of large ostriches and three brindled gnus, I climbed up the wooden side of the container and looked down at my patient. He glared up at me, ears back, and bucked with an irate squeal.

Normally the chloroform mask is put on a horse first and, once it is secure, the anaesthetic is introduced into the lower compartment. But I might have only one chance of getting near the head of the creature before all hell broke loose, so I had decided to put the chloroform-soaked swab in the felt mask before touching gloves with my adversary. Having done so, I climbed back up the side of the crate with the loaded mask in my left hand. The zebra was standing below and across me with his head to my left. Gently I tapped him on his bristly mane with my right hand. He threw his head up and tried in vain to get his teeth into me; the crate was just narrow enough to stop him bringing his head round. Quick as a flash I plunged the mask over his muzzle with my left hand and leaned way down with my right to bring the retaining strap over his ears. He bellowed like a bull, crashed, thrashed, kicked and tried to spring vertically upwards on all four legs.

The edge of the crate cut into my stomach as, red in the face, I leaned down into the container and clung grimly on. Suddenly the stallion reared, his forelegs scrabbling at the wood in front of him, and I felt the retaining strap of the mask slide crisply over his poll. Then, as the beast descended once again onto all fours, his weight combined with my desperate grip on the strap flipped me in the twinkling of an eye down into the crate. To Mr. Feng and his men standing anxiously round the crate, one instant I was there, the next I had vanished. The crate now contained one irate stallion zebra, its muzzle enveloped in a fuming bespoke

379

felt mask, and one veterinarian sitting side-saddle on the zebra's back, red-faced and winded. If the crate door had been opened at that moment, there would have rocketed out a duo that would have given the crowd at any rodeo the spectacle of a lifetime.

The zebra was still. So was I. Maybe, I thought, I can sit here until he goes under, like a cowboy having his horse shot from under him in slow motion. If I stood up I might slip down between my patient and the crate walls, or my movements might excite him again. All went well for a few moments, until the spinning world and the strange, overwhelming smell in his nostrils sent a wave of fear through the stallion's growing drowsiness. He made one final, instinctive explosion of effort. First crouching slightly and then powerfully extending his legs, he produced the buck of all bucks. For Mr. Feng and his men the earlier disappearing trick cleverly reversed itself. One moment there was just a box; the next a veterinarian rose like a malfunctioning Minuteman out of its silo and flopped in an awkward heap on the hard edge of the crate.

This spectacular double act produced a fresh crop of bruises round my midriff. Painfully I climbed down and sat on the ground, listening to the zebra's protests die away as the anaesthetic took good hold.

"My goodness!" exclaimed Mr. Feng as I panted and puffed and longed for the little old lady with the oil of wintergreen. "That was most spectacular, Doctor. I can see you have done that many thousands of times."

"Yes," I replied. Liar.

The sun was just beginning to pour a thread of molten gold along the horizon of the South China Sea, and tall grey pillars of cloud dotted the sky like poplars. There was no sound from the crate. I climbed up again. The stallion was down, unconscious. I poked him with my toe. No reaction. "Right, open the front of the crate," I shouted. "Pull him out as quick as you can."

Six Chinese dragged the patient out and I began my examination of the enlarged testis. One feel was enough. No hernia this, but a tumour. The whole organ was hard and irregularly shaped. Probably a non-malignant growth, but it had to be removed. The other testis seemed normal and the animal's ability to breed would not be affected. After checking his heart and lungs, adjusting the mask and telling one of Feng's men to make sure that none of the other animals in the enclosure interfered with my little field hospital, I washed and sterilized the operation site. That done, I made one incision, withdrew the diseased testis and tied off its massive blood supply with thick catgut in a special non-slip knot. To make doubly sure that there would be no disastrous haemorrhage once the beast was up and running, I placed a second similar ligature and then cut the testis free. As I would have done with a horse, I left the incision in the scrotum so that it could drain easily but packed the empty space where the testis had lain with a fly-repellent antibiotic powder. It was done. I took the mask off and after fifteen minutes the stallion groggily regained his feet and walked slowly off towards his mares.

"Now," I said to Mr. Feng, "let's see what sort of growth it was."

I knelt on the ground and sliced open the mass with my scalpel as Feng and his men crowded round. There was a distinct "ping" as my blade struck something hard as flint in the centre of the testis. I opened the incision with my fingers and the Chinese men gave one loud gasp of amazement. Out from the middle of the swollen organ fell a shining white object the size of a matchbox. There was no doubt what it was: a perfect zebra's molar tooth. It lay in the palm of my hand, complete with roots, glinting enamel and roughened cusps.

"A dragon's tooth!" exclaimed one man, gingerly extending a grubby hand and touching the object with the tip of one finger as if it might leap up and gnaw him.

"What beast is it that carries teeth in his loins?" murmured another reverently, spitting on the ground.

There was a babble of excited Chinese debate. One man saw the mark of the demons in the affair, another thought that if the English veterinarian had not been so foolish as to interfere the stallion would have sired the Chinese version of a centaur. The oldest man, Feng's gardener, claimed that the tooth should be planted at once, for perhaps this was the strange seed of which Lao-Tse, the venerable philosopher, had written and which might grow into the Tree of Knowledge.

Mr. Feng himself roared with laughter as he pulled his wallet from his hip pocket, extracted four or five notes and, flicking his lighter into flame, set fire to them. As the paper money curled and blackened into fragile ash he blew the fragments into the air with a puff of breath and another burst of laughter. "What fortune, Doctor!" he cried. "What fortune! You know what that is. You know. Oh, what fortune!"

Yes, I knew what it was, but during all the commotion I had not been able to get a word in edgeways. It was a tooth that had got lost. When the embryo zebra was a microscopic ball lying in the womb of its mother, the cells of which it was composed had started to sort themselves out. Those cells that were to become the brain and spinal cord took up their positions, kidney cells fell into line over here, liver cells got into a huddle over there, heart cells gathered at a point that would one day be the centre of the chest cavity and so on. During all this sorting out of a thousand and one different kinds of cell, some got lost, just like groups of schoolchildren making their way to their allotted coaches at the end of a school outing. This is how some kinds of non-malignant tumour develop, why bone tumours can grow in kidneys or, as in this case, teeth can bud in testes. Once a tooth cell, always a tooth cell. Magic? Yes: nature's magic.

Before I could try to outline this fascinating faux pas

of embryology to the exultant Mr. Feng, I had the distinct impression that the sky had fallen in. A split second before, I had been watching Mr. Feng prove inexplicably that he had money to burn. Wham! Now I was flat on the ground, my nose buried for the second time in a week in material more suitable for doing good to rosebushes. Worse, I was being thoroughly stomped on by heavy, clumping, scaly feet with iron-hard toenails. I was being gone over by an ostrich. The man detailed to keep an eye on the other animals in the paddock had left his post in the excitement of finding the tooth, and the male red-neck ostrich had decided to come looking for trouble. Now, beak gaping, ragged wings flailing in victory, he did his war dance on me. I could not help noticing that he lacked both the restraint and the skill of the little old lady and that instead of oil of wintergreen he used slimy white droppings. Stoically, hands once again covering my head, I took my beating until the ungainly bird was shooed away. As I climbed wearily to my feet I wondered whether the animal kingdom had put a contract out on me; there seemed to be no shortage of creatures from buffalo to zebra to ostrich that were bent on doing me in.

"You must stay for breakfast, Doctor," said my host, helping me to his bungalow. "I must discuss with you the good fortune you have brought me."

I began to feel the bruises on my bruises easing a little as a servant brought rice, eggs and lightly cooked vegetables to a lapis lazuli table. We drank the most delicate of pale jasmine teas with petals floating on the surface. "Tell me, Mr. Feng," I asked, "why did you burn the dollar bills?"

The Chinaman lit a cigarette and smiled. "Because of the tooth, of course," he said. "By the way, please pass it to me."

I pulled the tooth out of my pocket. I had hoped to keep it as a curio, a souvenir of the operation, but it was obvious from the way Mr. Feng lovingly turned it over in his fingers and then locked it in a bureau encrusted with lapis lazuli that he considered it well and truly his. His zebra, his zebra's testis, his miraculous tooth.

"The burning of the money was a traditional custom, a polite thank-you to the spirits of my ancestors. One must not forget the old courtesies, Dr. Taylor, even in these days of television and atom bombs." Mr. Feng still had not explained what he had to be so grateful to his ancestors about.

"The tooth is what pathologists call a 'foetal rest,' a tissue that was displaced during . . ." I began to describe the nature of the object. Mr. Feng waved a slim finger at me.

"Quite, quite," he interrupted, "but I think you do not understand how Chinese culture looks at such things. For a tooth to grow in the organ of generation, the source of life and potency, such a conjunction has profound implications. I could feel the energy of it when I touched it. I cannot describe what its abilities, its qualities must be, are."

"But you don't believe in magic, surely?"

He smiled benignly and looked at me over his spectacles. "What is magic? Today's science is yesterday's magic. There are powers that we Chinese understood when Western peoples were barbarians in wolf skins. Those powers existed then, they exist now. They are our heritage, the wisdom of the Middle Kingdom. Acupuncture, herbs—only now does the West begin to sniff round things our ancestors knew centuries ago."

"Well, what are you going to do with the tooth?"

"Quite frankly, Dr. Taylor, it will make me a millionaire."

"How on earth . . .?"

"I estimate it weighs, oh, forty-five or fifty grammes. Do you realize how much a Chinese with the necessary resources and need will pay for just a little of that tooth, say a milligramme or two, when it has been carefully ground into a fine powder? No? I tell you. At least one hundred and fifty pounds sterling! The power of my zebra's tooth is love, my dear Doctor, love."

I had operated on a zebra with a pathological testis and

384

presented my client with an aphrodisiac, the raw stuff of love philtres that would rake in a fortune from oriental gentlemen who were long in loot but short in amatory abilities. I gulped and thought of the hundreds of horse teeth lying neglected in the mud round the slaughter-house in Rochdale.

"Believe me," Feng continued, "when Tok Man in Medan hears about my zebra tooth, he will willingly pay five hundred dollars for some dust from it. He is a terribly worried man. A beautiful wife for ten years now and no sign of a child. You know, he has a sea cow in his garden just so that . . ."

My ears pricked up and I interrupted quickly. "Sea cow, Mr. Feng? He has a sea cow?"

"Yes, as I was saying, he has a sea cow caught by the fishermen. Now there is an animal that can turn a man into a lusty young lover again."

"How?" I asked, my attention riveted. Surely by a sea cow he meant a dugong, the strange vegetarian creature that started the mermaid myth.

"By collecting its tears, Doctor. The Indonesians say that a few drops from its eyes have never been known to fail."

Mr. Feng described the Medan sea cow; it certainly sounded like a dugong, a harmless, totally aquatic mammal that grazes on underwater weeds and grasses. The Australians had considered the possibility of farming the beasts, for the flesh is said to be utterly delicious. I had seen their cousins, the manatees, in Florida and California, but had never set eyes on a dugong.

"I would like to see this sea cow if possible," I said. "Is Medan very far?"

"An hour by jet. I will telephone Tok Man and I will give you the air ticket; after all, Doctor, today you have made me a millionaire." He went to the bureau and returned with a blue disc of lapis lazuli, bound with gold and with a rampant gold dragon in the centre. "And this is for you. The dragon will bring you luck."

It would take two days for me to obtain a visa so that I could fly out to Medan on the north-east coast of Sumatra, and I decided to see if I could pass them peacefully consuming gin slings in the bar at the Raffles Hotel and acquainting my taste buds with the unique (and as it turned out unexciting and wildly expensive) savour of shark fin and bird's-nest soup. With a bit of luck, hidden away in the fleshpots, I would avoid being stamped on by a yak or savaged by a tiger that had heard of the beastly conspiracy to do me in.

But the moment I arrived at the Lion City I was promptly thrown out. The hotel manager met me in the foyer with my bill and a pale and angry face. Apparently, ignoring my "Do not disturb" card, a maid had gone in to clean my room and on opening the door to the bathroom had been "attacked by a vampire bat". The maid had been given several large brandies and the day off, and the rest of the staff were threatening to walk out if the monster was not exterminated. The hall porter was crouched outside my bathroom door with a .22 rifle, hoping to shoot the bat through the keyhole. The manager had given strict instructions that on no account was the door to be opened, which made it pretty difficult for the gun-toting porter.

I paid my bill, bought a Pan Am flight bag to pack the flying fox in, cleaned up the bathroom and, feeling a bit like Count Dracula revealed, marched out of the hotel with all eyes upon me. I decided next to smuggle my companion into the Singapore Hyatt. After checking in, I set up my "vampire" once again in his private and now rather plushier bathroom and dressed his wounds for the second time. Although it might seem pointless when thousands of his fellows are being slaughtered or exploited at the need or whim of human beings, I still feel it is worthwhile to wrestle with the problems of one individual creature. An animal deserves attention for its own sake. That is another reason why zoo work satisfies me rather than the mass medicine of poultry or fish farming.

All the same, I had a problem with my adopted fruit bat. I did not like the look of the small Singapore Zoo, and I could not take him with me when I left in a couple of days. For thirty-six hours I worked hard at anointing and injecting his wounds while he consumed peaches and mangoes and made quite a mess of the Hyatt's marble bathroom. On my last evening in Singapore I packed him back into the Pan Am bag and took a ferry across the straits to Malaysia. At the dockside I hired a taxi and told the driver to take me inland to the first bit of dense forest. Once there I walked through the long grass into the trees, loaded a syringe with one more dose of long-acting penicillin and squatted down. The flying fox had his last jab, looked at me, squeaked and then launched himself out of the unzipped bag, up and away. Unsteadily he flew into the canopy of dark green and disappeared. I hope he made out. I walked straight back to the surprised taxi driver and told him to take me back to the boat. Strange fellow, this Englishman, I could see him thinking. All that way just to relieve himself!

Back at the hotel I rang Norman Whittle to report on my progress and to check that all was well at home. "I'm in the thick of the love potion business," I said, "and I'm off to Indonesia in the morning to see a mermaid!"

The intercontinental cable hissed for a few seconds as Norman digested my remarks. "Look, David," he said finally, "I don't understand a word of what you're saying. If you're lying drunk in some oriental bath house while I'm up to my ears tuberculin testing all Farmer Crawshaw's Friesians, covered in mud and muck with it raining non-stop for six days, we're going to have a little chat when and if you ever get home." He put the receiver down.

I went out specially then and there and bought a coloured postcard of a Chinese girl in traditional Cantonese dress.

It was the sort of card which if tilted slightly revealed the girl naked and unadorned. I sent it to Norman bearing the words, "Best wishes from the bath house. Hic!"

Next day I flew into Medan, a sprawling, seedy town of sleepy streets with houses stripped to the bare wood by the scorching sun, clouds of eye-stinging dust bowled along before a hot wind, and garish, squeaky trishaws. An enormous bald Chinese gentleman with the figure of a Japanese sumo wrestler, a purple shirt and candy-striped trousers was waiting by his car to meet me. "Welcome to Medan," said Tok Man.

We drove for twenty minutes before Tok Man pulled up beside a high wooden fence set in a grove of dense hibiscus bushes. It surrounded a compound set in rustling fields of tobacco and backed by a broad strip of yellow sand, with the dark grey ocean beyond. Through a heavily padlocked gate we entered a cool shaded yard with a bare earthen floor surrounded by hutches, cages and a variety of wooden boxes.

"I have only a few animals I keep for my . . . personal use," said Tok Man. "Feng Lo tells me you are interested in seeing my sea cow. Come, I will show you."

He led the way to a large coffin-like box in one corner of the yard. It had a stout grille set in the top. Looking in I could see the ungainly shape of a real-life mermaid, a dark brown, helpless roly-poly with dried and cracking skin and eyes that were caked and sore. It was a dugong all right and in terrible shape.

"Why do you keep it so?" I asked in dismay. "These are rare and precious creatures which need water; you see what is happening to the skin."

"Yes, indeed, they are precious, Doctor. Oh, how wonderful it would be if I could get more tears from the beast! Believe me I have tried, I have laboured, but I cannot make it weep."

I could hardly believe my ears. "But . . . " I faltered.

388

"You see, Doctor," interrupted the fat man, "if I can speak in confidence, I am a man in my prime with a wife who is a true jewel, but"—his voice hushed—"I have no children. It is a matter of great sadness and embarrassment to me. I have tried many things, and always I refuse to lose hope, but I remain . . . how do you say?"

"Impotent," I said.

He nodded glumly. "So now I try the creatures I have here."

"What exactly do you do?" I inquired, grimly fascinated.

He pointed to the various containers around us. "Over there I keep a bunch of snakes. Every day I slit the gall bladder of one and run its bile into a glass of wine. I think perhaps it will help."

"And the sea cow?"

Tok Man sighed. "Each morning I beat it with a bamboo in the hope of making it weep. But so far I have collected no tears. If only I could. Sea cow's tears are most potent." His face brightened. "Doctor, perhaps you can show me some trick of making it weep?"

I pinched myself to make sure that I was not lying in bed at home having a surreal nightmare. The pinch stung but I did not wake up. "It would be best if you released the sea cow," I said as steadily as I could. "I know no way of producing tears." In actual fact I did have a chemical, carbamylcholine, which I had used to increase the tear flow from crocodiles, but I was having no part of this sick affair.

"Ah well," said the Chinaman, "I suppose I must press on with the beating. It eats nothing and I must get some tears before it dies."

"Give it some lettuce and spray it with water," I said, grinding my teeth fit to shatter them as we left the compound, but I do not think he was listening.

I went back to the hotel in Medan where Tok Man had found me a room, but could think of nothing except the sad plight of the dugong. I had to do something, but what?

389

There was only one thing for it. At eleven o'clock I walked out of the hotel carrying just a little money and my small bag of surgical instruments, found a trishaw and with much difficulty explained to the driver where I wanted to go. By trial and error we came eventually to the compound in the hibiscus grove. Motioning the nonplussed fellow to stand against the high fence, I hoisted myself up on his skinny shoulders and pulled myself over the top. The moon was full and seemed to fill half the sky as I dropped down into the yard. No guard dogs, just a squadron or two of mosquitoes and the friendly carolling of tropical frogs.

The first thing I did was to prowl round the fence, looking for a way out. A shimmer of silvery water and a foul stench led me to a slimy ditch running under the fence towards the seashore. I went over to the dugong's box. It was too dark to see much inside it, but I could hear its soft breathing. I felt round the grille. It was secured by two bolted hinges and a piece of thick, twisted wire. A dog barked in the distance as a vehicle rumbled by. I tried not to think how Indonesian jails might appear to a European found guilty of burglary, but cold sweat ran down my forehead and stung my eyes.

With a pair of artery forceps from my bag I began to unravel the stout wire. Off it came, and a moment later I had lifted the grille and was stroking my first mermaid. This was no time for the finer points of animal handling. I pushed the horizontal coffin over onto its side and with a blubbery plop the dugong fell out onto the ground. Off I went round the compound again, until I found a length of sacking. Folded lengthways several times, this made a strip to put round the base of the dugong's paddle-like tail. "Come on, old chap," I whispered as I slipped the sacking round its quivering body, "this is no time to stand on ceremony."

I began to pull the 200-pound beast backwards over the rough, dry ground. It was back-breaking work and I knew that I must have been scuffing the skin on its underside.

After what seemed like an hour, with muscles indignant at my adding yet further insult to injury, I reached the murky ditch. Dismally I realized that I would have to go down into the slimy water and drag my mermaid with me through the hole in the fence. The mosquitoes had a field day as I slithered and strained first one way and then the other, basting myself thoroughly with ooze, algae and creepy-crawlies. At last I was through the fence. Sweat soaked my hair as I pulled the dugong through after me.

Next came a prickly ploughing through a stretch of reeds. I lost a shoe. Tiny bats skimmed silently across the moon. I cowered at every sound, expecting at any moment to be discovered. Then, mercifully, I heard the first soft hissing of the sea smoothing the sand. Stopping at the edge of the shore to rest, I sat down beside the dugong and put an arm round it. All animals like a cuddle, and I might never get this chance again. I touched the strange soft muzzle and delicate lips. Its gums were warm and velvety, its breath grassy like a cow's.

Then I was up and off again, down the gently sloping beach to the water's edge. At last I could remove the sacking and throw it into the black water. The dugong could smell the ocean and was restlessly moving its head from side to side. Wearily I bent down and rolled it over and over like a giant sausage until the surf caught it and the water bore it off the sand. Its crusty, flaking back was caught by the creamy moonlight as it orientated itself, floated on the surface for a second and then, with a wave of its paddle, dived beneath the foam. It was gone. Tired, wet and smelling like a compost heap, I trudged round the edge of the hibiscus grove and slapped my gaping trishaw driver on the back. "Back to the hotel," I said, gave him every rupiah note I had in my pocket and threw my one remaining shoe into the gutter.

Tok Man arrived in the hotel lobby next day with bad news. Vandals had broken into his compound and stolen his sea cow. "Some people will eat anything," he fretted. "And my wife is scolding me more than ever. She doesn't seem to realize I want children as much as her. It's a curse on me. Today I will slit the galls of ten live snakes and drink their bile with wine."

I should have released the snakes as well, I thought, but he would easily have got some more. Perhaps . . . I decided to give him some advice.

"Look, Mr. Tok," I said, "I work with wild animals and, though I do not talk about it usually, I do know of one substance which, if taken very carefully—not too little, not too much—can produce an effect a thousand times stronger than snake bile or sea cow's tears. It always works. If I let you have some of this drug for your personal use, will you promise not to let it fall into the wrong hands?"

For a moment I thought the corpulent fellow was going to kiss me. "Of course, certainly, yes, yes, *yes*!" he gurgled. "How much do you want for it?"

"Nothing," I replied. "It is unprofessional and unethical for me to supply you with it. I do it only as a favour."

Tok Man was beside himself. I went up to my room and opened a tin of orange, sugar-coated vitamin B tablets. Counting out one hundred, I put them into an envelope and went back downstairs.

"Now, take one tablet at exactly eight o'clock in the morning and one tablet at nine o'clock at night," I instructed. "They always work, without fail. But you must not mix them with anything else. No snake bile, no sea cow's tears. They must be allowed to work alone."

Tok Man looked at the envelope he was clutching as if it was a bag of fine black pearls. "Doctor," he exclaimed, grabbing my hand and shaking it furiously, "I cannot thank you enough." He thanked me all the way to the airport and kept shouting his thanks as I went through the departure gate.

Well, I thought, if he believes what I say hard enough,

those harmless little vitamin pills will do their stuff, a lot of poor reptiles will be spared being gutted alive, Mr. Tok will not need to replace his truant sea cow and the only loser will be Mr. Feng, who will have one less customer for his ground-down zebra's tooth. And that was how it turned out, for two months later, back in England, I was to receive a cable from Tok Man in Sumatra: DEAR DOCTOR WONDERFUL. EVERYTHING MARVELLOUSEST. WIFE VERY MUCH PREGNANT.

But now, as I flew between the cloud stacks suspended over the Malacca Straits, I looked down and wondered how the dugong was faring and whether it was at that moment gorging its empty belly on succulent bunches of submarine sea grass. I thought of a fruit bat and a zebra stallion and then of the cats, dogs and cattle that I might have been busy with at that very moment in the familiar streets and fields half a world away. Safe and comfortable respectability in Rochdale, or challenge and fulfilment? Mr. Tok's dugong or Mrs. Partridge's arthritic corgi?

The decision was taken as the plane touched down again at Singapore Airport. As soon as I got home I would make my peace with Norman Whittle and break the news. I was going to take the plunge and set up my own practice to work only with wild animals from now on. There was no going back.

Going Wild

More Adventures of a Zoo Vet

One

Have you ever seen a black polar bear? The first one will be worth a fortune, and it looked as though Belle Vue might have struck lucky. The coats of their polar bears were becoming darker and darker, giving a fair impression of bottle-blonde barmaids who had been slack and let their hair-roots grow through the bleach.

Belle Vue was the city zoo in Manchester, set in an old Victorian pleasure garden, where I had taken my first steps in wild animal medicine and to which I was still veterinarian. My family often found themselves involved in my work there, especially my wife, Shelagh, who had helped me pull back from the brink of death two new-born polar bear cubs after their mother had deserted them.* One summer Sunday a few months later, she and I watched delightedly with our two daughters as the cubs, vigorous and lively now, played by the edge of their pool.

It was Shelagh who first noticed the bears' colour. 'The babies are lovely,' she said, 'but the others are just plain—well—filthy!'

My daughters agreed and wagged admonitory fingers at me. 'The polar bears are turning brown like Mum says,' chirped five-year-old Lindsey. 'Why don't you give them a good bath in Omo?'

'In my view,' opined Stephanie, with the solemnity of a nine-year-old newly embarked upon biology studies at school, 'they're mutating into brown bears.'

*See *Doctor in the Zoo*

I had to admit that there was something in what they said. Only in picture books are polar bears portrayed as being white as snow; in their native Arctic they are actually a creamy colour. But compared with the shining pearly coats of the bears I had seen at other zoos, and even allowing for the Manchester atmosphere, our bears were not the right colour. I raised the matter with the zoo's director, Ray Legge.

'Funny you should mention it,' he said. 'I've watched this darkening of the fur for a couple of weeks now. I wondered if my eyes were playing tricks.'

'My girls said the colour reminded them of caramel cream.'

'That's it,' Ray replied. 'Caramel describes the shade exactly. What's more, it gets deeper every day. At this rate, within two months you won't be able to tell them apart from the real brown and black bears.'

What could be the reason? The animals had a deep pool of sweet water in which they swam during daylight hours and they were hosed down regularly. Surely this was more than just grime.

'Let's dope one of the most café-au-lait individuals,' I suggested, 'and have a look at the skin.'

On close inspection, the skin of the slumbering beast appeared to the naked eye to be healthy, the coat was thick and shining and the animal was generally in tip-top shape, yet without doubt the hairs were more like those of a seal-point Siamese cat. I took a small bunch of hair clippings for microscopical examination, and in due course these revealed, loosely speaking, that the polar bears were growing seaweed! Under the microscope thousands of minute brown plants could be seen clinging to each hair. These algae, the sort of primitive vegetation that forms the green scum on pond water, are the smaller relatives of the various types of seaweed. In the case of the polar bears, they were not invading the hair and causing disease as, say, ringworm fungi do; they were just camping out and multiplying in the warm, moist forest of the bears' coats.

It was the same little plant which made the stone steps at home as slippery as oiled ice in damp weather. Shelagh tried to keep it at bay with scrubbing brush, chlorine solution and copper sulphate crystals, but her methods were never successful for very long and anyway could not be applied to living animals. After a long hunt I found a chemical manufactured in the USA which was lethal for algae but completely non-toxic for every other living animal or plant except, oddly, rice sprouts. As there are no paddy fields in Belle Vue I felt safe in using the stuff, which we sprayed over the bears and added to their pool water. Within three weeks our Manchester polars looked as if they had just come back from the laundromat. It is not true that bears are pure white only in picture books; maybe in the Arctic they are not white as snow, but they were for a time in the icy wastes of north-west England.

A small, whitewood coffin lay on the back doorstep. The sunlight glinted off the brass knobs, brass handles and oblong brass plates with which it was fitted. I stood looking down at the doleful box, my hand frozen in mid-air on its way to pull my keys from my jacket pocket. The family had appeared hale and hearty at breakfast a few hours before, as far as I could remember I had never brushed with the Rochdale branch of the Cosa Nostra if it existed, and my wine-merchant would have had difficulty in fitting my monthly order into the rather shallow sarcophagus even if he had for some reason started to deliver his wares in so funereal a fashion. The brass plate on the coffin lid was unengraved but the corner of a piece of white paper had been slipped under it. Stooping down, I read the words scribbled in pencil on the protruding part: 'Having a drink at White Lion. L. Fazakerly, Undertaker.' I was intrigued. Shelagh was out shopping, the girls were both at school. I decided to go down to the pub for a beer and find out why Mr Fazakerly had taken to leaving samples of his craft on my back doorstep.

It was 1968 and I had only recently taken the plunge and left general veterinary practice to set up on my own as the world's sole independent, full-time veterinarian for zoo animals and other wild, exotic creatures. Working from my home on the outskirts of Rochdale, the most unlikely and unexotic cotton-mill town in drizzly north-west England, I had not found the first few days of my new venture very encouraging. As part of a bustling practice in Rochdale for the previous dozen years, I had been gradually expanding my wild animal work: from seeing the odd parrot or lizard once in a blue moon, I had taken over the care of the animals at Belle Vue Zoo on behalf of the partnership, travelled increasingly to patients all over the world, and gained my Fellowship of the Royal College of Veterinary Surgeons in the specialised area of zoo primate diseases. But during all those years I had been backed up by my partner and assistants in the practice, there had been a full range of surgical and diagnostic equipment in our clinic, I had been able to fall back on pigs, cattle, dogs and cats when ailing armadillos and infirm elephants were hard to come by, and there had been a secure, regular income from the practice of medicine round the cobbled streets and rainswept Pennine farms of this grey and gritty industrial town.

Now all my connections with my old practice had been severed. A legal document dissolving my partnership had been drawn up and I was forbidden to treat anything other than exotic species within a ten-mile radius of Rochdale Town Hall. There were three named and specific exceptions to this. One was the stock owned by Farmer Schofield, my next-door neighbour, and then there were two dogs which I had personally attended to from puppyhood to old age. They were old, old friends and everyone had been agreed that the animals might not take kindly to a switch of physician so late in life. So the lawyers, in dissolving the partnership, had taken solemn and formal note of my two remaining pet patients: 'Bouncer', a beagle owned by the Brown family, and 'Fly', a spaniel belonging to Mr and Mrs Phillips.

I had also brought with me from my previous practice veterinary responsibility for the large collection of zoo animals at Belle Vue, but otherwise it was a matter of waiting for the telephone to ring. It did ring, and often, but invariably the caller was someone with a horse, a cat, a cow, or something else that was not in any way outlandish or untamed or might fall into my new province of 'exotica'. Already I had begun to wonder what had happened to the population of unusual pet animals out there. I knew that there were parrots and bush-babies and snakes and monkeys around for I had treated many of them in my old practice, but where were they now? Had they all been blessed simultaneously by uncommonly good health or had they been decimated, unknown to me, by some undiscriminating pandemic? Had folk with a penchant for cobras in the greenhouse or otters in the bathroom recanted and taken up pigeon-flying or suddenly seen the virtues of Siamese cats? Had they forgotten about me, now ready, willing and anxious to devote myself to their bizarre beasts or had they, more likely, never heard of me? Professionally prevented from advertising my presence as a zoo vet, I sat in the white-tiled dairy of my farmhouse that Shelagh had converted into an office, and began to consider whether my planned exotic animal practice was not only invisible but illusory.

To resist such gloomy fancies I filled my abundant spare time with reading, losing myself in piles of books and manuscripts about the care and treatment of wild creatures, which I found in the University library at Manchester. And now, coming home for lunch after a morning poring over such esoteric works as *Captain Bob's Experiences with Walruses, 1888–95*, I had found the undertaker's macabre visiting card.

The snug of my local pub, the White Lion, was almost

empty when I entered. Mr Fazakerly, whom I had heard of but never met, was instantly recognisable as he leaned against the copper-topped bar with a pint of bitter before him. Black jacket, faintly striped dark grey trousers, white shirt and black tie, the whole outfit clothed a slight and stooping figure surmounted by the pale face of a Low Church ecclesiastic and the Brylcreemed hair of a British Rail buffet car attendant. Coal-black eyes flanked a waxy, pointed nose.

'In nomine Patris, Filii . . .' the unmistakable undertaker was intoning as I walked over. I saw that he had a saucer of mussels in front of him, and that with one hand he was shaking drops of tabasco sauce from a small bottle over the plump bodies of the molluscs.

'Mr Fazakerly?' I asked.

The undertaker nodded but continued his invocation: '. . . et Spiritus Sancti.' When he was satisfied that each mussel had been splashed with the red sauce, he picked one up between black-gloved fingers and popped it into his mouth. Then he beckoned to the landlord before turning to me with a thin smile as delicate as hoar-frost on a thread of gossamer.

'Dr Taylor? Will you have a drink? How about a mussel?'

'Thank you,' I replied. 'I got your note on the, er, the box. What's it about?'

Mr Fazakerly wagged one glistening leather finger at me and drops of tabasco and mussel juice ran down onto his curling shirt cuff. 'Casket, Dr Taylor, casket, I beg you.'

'The casket, then, the one on my doorstep,' I went on correctly. 'Is it meant for me?'

The undertaker's whole face miraculously reformed itself into the spitting image of a saint or martyr as conceived by an Italian Baroque artist: the diagonally uptilted face, the lowered eyelids, the half-open, inverted crescent of pale lips, it was all there. He pressed his gloved palms gently together and breathed his next words towards me. 'The bereaved gave me your name, Dr Taylor. Normally we would not need assistance, but as this is a, well, rather unusual loved one. . .'

402

'Something's died?' I whispered awkwardly over the rim of my tankard.

'Some*one*, yes indeed. Sorely to be missed, I'm sure. A good, a loyal, an abiding friend.'

'Who?'

Mr Fazakerly cleared his throat and looked at me solemnly. I expected any moment that he would reach out, grasp my shoulder resolutely and support me as he delivered the sad tidings. 'Phillips—Lumbutts Lane. . .' He hesitated for a moment as if to give me a chance to take it all in, then he went on, 'The dear spaniel, Fly by name, I believe.'

Fly Phillips; so that was it. The epileptic spaniel with an incompetent mitral valve, who had uncomplainingly gobbled down each day a shower of multicoloured capsules, digitalis, tocopherol, primidone and phenytoin, was dead. Half of my remaining canine practice had passed on.

'How did it happen and how do you fit in?' I asked.

Mr Fazakerly looked about to break into tears. 'The loved one. . .'

'The dog,' I interrupted tetchily.

'. . . died suddenly in its sleep this morning. Mr and Mrs Phillips called you but you were not at home, so they contacted us.'

'To bury him, I presume?'

'No, Dr Taylor, to prepare him.'

Now I was stumped. As far as I knew, the Phillipses were not any sort of religious eccentrics. They were devoted to their pet, but I had never heard them mention anything special that should happen to Fly after he died. They were well-off, and I could imagine them forking out the cash to have the dog properly buried, but what was this about preparation?

I wondered if Mr Fazakerly, despite all this solemnity, was playing some sort of joke, fuelled by the White Lion's best bitter. Grinning, I thumped my companion in the ribs. 'Come on,' I said, 'you can't be serious. What do you mean by preparing him?'

Mr Fazakerly did not allow his pious expression to slip so much as a millimetre; there was no hint of a smile, no relaxation of his frown. 'Dr Taylor, the loved . . . that is the dog, Fly Phillips, is to be buried in a plot at Mumbles on the Welsh coast, where he used to run on the cliffs as a puppy. Mumbles is over two hundred miles from here. My firm has been asked to embalm him.'

'Embalm the dog!' I exclaimed. 'You must be pulling my leg.'

The undertaker sighed and looked round conspiratorially to make sure that he was not being overheard. 'Not at all, Doctor. He is to be embalmed in a running position, albeit lying on his side, with his ears tastefully disposed as if blowing in the wind as he gaily bowls along.'

Astounded, I could still detect no chink in the undertaker's grave countenance. To give myself time to collect my thoughts, I invited him to have another pint.

'No, thank you. We can't possibly discuss matters further here. Let's go to your home. I'll meet you there.'

We left the pub and I climbed into my car. As I pulled out onto the main road moments later, I glanced into the driving mirror. A few yards behind me was cruising a highly polished Daimler hearse with Mr Fazakerly at the wheel.

Back at the house, the coffin was still lying on the doorstep. Soundly asleep on top of it was Lupin, my cat. There was nobody about although Henry, our pet goat, with his head as usual poking inquisitively through the market-garden gate, did seem to be straining his ears in our direction. The undertaker eyed Henry and motioned me away out of the goat's earshot.

'The dog must be embalmed, as I explained. I have all my equipment and materials with me, but as you will appreciate, my, er, subjects are normally humans. Of dogs I have no anatomical knowledge. That is why I need you to help me achieve a perfect closed circuit.'

'Closed circuit?'

'Yes, indeed, the touchstone of one in my profession, Dr Taylor: absence of bubbles.'

Mr Fazakerly had lost me again. What had all this flatulent talk to do with circuits and dead dogs? I decided to push on and tackle the bubbles when they appeared.

'So you want me to help you at the embalming?' I said.

'Yes.'

'Where is the body?'

'In the casket.'

I looked across at Lupin, blissfully unconscious with his head resting on the twinkling brass plate.

'Couldn't we have done this at your premises?' I asked. Fazakerly's Chapel of Rest was a sizeable building near the Town Hall.

The undertaker looked alarmed and tut-tutted. 'Oh, I'm afraid not, dear sir. We have our other loved ones and their bereaveds and their bereaveds' feelings to think of. I mean, if it got around the Freemasons and the Catenians and all the rest of our clientèle that Fazakerly's wasn't exclusively for, er, homo sapiens. . . Oh no! Quite out of the question. Hence the need for some degree of secrecy.'

A few minutes later Henry the goat watched soberly as Mr Fazakerly and I carried the coffin into the shed that I was planning to use for autopsying the cadavers of exotic birds, reptiles and small mammals which would, I hoped, soon begin to arrive by post from all over the world. Mr Fazakerly went back to the hearse and returned with a large black box which he placed on the floor near the examination table. Then he unscrewed the brass knobs of the little coffin, took off the lid and brought out the body of the cocker spaniel. I was intrigued, and waited expectantly for the undertaker to begin his arcane rites.

Fazakerly opened his black box, which was split into two equal halves. One side contained two large glass flasks, one empty and the other full of clear, pink liquid; there were also coils of rubber tubing and a shiny, dagger-like instrument.

The other side of the box was crammed with cosmetics: creams, powders, make-up sticks, eye-liners, rouges.

'Leichner,' said Fazakerly proudly, when he saw me staring at his collection. 'We always use Leichner—nothing but the best for Fazakerly's.' He fished in the box and pulled out a lipstick. 'The latest spring fashion—crusty pearl. May I offer this as a present for your wife, Doctor? Or would she prefer some gunmetal mascara?'

Hastily, I made up some story about Shelagh being allergic to the stuff.

Fazakerly returned the cosmetics to their compartment, then put the two flasks, the tubing and the dagger instrument on the table near the body. 'In order to preserve the loved one's appearance and presentability for the inspection of the bereaved between now and the interment in Wales,' he began, 'I shall now replace all the loved . . . the dog's blood with this pink solution of formalin in water coloured with cochineal. In humans I would set up an airtight closed-circuit pumping system by attaching one rubber tube via a glass cannula to an ankle vein. This tube leads into the empty flask, and a second tube links the empty flask to the one containing pink fluid. A third runs from there to this trocar'—Mr Fazakerly picked up the dagger-like instrument—'which is inserted by a deft thrust through the upper abdomen and diaphragm into the left ventricle of the heart. By squeezing this rubber enema pump clipped into the system, I can cause blood to enter the empty flask and be replaced via the heart and arterial system by the suitably coloured preserving fluid in the other container.'

Mr Fazakerly's enthusiastic exposition of his art had left him slightly breathless. He turned to me. 'So now you see why you are required, Doctor. Since my anatomical knowledge extends only to the human, you must find me an ankle vein on the dog and, more importantly, the left ventricle. I needn't say how vital it is that the loved one isn't mutilated unnecessarily.'

406

I thought about it. The 'ankle' vein would be no problem, and it took only a second to attach the first tube to a blood vessel below the right hock joint. The precise point at which to insert the dagger-like trocar was far trickier. Fazakerly was right. For his pumping system to work efficiently without air entering the system, the trocar had to be placed absolutely correctly; anywhere else and the strange postmortem circulation of liquids just would not take place. The problem was that a dog's heart is quite small, and the left ventricle forms only one quarter of the heart. Its position in the living animal is fairly precise, but it is much less easily located from outside after death and least of all with a big instrument designed for the larger human species.

After much careful consideration I selected a spot and inserted the undertaker's grim weapon. He connected all the tubes, checked for obvious leaks and began to pump vigorously. I watched the two flasks with fascination, feeling a bit like Igor, Dr Frankenstein's idiot assistant.

Some dark blood fell into the empty flask, while the level of pink fluid in the other fell slightly. Then, with a friendly chuffing sound, the empty flask began to fill with great big pink bubbles. All the tubes began to gurgle and vibrate.

'Holy Harry!' exclaimed Fazakerly irritably and pumping ever more furiously. 'Look at those bubbles. The circuit's faulty. You've got it wrong!'

It was not much use explaining that cardiac punctures on stiff and lifeless cadavers were hardly everyday work for veterinarians, so I began to fiddle with the tubes, made sure the connections were tight and adjusted the position of the trocar. My anatomical expertise and reputation were at stake.

The undertaker pumped some more and the froth multiplied. Bubbles danced prettily and inexplicably through the pink embalming fluid which was now certainly not going down. Mr Fazakerly positively growled at me. He couldn't have looked more deadly serious. He pumped on with wild abandon. Suddenly, the flask containing the fluid hiccupped and blew its lid off. Smelly formalin ran over Mr Fazakerly's black boots.

'There—you see! Look at that! That's never happened in all Fazakerlys' seventy-eight years!' He lowered his voice to a passionate whisper. 'Imagine what our bereaveds would say if that happened in the home!'

My future as a mortician's apprentice had never looked bleaker, but try as I might, I could not re-adjust the trocar in a way that started the exchange of liquids. Air was entering the system somehow. We both waggled the tubes, pushed and pulled, but it was no use. Eventually the undertaker reluctantly suggested that I operate on the dead animal, correctly place and sew in the trocar and then stitch everything up neatly beneath the long hair. For the first time since I was a student I practised surgery on a dead animal, but an hour later I had managed to link up Fazakerly's confounded plumbing system and the fluids began to flow. Fly was embalmed.

Mr Fazakerly was by now a trifle less indignant. He bent down to his black box again and rummaged among the cosmetics.

'You're not . . .' I began incredulously.

'I am indeed,' he replied, straightening up with a fistful of tubes and waxy sticks. 'Fazakerlys' are rightly appreciated for their thoughtful and realistic attention to every detail.'

Still keeping his gloves on, he began to reflect the lips of the dead spaniel and to reinforce the pale pink tinge produced by the embalming fluid with a liberal application of coloured cream. A glazed, partly-open eye was given a liquid glint by dropping in some glycerine, and the dried-up nose was freshened into the counterfeit dampness of health through the vigorous application of Nivea cream.

When my companion was satisfied with his artistry he stood back to admire the overall effect. 'Hmm. That seems fine,' he said. 'D'you see how I've got the shading of the tongue just right?' It was indeed a glorious salmon pink.

'I've done the make-up for Littleshaw Amateur Players for years, you know.'

Not with the same black boxful of cosmetics, I hoped.

It was time to box Fly's remains, now eternally glorious. The little coffin was neatly lined with white satin. We placed Fly inside. 'Now for the final effect,' said the undertaker. He flapped the two ears up over the head and, straining with all his might against the hold of rigor mortis, gradually persuaded the fore limbs to creak forwards and the hind limbs to groan backwards. Fly was silently galloping over the heath.

'There,' said Mr Fazakerly. With a sigh of satisfaction, he put the lid on the coffin and tightened the screws. 'The bereaveds will be satisfied and reassured, I think,' he said solemnly. 'Now, Doctor, would you be so good as to help me carry the casket out in proper fashion? In case there's anybody about, I don't want Fazakerly's to be thought capable of levity or lack of propriety.'

I guessed correctly what he meant. With Mr Fazakerly at the front and me at the back, the coffin was hoisted onto our left shoulders. When the undertaker gave the word the cortège trooped out of the shed and, at a pace that Fazakerlys' over seventy-eight years had no doubt found appropriately sedate and impressive, bore its burden towards the waiting hearse. Only Henry looked on as we slid the coffin in and Mr Fazakerly gravely shut the doors.

'Well, good afternoon then, Doctor,' said the undertaker, shaking my hand and leaving my fingers smelling of pickled mussels, formalin and greasepaint. 'I'll leave you my card. Perhaps Fazakerlys' can be at your service some time.'

After he had driven off at a sedate speed, I gave the business card to Henry, who quickly gobbled it down. 'Do you think that might have been some sort of ill omen for the future?' I asked the old goat.

Henry said nothing but his wise eyes, with their pupils like ever-open letter boxes, twinkled. No, it was going to be all right.

Two

Autumn was upon us shortly after Fly, the embalmed spaniel, had been lowered to his rest overlooking the Welsh coastline. Autumn in Manchester meant chill, clammy air and sulphureous mists that stung the eyes and clutched at the throat. It was the time for smog, the yellow blend of water vapour and industrial smoke, and smog time was always busy for the veterinarian of a city zoo. Each year as October came round, cases of disease and death among the animals at Belle Vue began to soar. Peacocks hacked away like chain-smokers, tigers heaved their chests with the desperate concentration of asthmatics, and chimpanzees wiped running eyes and nostrils with the backs of hairy hands. And animals died. Some, experiencing all this for the first time, died quickly from pneumonia. Others, the time-servers, finally gave up the struggle against fibrous lungs and chronically enlarged hearts and wheezed their last. Most animals do not live long enough to develop the chronic degenerative changes seen in humans, but at Manchester, in the bodies of big cats, rhinoceroses, apes and the like, I saw all the post-mortem signs associated with old human city-dwellers.

That year, not only was the smog particularly bad, but Winter must have been snapping at Autumn's heels. The leaves browned, fell and were whisked away by the moist wind, and within a few days precocious atoms of ice silvered the bare trees in Belle Vue's Victorian gardens. What was more, as if Matt Kelly, the zoo's Irish head keeper, was not busy enough breaking the ice on moated paddocks to prevent inmates walking their way to freedom, the small boys

410

who daily invade the zoo grounds free by scaling unscalable walls, outrunning corpulent gate keepers and various other means, became unusually active: perhaps it was the early frost that kept them on the move.

Worse still, there was a positive epidemic of animals going 'over the wall' in the other direction. The keepers had neglected to re-clip the flight feathers of the flamingoes at six-monthly intervals, and on a suitably windy day a gang of the gorgeous birds took off and cleared the zoo walls, never to be seen again. With even less chance of survival unless they could reach some centrally heated building, complete with a supply of mice for food, a posse of young rattlesnakes set forth from the reptile house one day after sneaking through a broken pane of glass. When he found seven of the venomous reptiles absent without leave, the keeper in charge decided to keep quiet about it in the hope that either they would turn up or the low temperatures outside would finish the little wanderers and so remove any threat to the local population. If it were known that such creatures were on the loose, he could foresee a drastic reduction in the numbers of visitors coming to the zoo to walk round the exhibits with their children on a Sunday morning. This in turn would undoubtedly lead to the zoo director giving him the boot.

The keeper tried to conceal his loss by stuffing rocks, logs and vegetation of all sorts into the rattlesnake vivarium, so that what had been a fair simulation of the dry, sun-baked environment of a Californian rattler, with coiled serpents easily seen against a sandstone background, was transformed into a dripping, dense and inappropriate jungle, in which the rattlesnakes could rarely be glimpsed, let alone counted. This trick worked until two little girls, coming through the main gates on their way to the fairground, came across a pretty, if rather sluggish, little snake wearily making in the general direction of the bus stop. They picked it up, were quick to spot that it was not a worm, were relieved to see that it had not got a V-mark behind its head—the little

411

girls had been learning about Britain's only poisonous snake, the adder, at natural history lessons—and popped it into one of their purses. Their brother would just love to have a grass snake as a pet.

Later that day, back at home, Dad wound the little snake round his fingers, remarking how the warmth was making the little fellow much more agile and alert. Then he noticed the curious rings of loosely jointed dried skin at the tail. For some reason, although he was a builder's mate and this was the middle of Manchester, something worried him about those rings and he reached for a copy of *Pears Cyclopaedia*. Two minutes later he broke into a sweat and dashed to phone the police.

Matt Kelly, the head keeper, was the one who had to clear the mess up, calm down the builder's mate and his family, defuse the concern of the constabulary and divert the Press with blarney. He then fired the reptile keeper.

To add still more to our troubles that autumn, the numbers of animals being bodily purloined rose dramatically. All zoos have stock stolen from time to time: a guinea-pig or two from the Pets' Corner, tortoises from the reptile house, birds particularly parrots and cockatoos, and a variety of small mammals. Although it appeared that 'fences' did not want to touch gorillas, tigers or ostriches, that autumn saw some sizeable creatures disappear. One almost had to admire the thieves who got clean away with a five-foot alligator of irascible temperament in broad daylight, while the two little urchins who were collared half a mile from the zoo, breathlessly lugging home a trio of outraged coatimundi bundled inside a sack, must otherwise have led sainted lives not to have been severely injured by the hard-biting beasts.

Matt Kelly had hardly finished giving the crestfallen young culprits a lecture which, despite his soft Irish brogue, set their ears burning, when he was summoned to the scene of more animals gone a-missing. Two valuable De Brazza monkeys had vanished from the monkey house and the monkey keeper was certain that they had been stolen. A party had been round just before they had gone, a boisterous bunch of noisy schoolchildren. Matt quickly inspected the De Brazza cage; just possibly someone could have forced apart the vertical wires that formed the front. But how could they have grabbed hold of a big, tough species that could bite harder than a dog? Still, Matt had known it happen in the past—a jacket thrown over the animal, or even bare hands and bravado and never mind the bites and the blood when showing off in front of your pals. Before now the head keeper had stopped a coach laden with children before it left the park and had retrieved from under a seat a penguin with its powerful beak safely immobilised by rubber bands, and a wallaby hog-tied by a blushing schoolgirl's black lisle stockings. Anything could happen.

Matt rushed off to the car park with the monkey keeper. They were too late; the school party's coach had gone. The school was traced and its headmaster contacted, but the pair of monkeys, to my mind the most attractive of all primate species with their olive coat, brown and white face and goatee beard, were not forthcoming. Matt cursed and worried. Both of us could imagine the two monkeys stuffed into a dark, cramped rabbit hutch somewhere in Greater Manchester and pressed to take a diet of sweetmeats and peanuts.

The next crisis of that eventful autumn for Belle Vue was not long in coming. Someone was pinching food. Fruit, vegetables and other things were being stolen, particularly from the great ape house, the modern, self-contained unit which housed the chimpanzees, orang-utans and gorillas. Len, the senior great ape keeper, was up in arms about it. Food pilfering by keepers is an unpleasant but not uncommon problem facing all zoos, but a particularly severe outbreak at Belle Vue a few years earlier had led to the most rigid controls being imposed there. Ration sheets were printed for each species, and a cook dispensed all the food to the keepers.

The system recommended by Jimmy Chipperfield at his safari parks of chopping all fruit before sending it from the stores was adopted—nobody wants to take home a pocketful of sliced apple or pear—and I personally presented the zoo with a fruit and vegetable chopper of the sort used by farmers for mashing turnips.

I discussed this latest problem with Len and Matt Kelly. 'Whoever's doing it, they're damned sharp at it,' said Len, as he told us how some 'hands' of bananas had vanished during the tea break. 'Funny thing is, I didn't pass any keepers on my way back from the cafeteria.'

The great ape house stood apart from the other units, so anyone entering or leaving the house would have had to cross an area of open ground. The nearest unit was the Pets' Corner.

'Mebbe it's that new feller in there, the one that's lookin' after the goats and the donkeys,' growled Matt. 'Oi'll wander over and root around.'

But Matt found nothing to incriminate anybody in the Pets' Corner in any way—no banana skins in the dustbin, nothing secreted in the staff rest room. Two weeks passed. Each day one section or another reported losses of food. Apples here, tomatoes there, but always Len's great ape house was hardest hit.

Then came the nastiness. First it was a fountain pen that went, then a cigarette lighter. Finally, when a packet of cheroots disappeared while Len nipped over to the men's room, the great ape keeper had had enough. He stormed into the director's office, white-faced behind his spectacles.

'Get the police in,' he demanded. 'This light-fingered sneak-thief's gone too far.'

A report was made to the police and a detective-constable made a perfunctory visit, but there was nothing to show him and even less to be done, except to keep a sharp eye open.

'Oi'll have him. Oi'll catch him with the stuff on him one of these foine days,' proclaimed Matt after Len's lunch, a packet of sandwiches, vanished into thin air. 'Oi think the bloighter's havin' us on, teasin' us.'

It made sense. Pinching juicy peaches or even a lighter was one thing, but having designs on Len's meat paste sandwiches suggested more mischief than criminal dishonesty.

Despite a high level of vigilance, Matt and his men made no progress in identifying the miscreant and the crime wave grew. Night attacks became more frequent than ones during the day, and the fact that there was no forcing of locks or windows anywhere confirmed our suspicions that a keeper with a key was behind it all. When the real malevolence began, it all seemed to be aimed at the unfortunate Len.

'This—this imbecile, this kleptomaniac has a grudge against me,' he moaned bitterly to me one day, as we wrestled with a baby chimp that needed his polio jab. 'Vindictiveness, that's all it is. It can only be a keeper who thinks I've done wrong by him.'

'Why, what's he done now?' I asked.

Len drew in a great breath and then spat out the words with ripe indignation. 'Crapped in my tea!'

'I'm sorry, I don't understand.'

'Crapped—defecated—in my tea!'

Trying to keep a straight face, I asked 'What, how, when?'

'This morning, at eleven o'clock. I brewed up in the ape house instead of going to the cafeteria, poured a cup for me and one for Harold.' Harold was the patriarch of the orang-utans at Belle Vue, a red-haired potentate with a figure like a Sumo wrestler, who relished a mug of sweet, milky tea. 'I took Harold his, came back to my room, picked up my cup and there it was, floating on the surface.'

I cleared my throat. 'Could it not have been, say, chimpanzee or orang excrement?' The great apes generally are enthusiastic and skilled throwers of faecal matter. Some, such as an orang at Rhenen Zoo in Holland or a male chimp at Dudley, are so adept at inswingers and so accurate, even when bowling backwards, that it beats me why they have not been snapped up by the MCC cricket team or transferred for a fat fee to the New York Yankees.

Len sniffed. 'It could not,' he said. 'No apes were loose. The cup and the table it was on are twenty feet or more away from the nearest animals, which are separated from the passageway leading to my room by a brick wall anyway, and the stainless steel drawers that are set in the wall for passing food through were closed. The only animal that could have had access to my tea was a human!'

'I suppose it could have been a chimp stool that he picked up and dropped in,' I ventured.

'Still a dirty, filthy, perverted sense of humour,' Len scowled.

The next day the invisible thief and defiler of teacups, if they were one and the same person, struck again. This time it was another batch of Len's sandwiches, not stolen but left crowned with a noisome offering. To add insult to injury his daily newspaper had been removed. '*Daily Mirror* gone and crap on my lunch,' Len roared at Matt and me as we tried not to laugh.

As usual there had been no sign of the villain, but interestingly the deed had been done while Len was feeding his animals elsewhere in the house with the outside door to the passageway leading to his room securely locked. Len was also quite certain that the catch had been dropped on the Yale lock when he closed it. Even if the culprit had a key to the house, it would have been useless with the catch down. The only logical answer, if Len was right, was that the villain had been in the house all the time.

I decided to look again at the scene of the crime. Len's room was a bare, smooth-walled place with an empty isolation cage against one wall and a single door. High on the wall facing the door was a window that flapped back on runners, leaving an opening too small for a human to climb through. The only furniture was a small sink with a gas ring, and the table. I looked around. Just possibly someone could throw objects from the outside up and over the window when it was open, but aiming would be impossible. I looked up at the ceiling and at the large, galvanised central heating duct which ran across the width of the room. Then I noticed something. The vent for warm air was a slotted grille in the duct, and it was situated directly over the table.

The great ape house's revolutionary system of channelling warm air to all the exhibits through the galvanised ducting had proved very successful until it was found that thick growths of mould had begun to sprout on the inside of the metal tube, encouraged by the warm, moist air. I had been consulted with an eye to possible health hazards from fungus spores being inhaled by the animals, and had managed to solve the problem by getting Len to spray a non-toxic fungicide into the airstream once a week. I recalled climbing up on a chair and looking into the mould-caked ducting through a manhole. Sure enough, every few yards there was a manhole covered by a disc of metal that was secured by two wing-nuts. The manhole in Len's room was firmly sealed. I walked back down the passageway and looked up at the ducting. Another manhole, sealed. Then another, its covering plate slightly askew and leaving a gap at one edge. Halfway down the passage was one manhole where the cover was completely off. I looked up at a round black hole from which a draught of warm air blew gently down.

'Get a torch, Len,' I said. 'I'm going to have a look up there.'

When at last a torch was found, Matt produced a stepladder and I climbed up to the hole. There was just enough room for me to get my head and one arm in. I switched on the torch and shone it down to my left. An empty black tunnel, dusty but no longer choked with mould, stretched down to the end of the house. Wriggling round, I pointed the torch down the length of ducting extending over Len's room.

The torch beam ran along more sheets of grimy black

metal, then suddenly it was shining on a colourful, twinkling tableau at the far end, a cross between Fagin's den and Aladdin's cave. There, blinking in the beam of light, caught red-handed with surprise and apprehension written all over their faces, skulked the two missing De Brazza monkeys. They crouched on a bed of paper, shredded cheroots, dried vegetable peel and nutshells, surrounded by fruit of every kind, some fresh, some half-eaten. Bags of nuts, dog biscuits, potato chips and bars of stolen chocolate were near at hand. Amid the debris the polished metal of a lighter and a fountain pen glinted.

'Gotcha!' I said quietly, and climbing grinning down the step-ladder.

'Who's up there? Let me get at 'em,' shouted Len, rushing forward to take my place. There was a silence, then his wrath turned to chuckles as he came face to face with his perse-cutors at last.

The episode drew to a swift close. The De Brazzas were injected by dart-pistol with phencyclidine, a quick-acting anaesthetic, and when they were unconscious I raked them back to the manhole using a shepherd's crook lashed to the end of a long pole. Matt hauled the two dreaming felons back to their quarters in the monkey house, while Len cleared out the den in the ducting. The total weight of the cache of food and other items was seventy-eight pounds.

I was surprised that Len, while sitting in his room, had not heard any noises in the duct above him; heavily-built speci-mens like De Brazzas would surely have made a racket moving around on the thin metal floor of their hideaway. But the senior keeper had noticed nothing apart from the gentle scurry of mice, a sound to which he had long been accus-tomed. We could only assume that the monkeys, like prison-ers of war on the run, had lain motionless amid their booty as long as the 'enemy' was present below. It was surely acciden-tal that they had fouled Len's tea and sandwiches in obeying calls of nature close to the air vent. But what had happened when there were no humans about, particularly at night? They must have dropped from the manhole, moved up the passageway to Len's room and left the house through the gap in his permanently flapped-back window. From there it would be easy to enter almost any other building in the zoo through holes, skylights or broken windows. De Brazzas have a distinguished, aristocratic countenance and, loping over the flower beds with armfuls of edible swag, they would have been the nearest thing in the monkey world to Raffles and Bunny.

Three

It might have been a scene from a film about the Green Berets: I was John Wayne with an M16 carbine crouched at the open door of a helicopter gunship as it whirled low over the bush. Not quite, but I was hanging from my straps with the down-draught from the helicopter rotor arms blowing cold around me and my eye jammed to the sights of a rifle. I had drawn a shaky bead on something on the sunbaked ground forty feet below.

'Right ho, Doc, let her have it!' shouted the pilot, levelling the chopper out.

I squeezed the trigger gently. There was an almost inaudible crack and a spot of blue suddenly appeared on the offside haunch of the zebra mare galloping flat out through grass dark with our insect-like shadow and pressed flat by our rushing wind.

'Got her!' I bellowed, and we curved abruptly so that my doorway was full of the rich blue of the African sky studded with a scatter of vultures turning idly like paper mobiles suspended from a ceiling and keeping an eye on the flash of our red strobe lights. Although it was high noon, we had four strobes working; vultures dozed off after lunch, it seemed, as they sailed on the thermals, and the idea of intense flashes of light from the helicopter was to interrupt their morbid reveries and protect us from collision.

A minute later we settled down onto the scrubland in a cloud of yellow dust. Not far away the zebra mare was buckling at the knees, nostrils flared, eyes unseeing. Tidily she collapsed and rolled onto her side. Louie, the pilot, was already giving directions over the radio that would bring the boys in the truck over to us, while I ducked under the slowing rotor blades and ran with my tool-box towards the zebra.

Not a war film, not jet-set hunting even, at least not of the killing sort. I was in East Africa, on the Kenya-Tanzania border about fifty miles south-east of Arusha, collecting a group of zebras for Mr van den Baars, a Dutch animal dealer and one of my best customers. Instead of the pole and lasso handling from a pursuing truck, we were trying out the more sophisticated technique of air-to-ground missiles: blue-tufted flying syringes fired by compressed air from a dart-rifle and loaded with etorphine, a powerful, reversible anaesthetic.

It had been a very successful week, with thirty zebra captured, no deaths, no fractures, no men injured and only eight flying syringes, worth around ten pounds each, lost through misses. It had also been a helluva good time, with cold beer at the Nairobi Hilton every evening and slivers of roast lamb eaten before sunrise with Masai herdsmen after we had put the helicopter down beside one of their lonely circular corrals of thorns. Back home, the hills round Rochdale were showing their first sprinkling of December snow.

When the truck rolled up quarter of an hour later, the sleeping zebra was lifted easily by half a dozen cheerful Africans into a wooden crate. Just before dropping the slide to shut her in, I injected a syringeful of antidote into her jugular vein. She would be on her feet within minutes. Later in the day the whole bag of zebra would be on their way via Nairobi to quarantine in Mombasa, and after a couple of months there, they would make the three-week journey by sea round the Cape to Rotterdam. The mare was the last of the consignment.

Louie, a young white Kenyan with red hair and beard and a skin like burnished bronze, sat in the shade of his chopper with a grin on his face. He squinted after the dust cloud that was the wagon bouncing its way back to Nairobi and unscrewed a bottle of pomegranate juice.

'Well, Dave,' he said, with the rather old-fashioned turn of phrase to which I had become accustomed, 'I fancy all is hunky-dory. A spiffing week, I'd say.' For someone who was considered one of the toughest bush pilots in East Africa and had survived two serious crashes during the Mau Mau troubles, Louie talked like an Etonian officer cadet. 'What do you want to do for the rest of the day?' he went on, passing me the bottle. 'Care for a spin towards Meru? We might get a peek at some of those poacher johnnies.'

Elephant poaching was rife. We had dropped down a few days earlier beside the bloated corpse of a big bull that had died slowly from a gut shot. His tusks had been hacked from him while he lay dying and would by now be on their way to the Nairobi dealers who would turn them into souvenirs for genteel blue-rinsed ladies on package tours from the Home Counties, Connecticut or Cologne. Yes, I would dearly like to come across poachers in action, even though it was costing my client eighty pounds an hour to keep the helicopter in the air, and even though the poachers were reputed to be hard cases who would exchange fire with police and game wardens and pump rifle slugs at whirly-birds like ours that intruded on their rapacious forays.

'Top hole. Let's get the old girl wound up,' said Louie happily when I agreed.

The engine thumped into life, and soon we were scything through the air, our skids almost touching the tops of the acacia trees. There was not much life about: a small cluster of elephants sheltering from the midday sun, a lone warthog scooting angrily from a mudbank as we went milling by, a clay-red Masai in a ragged shawl leaning against the trunk of a baobab with the elegance of a Roman senator.

'I can remember when the game hereabouts was thick as locusts,' shouted Louie, 'but look at it now. Over-hunting,

422

poaching, indiscriminate burning of tree cover. It's a bally shame.'

I looked down at a rare trio of whiskery wildebeest. Only a decade ago they would have been like lemmings around here at this season of the year. All at once we passed over a handful of zebras trotting apprehensively beneath our shadow.

'Some poppets among that lot,' bellowed my pilot. 'Still, we've got our quota.' He pulled the helicopter round into a tight circle and we ran back to look at the zebras head-on.

The lead stallion had had enough of this uncomfortable aerial attention. He wheeled about and broke into a fast gallop, the rest of the herd keeping up with him. There were ten altogether, including three young foals. We followed, hovering, as they raced along. I could not hear the pounding of their hooves but they were raising plenty of dust. There were trees ahead, leafless, twisted skeletons of acacia killed by a grass fire. As the zebras charged towards the trees they split into two groups, one passing the gnarled white trunks on the right, the other on the left. Once past the trees, they re-united into a compact band—except for one of the foals. From our seats in our floating plastic bubble, thirty yards behind them, we saw it gallop full tilt towards one of the acacias. It was twenty feet from the tree, going straight as an arrow. Ten, eight, still flat out. The machinery above us drowned the sound of the thwack. There must have been one, for the young zebra slammed hard and unswerving into the bleached wood and fell instantly as if pole-axed.

'Land!' I yelled, but Louie was already closing the throttle. He touched down light as a feather. The zebra herd had disappeared as we both ran across to the little body lying beneath the tree.

I knelt down and put my hand flat on the foal's chest. It was alive, for I could feel the heart thumping under my palm. I raised its head. Its nose was bleeding. I pressed cautiously over the head bones, but there was no detectable fracture. It was a youngster of around three weeks, concussed, out for the count.

'Darn queer how it ran slap bang into the tree,' mused Louie.

I lifted an eyelid to test the corneal reflex. Then I lifted the other.

'Damnation, just look at that!' I exclaimed, pointing to the eyes. 'There's your answer.'

Louie bent close as I indicated the blue-white spots deep within each of the eyeballs. They were true cataracts. The baby zebra was as blind as a bat.

The foal blinked and shook its head feebly. It was coming round.

'What are we going to do with the little blighter?' asked Louie.

At that moment I was not at all sure of the answer. 'Get my gear, please,' I said.

Louie loped back to the helicopter for the workman's tool-box in which I carry a full set of emergency equipment when on safari—whether in Africa or on English moorland. I gave the foal an injection of valium and betamethasone. We sat on the baking ground, watching as it wobbled into a sitting position.

What to do? That was indeed a poser. It was amazing that the animal had survived so long. I assumed that they were congenital cataracts, present at birth. The foal's dam must have taken good care of it, keeping a watchful eye to see that it did not stray too far from her side. It must have used touch and smell to feed, and hearing to move when the others did. But its future in the bush was predictable and sure to be brief. Taken by a hunting dog, hyena or lion, drowned at a waterhole, breaking its neck by falling into a dry river bed; one of those or something similar was the foal's certain fate today, tomorrow—soon, anyway. To be young and sightless when death came out of the long savanna grass or the red

424

mud or the parched rock: life in the bush is devoid of pity and only the fittest survive.

Louie and I both knew this, but we were involved now, and we also knew we had to make a decision on the wild animal's behalf. Let it go? Maybe it would be found again by the herd. Kill it? I had a bottle of barbiturate in the box. I looked again at the unseeing eyes. A sunbeam caught one of the pupils and it narrowed fractionally. There was a faint light reflex, then, which meant that a normal retina probably lay behind the opaque lens.

'What are we going to do?' repeated Louie, looking concerned.

I made up my mind. 'Take it back with us,' I replied.

'Super idea.' Louie brightened at once and helped me carry the drunken-looking foal to the helicopter. 'But what are you going to do with him, old boy?'

That I was not so clear about. Get him back to Nairobi first of all. Then what? He could be artificially reared easily enough on cow's milk diluted with lime water and sweetened with lactose: I had done it several times at zoos in England. Maybe John Seago, the Nairobi animal catcher and a man with a deep feeling for all kinds of living things and infinite patience, would take the foal on. But the eyes, they would not clear spontaneously. What about them?

'Call up the Seago organisation,' I shouted when we were in the air. 'See if they're prepared to foster it after an operation.'

Louie got busy on the radio. When I was in general practice I had taken a special interest in ophthalmology, done a post-graduate course in eye surgery at Manchester Royal Infirmary and extracted a number of cataractous eye lenses from domestic dogs. I had never tackled a single case in a zoo animal.

'Seago and his partner are away for the next few weeks on a catching expedition,' Louie informed me after a while. 'What about keeping it at my place?'

I thought about it as we whirled towards the outskirts of Nairobi. Maybe van den Baars would accept the youngster if the operation went well. Louie had a big farm with lots of good loose-boxes. I decided that if the Dutch dealer would agree to have the foal added to his shipment, I would operate and the little animal could go down to Mombasa after a week or two. I would only be in Kenya for another fourteen days, so I would have to get cracking immediately. After I left, maybe one of the local veterinarians would keep an eye on the patient—if the surgery was successful. There were a lot of 'ifs', particularly in removing the lenses from an animal's eyes.

Back at base, the truck had not yet arrived. The zebras caught earlier in the week were munching alfalfa inside high wooden corrals. While Louie arranged the quartering of the foal in a cool loose-box at his farm, I went to phone van den Baars. As I had anticipated, the bluff Dutchman was pleased with the success of our helicopter hunt and readily agreed to take a chance on the little fellow. Now I could make arrangements for the operation, although the prospect made my spine tingle with a mixture of fear and excitement.

When I went back to the loose-box, a young Kikuyu with buck teeth and a smile from ear to ear was leaning over the half-door, looking at the foal. The animal was on its feet and wandering dreamily about.

'Jambo, Doctor,' said the African. 'I am Augustine. Mr Louie says I am to help look after the young one.'

'Have you taken care of young stock before, Augustine?'

'Yessir. Waterbuck, impala, Tommies, leopards, many things.'

'You'll do excellently. Now please make up a feed for it like this.' I gave him instructions and he went off for the ingredients and feeding bottle at a jog.

I took Augustine's place at the half-door, and watched the little zebra walk smack into a wall. He was moving so slowly he came to no harm, but it was clear that I would have to operate within forty-eight hours. First I wanted him to get over his shaking-up in the bush, and I also needed the time to dilate his pupils as much as possible with atropine ointment to give me a wide opening to approach the lenses. Augustine bottled the milk mixture into the foal with firm yet gentle expertise. It looked as if the baby—we decided to call him Tatu, Swahili for 'three', because he had three black spots on his forehead and was three weeks old—had found a capable foster parent.

Louie and I drove into the city. Although I had my pack of basic surgical instruments in my tool-box, they were not suitable for eye work. I needed special scalpels, forceps, needles and silk thread among other things. First stop was the main hospital, where I explained my problem to the consultant ophthalmologist. A pawky Scotsman with a broad Glaswegian accent, he had been an MO with the old King's African Rifles.

' 'Fraid there'd be the dickens of a row if I was caught lending out the theatre equipment,' said the surgeon, 'but what I can do is let ye use my old field kit. It's a bit antiquated but ye should be all right.'

He produced his set of instruments. They were collector's items: ivory-handled, thin-bladed cataract knives, loops and hooks for teasing out lenses, and tiny needle-holders. All matching, they lay in padded velvet within a brass-inlaid mahogany box.

'Take them and welcome. Hope ye're successful,' he said. 'After all, we Glesga graduates must stick together, mustn't we?' The surgeon insisted on our having a dram with him and talking about our Scottish alma mater before we left.

Next I called on a veterinarian who had a sizeable horse practice around Nairobi. He willingly agreed to watch over Tatu's post-operative care when I went on my way the week after next.

All was arranged. Now all I needed was a large helping of luck—and no nasty surprises lurking in a zebra's eye to

427

booby-trap me on what was, as far as I could tell, the first cataract operation on the species.

Two days later, Tatu was strong, lively and highly strung. His pupils were nicely dilated. I decided to operate in the cool of the day before the flies clocked on. With Augustine and Louie each holding one end of him, I slowly injected a dose of xylazine solution into his jugular. After three minutes Tatu was sleeping soundly and I dropped local anaesthetic copiously into each eye. When I was satisfied that all sensation had been dulled to nothing, we lifted the foal onto a table set up outside his loose-box. The light from a pink and silver sky was good.

Many folk imagine the eye to be a terribly frail organ that must be handled like a soap bubble. In fact it is a tough and resourceful piece of equipment that can be tackled surgically with the same basic techniques of cutting and stitching—needle and scissor work identical to that of the seamstress—which are employed on humbler areas of the body.

One cut opened the transparent and remarkably thick cornea along one-third of its circumference. Now for the tricky bit. The lens lies behind the pupil, suspended on tough strands of rubbery jelly. First I had to get a grip on the lens, a task rather like grasping a miniature greasy pig. I managed it with the help of a small rubber bulb and a metal pipe which stuck to the lens by suction pressure. Now to free the lens. I wiggled it very gently. It did not want to break free from its strands, so I would have to try dissolving the attachments with an enzyme. I injected a little of the chemical around the lens with a blunt needle, then waited for five minutes which seemed like five hours. Then the wiggling again. Marvellous! The enzyme had done its work, the lens came free and I lifted it out of the eye on the end of my suction tube.

Anxiously, I looked into the completely bloodless wound

in the eye. I was relieved to see that the thick jelly behind the lens had not tried to follow the lens out—a crucial matter. Now all that was left was to stitch the corneal incision with silk. The collapsed front of the eyeball would quickly fill up with water again if I made a watertight seal. In twenty minutes it was done. Dr Stewart-Scott, the Manchester surgeon who had let me attend his cataract operations on human patients, would have finished it in a quarter of the time. Still, I was as pleased as Punch. One eye done with no signs of trouble, now for the other.

We gently turned Tatu over and I began all over again. Augustine watched, wide-eyed. Louie dropped sterile saline into the foal's eye from a bottle every half-minute. It was beginning to warm up; I could not have the eye drying on me. The second eye went as well as the first had done. An hour and a half after I had knocked him out, Tatu was cataract-free.

'Whizzo, old boy,' crowed Louie as I plastered antibiotic cream into both eyes before we carried the unconscious foal back into the loose-box.

'Okay, okay, okay,' chuckled Augustine.

'Let's wait and see how he looks tomorrow before we start getting excited,' I said. 'Meanwhile keep him in the dark.'

Next day it was raining heavily when I went to look at Tatu's eyes. Augustine was standing outside the loose-box looking drenched and very miserable.

'Good morning, Doctor,' he said as I came up to him. 'Before you go in'—he cast his eyes down and I saw that there were tears as well as rain running down his face—'I have unfortunate news.'

My stomach turned over. The foal must be dead—post-operative collapse of some kind. Yet xylazine was normally so safe and reliable.

'What is it?' I asked, not daring to open the half-door.

The African kept his head down and spoke softly. 'I think, Doctor, that all was in vain. The cataract is back, worse than before in both eyes. I have seen it when I fed him this morning.'

Partially relieved, I flung open the half-door and looked inside. Tatu was standing quietly in a corner. 'Grab him quickly before he can hit anything,' I told Augustine.

The African went in silently and seized the foal around the neck. When he had backed its rump into a corner I went in and took out my pencil torch. The narrow beam of light played over the foal's eyes. True enough, they were blue-white again, all over; it was impossible to see the depths of the eyes. There was no sign of blood and the eyeballs had plumped up to their original shape. First class!

I slapped Augustine hard on the back. 'Don't alarm yourself, my friend,' I said. 'That's not the cataract back. Without lenses you can't get cataracts. The haziness of the cornea is quite natural after it's been interfered with. It will clear gradually over the next week or so.'

Augustine looked up at me and the ear-to-ear grin re-appeared. More tears—of relief—trickled down his cheeks.

'Now go and get dried,' I ordered.

As the days passed, Augustine fed the foal, put cream in his eyes and generally fussed over him. The animal was taming surprisingly quickly. Each day I looked at the patient, and slowly the opacity of the cornea began to clear without any sign of infection or other complication. By the fifth day I got my first glimpse of the deepest part of the eye, the retina. It looked good, but I kept the pupils dilated with atropine and would not let the zebra be exposed to anything but the dimmest light. The acid test would come when I stopped the atropine and took out the stitches on the tenth day. Until then I had the other animals to blood sample and see loaded for Mombasa, and arrangements to make for a visit to Israel on the way home that van den Baars had just requested.

'What are you going to do if it failed?' said Louie, as we sat drinking Beck's the evening before I was due to take out the stitches. It was worrying him, too. I did not know what to say. I asked the bartender for an olive or two and he obliged by bringing a couple and adding them to my beer. Fishing them out, I looked at Louie and answered, 'Put him down, of course.'

Just before sun-up the next day the air was heavy with the perfume of frangipani blossom. Jays were quarrelling in the hibiscus shrubs around Louie's farm. The stupendous African sky dwarfed the land, pressing down on the flat brown buildings, the ochre soil, the close horizon. Augustine brought Tatu out onto the hard ground. I could not take chances nipping the sutures out of his eyeballs, so I gave him a knock-out injection of etorphine. When he was unconscious I squinted into his eyes through my ophthalmoscope. The interior of both eyes looked fine; I could trace the winding paths of the retinal blood vessels. The pupil constricted slightly as the light from the instrument hit the back of the eye—very good! There was still a fuzzy line of blue-grey where the eyes had been cut, but that should soon vanish after the stitches were gone. With forceps and scissors I picked up the knots of silk, cut them and pulled the sutures out. A shot of antidote and Tatu was back on his feet in five minutes.

Now for the test. There was an empty corral nearby. 'Put him in there,' I said to Augustine. 'Let him go and we'll watch.'

The little foal was pushed through the gate, then Louie, Augustine and I sat on top of the fence anxiously observing his movements. Tatu moved slowly around the enclosure. There were adult zebras next door. He could hear and smell them, and he seemed to be looking in their direction. When I called out loudly, he turned his head towards the sound. He was looking at me, wasn't he? Or was it just reaction to the noise? Tatu skipped a few steps, then he stood still, little nostrils distended, sniffing the morning air.

Suddenly something happened which was predictable but

431

which I had utterly forgotten about: the first fiery ray of the rising sun cleared the ground to the east. It flashed through the limpid air, a bolt of gold which spread over Tatu's left side. Then, to my spellbound delight, the little foal turned his head to look at the flash. He blinked, dazzled.

'He can see, he can see!' cried Augustine.

Louie whooped and whooped, while I scrambled exultantly down the fence, missed my footing in my haste and slipped, spraining an ankle badly. Augustine was still yelling, 'He can see,' as I limped into the corral and went cautiously towards the foal to make sure that we were not kidding ourselves.

Tatu dodged out of my way, pranced towards the fence and quite definitely checked when he came within two feet of the wood. Then he turned nimbly away. I was convinced —Tatu could see. Probably his vision was only fuzzy, for without a lens the eye cannot focus and in the wild he would still be greatly handicapped, but in a zoo or safari park he would be as good as the next little zebra.

For the first and only time in my life so far I had champagne for breakfast. Louie cracked a bottle of Mumm and by nine o'clock we were definitely tipsy.

With Tatu's eyes looking good, I prepared to leave Kenya for Israel. Louie arranged for Augustine to go with the foal down to Mombasa when the time came and to stay with him until he was shipped. On board ship there would be an experienced man from van den Baars' organisation to take over.

'See you in Rotterdam, young feller,' I said, as I took one last look at the zebra and waved my ophthalmoscope in front of him. He did not answer with words of course, but he said all I wanted to know by following my moving hand with his large, brown, shining eyes.

Judaism, like Christianity, sees Jehovah as mainly concerned with the pesky behaviour of one of the non-arboreal

432

primates that He knocked together on one of His off days. There are few references in the Old Testament to charity towards other species, and Hebrew theology dwells more on the ritual slaughter and butchery of lower creatures. But animals are involved in other aspects of man's concern to keep himself and everyone around him in God's good books—whether they like it or not.

The El Al plane from Nairobi took me into Tel Aviv. Van den Baars wanted me to do some tests on a quartet of Somali wild asses which were in quarantine near Elat on the Red Sea, and which were suspected of carrying swamp fever microbes. It took only a few days, and when I had finished I went by road on the spectacular route past Sodom, the Fortress of Masada, through the rolling Judaean hills to the Old City of Jerusalem where I had lunch of stuffed pigeon in the shadow of the golden-domed Mosque of Omar, and finally back to brash Tel Aviv to pay a call on my old friend Dr Abram, director of the zoo. Tel Aviv's city centre animal park is small and sadly in need of renovation, but the inmates thrive remarkably well.

On my first visit, a couple of years earlier, Dr Abram had proudly shown me his new-born baby Indian elephant and the second crop of flamingo chicks to be hatched within twelve months from the same parents.

'Everything in the garden looks rosy,' I said as we walked round. 'You must be very pleased.'

Abram smiled wryly. 'Yes and no,' he answered. 'You know it is Passover now, when the rules of kosher are even stricter than normal for the observant Jew?'

I knew all right. I had been craving in vain some of the delicious pitta bread baked everywhere in Israel except during the Passover, but had had to make do with piles of insipid matzo biscuits, and I had become accustomed when asking for wine in a café to being hustled into some tiny back room and served the taboo beverage in speak-easy secrecy.

'Well,' Abram went on, 'Israel is a theocracy where the

Rabbinate possess real power, and I'm having some bother with them.'

'How?' I knew the director to be a kind and tolerant man with liberal religious views.

'As you know, I feed my herbivores a balanced diet containing bread and broken biscuits together with grain, legumes and fresh greenery. It's high in protein and you can see that the animals fatten and reproduce splendidly on it.'

'So what's the problem?'

'Someone has given me away, and I've had a high-powered deputation from the Rabbinate in my office. They have said that all leavened products must be withdrawn from the animals' diets forthwith or they'll see that the zoo is closed.'

'No bread or non-kosher cereal ingredients, then?'

'That's what they say. I've fought the edict, but they have a spy in the gardens each day going round looking in the food troughs. They've put pressure on my keepers, too, not to feed the stock. Not a scrap of bread or hametz, forbidden food, must be on the place, and I must sign a certificate agreeing to be a good boy in future and to observe all the Passover kosher rules for my herbivores. My diets must be changed; they leave that to me.'

Dr Abram and I spent several hours re-adjusting the feeding programme to available unleavened alternatives that would nourish the stock as well as their previous menus but would not shock the temperamental stomach and intestinal bacteria of the animals, producing diarrhoea or even worse. Rabbis know nothing of the subtle and deadly disease, bowel oedema, that can kill pigs suddenly when the tiniest alterations to their diet are made; similar ailments can wipe out zoo animals.

We completed our Passover diet for the zoo and Abram prepared to put it into action. Next day he pointed out a bearded, black-dressed individual who was moving methodically from pen to pen, peering into the feed troughs and ocasionally leaning over to rub a handful of the provender through his fingers.

'There goes the shochet, the official sent by the Rabbinate to see that the Cretan goats and the camels and the elephant aren't upsetting Yahveh.'

Yahveh was good to us. Only a few of the animals developed mild 'rabbinical diarrhoea' as we named it. The rabbis kept a careful watch on the zoo for years after that, with meticulous daily inspections during the holy season. Finally the religious authorities put Dr Abram on trust, although still at the start of each Passover he has to sign an affidavit in which he swears to bring up his wild beasts like good Jewish boys. Oy vey!

Four

My new life had its minor compensations; for one thing, night calls became few and far between. Zoo animals are locked up in the evening and rarely looked at during the next twelve hours. Unless an already sick individual needs attention or an important birth is anticipated, ailments and accidents that happen in the hours of darkness are not discovered until the keepers clock on at eight in the morning. General practice had been teeming with dogs run over just as the pubs closed, cats that threw fits in the early hours and woke a startled household and, of course, farm visits. Nature seems to choose the quiet depths of the night for nudging calves and foals out of their submarine slumbers in the womb and into a journey that sometimes goes badly wrong. At such times farmers or stable lads tend to be around, for their experience and intuitive stockmanship somehow enables them to smell trouble and to sense the imminence of birth. Among zoo keepers, despite their passion for and deep interest in the species under their care, such intimate closeness with their animals is the exception.

As a result, my glummest hour of the day now became that between 7.30 and 8.30 am. It is still so. As like as not, a shrill telephone bell at this hour heralds tidings of a warm corpse discovered when the house was opened up. If I can finish off my scrambled eggs and coffee and launch a sally at the *Daily Telegraph* crossword without the phone putting paid to these bastions of my day, you can be absolutely certain that, apart from an ancient monkey or emaciated snake that has long been on the critical list, the birds and beasts at zoological

436

collections dotted all over Europe have passed a peaceful night without anybody of importance shuffling off his brutish coil.

It was a dreaded breakfast phone call, one bitter January morning, which summoned me urgently to Belle Vue. The twenty giraffes in the quarantine premises were in trouble, and four of them were doing the most sinister thing a giraffe can do: lying down and not getting up either because they could not or would not. It was the simplest but deadliest of symptoms, and Matt Kelly had often told me when I was a student, 'Boyo, if a giraffe goes down it never gets up!' I knew that he was not entirely right, for I had seen giraffes recover after being down, but he was as near right as made no difference.

Although the giraffes with problems on this occasion did not actually belong to Belle Vue, they were the zoo's responsibility. They were new arrivals into the country and were being quarantined there in two red-walled blockhouses. Once the giraffes had finished the quarantine period, the dealer who had rented the accommodation and other facilities from the zoo would sell the animals to collections all over Great Britain. They had arrived in Manchester on a foggy October day, having been in the heat of Mombasa three weeks before. No-one in their right mind brings African fauna into Britain after September, but the cut-price East German freighter booked to carry them had been delayed for weeks in setting sail from East Africa. It had been gross folly on someone's part to consider loading the animals on the delayed vessel but, as usual where commercial interests are involved, time is big money. To over-winter the giraffes in Africa would entail considerable expense and so someone gambled—with the dumb animals' lives. The journey had been made even longer by unscheduled stops at ports on Africa's west coast, and the animals' feed ran short. The giraffes slimmed considerably en route and lost some of their protective layers of fat.

I drove up to the quarantine area and joined Ray Legge, the zoo director, and Matt in one of the blockhouses. Two giraffes were lying on the straw, surrounded by a forest of legs. Their companions stood looking lugubriously down at them. It was freezing hard outside and little warmer inside; there had been a power cut during the early morning and the temperature in the house had plummeted. The walls were thin and provided meagre insulation, so when the hot-air blowers failed, the contained heat leaked rapidly away. The picture was the same in the other blockhouse, where another couple of animals lay limply on the ground.

I examined the recumbent giraffes. They looked sleepy, with drooping upper eyelids, their pulses were abnormally slow, their ears flopped like spaniels' and they made no effort to rise. Some of the standing giraffes also had unusually limp eyelids and ears. The temperatures of the ones on the ground were way below normal at the mid-nineties Fahrenheit. While I cautiously worked over my patients I kept a wary eye open for the flailing kick of one of the nervous beasts who towered above me, silently supervising the examination. The three of us made all our movements slowly and talked softly; if the standing animals panicked and began to mill around in the confined space, I would be pounded into the ground in an instant.

There was no evidence of infection, and I had no doubt that I was handling my first cases of hypothermia—chilling, or exposure—in giraffes. Manchester's winter frosts and bitter winds had gripped these unacclimatised creatures. If only they had had an English summer to give them time to adjust, to grow longer coats, to store up fat.

'What do you think?' asked Ray anxiously. 'The emergency blowers are being brought over this minute. Is there anything else to be done?'

In general practice, I had brought round cows dragged out of icy reservoirs by vigorous, commonsense treatment. I had once given a prescription to an owner of a horse that was found half-buried in a snowdrift so that she could get a bottle of whisky from the local pub outside licensed hours and pour it down the animal's throat. The pub's landlord had accepted the prescription. I decided to try the methods that had proved successful in domesticated animals, since there seemed no reason why they should not work just as well on giraffes. 'Blankets, sacks, more straw, some clean yard brushes, two bottles of good rum from the bar,' I ordered. 'While you're getting that, I'll give some injections.'

The droopiness and slow hearts of the animals worried me. Circulation seemed to be failing and the extremities were icy. I took some bottles of millophyline and Pastrum out of my bag. These circulatory stimulants should make a difference, and to get maximum effect I would shoot them straight into a vein.

Finding the jugulars of giraffes is dead easy when they are lying down. I knelt by the first animal's chest and curled myself up to avoid sideways lunges of its head. The giraffe did not seem to notice the needle and soon the stimulant liquids had all swirled away into its bloodstream. I kept a hand on its pulse and listened to the mighty heart through my stethoscope. After a few seconds, when the drugs first came into contact with the heart muscle, I felt and heard the pumping action increase in speed and volume, but the effect seemed to fade rapidly.

As I completed the injections, Matt and Ray arrived with the equipment I had asked for.

'Right,' I said. 'Now pour some of the rum over the legs and hindquarters and start brushing it in vigorously with the brushes. Make sure your movements are all upwards towards the heart.'

Matt shook his head sadly as he splashed the rich liquor over the first animal. 'Can oi have a pull too, Doctor?' he asked.

'Yes—when they're on their feet and not before,' I answered with a grin.

They both worked away at the rough massage while I set about giving inner warmth to the nearest giraffe. Holding the animal's muzzle under one arm was not difficult; it seemed too weak to struggle. With my other hand I carefully pushed the neck of the other rum bottle between its lips, through the gap separating its front and molar teeth, and let the alcohol slip over the back of its tongue. When a quarter of a bottle had disappeared I moved on to the next patient. Although I kept checking circulation, there was little sign of improvement. The giraffes retained their bleary, morning-after-the-night-before expressions. I gave them more shots of stimulant, and once again there was a short-lived boost in the circulation.

My vague worry was now a distinct feeling of apprehension. When Ray and Matt had worked up a good sweat brushing the animals' legs, we covered the recumbent beasts with a loose sprinkling of straw and then laid blankets and sacks over the top. The air spaces supported by the straw between the giraffes' skin and the blankets would make a warm, insulating layer. If these animals reacted like bullocks, they would be chirpy and warm as toast in no time—*if* they reacted like bullocks.

We went for a cup of coffee in Ray's bungalow and discussed ways of combating future power failures. An hour later I returned to the giraffes and was horrified to find that there were now three animals down in the first blockhouse and five in the other. The ones I had already treated were worse, if anything, and the newly prostrate beasts were showing the identical signs of failing circulation and drowsiness. By now I was thoroughly alarmed, Ray was white as a sheet with worry and Matt was muttering colourful Irish imprecations under his breath.

'It's like oi've told ye,' opined the head keeper, nodding grimly. 'Giraffes never get up!'

The two of them set to work rubbing and brushing with further supplies of rum, while I tried anti-shock drugs, filling

440

giant, 60-cc syringes with cortisone and anti-histamine solutions and jabbing clammy buttocks. The air blowers, reinforced by portable heaters, were pumping hot air into the buildings in gusts that swirled about us. Surely, if only the giraffes would hang in there for a little while longer, they would feel the rosy glow of vitality.

Not so. As we stood and watched, first one and then another adopted a posture of the head and neck that I knew to be a near-precursor of death. Curling their necks round and tucking them into their sides, they gazed with half-shut eyes at their rear ends. By pulling we could straighten an animal out again, but as soon as we released our grip, it insisted on returning to the curled-up position. I was almost desperate, but I had a few shots left in my locker. I sent for glucose powder, dissolved it half a pound at a time in hot water and bottled it into the giraffes as another source of calories. When that failed I transfused dextrose solution into the jugular, using Matt and Ray standing on chairs, their arms outstretched painfully high above their heads for long periods, as holders for the slow-dripping bottles. At least no more animals were going down, but the eight prostrate giraffes started to fade into semi-consciousness. As a last frantic resort I attempted to heat them up centrally by pumping water warmed to just above blood heat into the bowels through a stirrup pump and a greased rubber hose inserted as far as possible into the anus.

No matter what we did, the eight giraffes were slipping inexorably away. Nothing had the slightest effect. One animal quietly died, then a second and before long a third. Night came and then another morning and the three of us worked on without sleep, moving from one blockhouse to the other, going through the motions of rubbing, drenching and injecting but knowing that all was in vain. That afternoon the last of the recumbent giraffes died. Not one of them showed an iota of pathological abnormality when I wearily tackled the huge task of autopsying them, alone in a cold and

441

windy yard. The twelve remaining animals were given supplements of glucose in their drinking water; it was the best I could do.

Exhausted and demoralised, I set out at last for home. My drugs, all our efforts, had proved utterly impotent and eight giraffes out of twenty had been lost. Even those that had collapsed whilst I was on the premises had eluded me. I was playing in the big league of animal medicine now, I thought, and it looked like I wasn't up to the standard of the game. I had taken on a bunch of big boys from overseas—and lost.

During the next few days I was not called out anywhere. I had plenty of time to sit in my favourite room of the Jacobean farmhouse that was our home. It had windows piercing the thick stone walls on three sides and overlooking a raised garden where rhododendrons and roses crowded round a little pool which I had installed and stocked with frogs and ramshorn snails. Sprawled on the couch, I would immerse myself in the baroque music of J. S. Bach, Telemann and Couperin which, combined with the peaceful surroundings, was an unfailing washer-away of depression.

The room was my think-tank, too, and there I ruminated for a long time over the shambles of the giraffes. As far as I could learn, no-one had reported dealing with hypothermia in the species before. I was puzzled by the lack of response to normally effective stimulant techniques: it was as if the circulation system of these animals, which we knew to be specially adapted to forcing blood up and down long legs and necks, passed a point of no return and collapsed remarkably quickly.

Such physiological considerations were not the only ones which troubled me. There was a gnawing sense of guilt on several levels. First, I had to face the fact that my treatment had met with complete lack of success. Had I missed something in the diagnosis? Or in the therapy? Then at another level I pondered over my position as someone working for an organisation that did daft and irresponsible things like letting giraffes get cold. I had not personally given the OK to load the animals onto the boat in Mombasa, nor had I selected the blockhouses as quarters for the new arrivals, nor had I played any part in installing the vulnerable heating system, but I was part of the business, a supporter of the machine that made cash out of captive animals. At yet another level I questioned once again, as I had done a thousand times and still do every day, whether I as a human being had any right to assist in any way in the bringing of wild creatures forcibly out of their rightful habitats. I was glib with plausible justifications: education, scientific study, conservation, enrichment of the lives of those who cannot afford to travel to the Serengeti or Galapagos. But such sophistries neglected the moral argument, and that was the one that tugged and still tugs. My brother the warthog? Yes, that did ring a bell deep inside me. Yet is seemed at the time, as indeed I suspect it still does, too easy to let Handel's glorious trumpets and mighty organs drown such uncomfortable thoughts.

I decided to use some of the long hours when the telephone did not ring in improving my command of some foreign languages. Already I had had awkward moments of mutual incomprehension when speaking, sometimes on urgent emergency matters, to clients and veterinarians overseas. There was the Italian with the private zoo who had a smattering of English and, I was convinced, a much-thumbed copy of *Roget's Thesaurus* instead of a dictionary, into which he delved with reckless enthusiasm before sending me one of his express cables. 'SUCCOUR PLEASE,' one ran. 'AM HAVING MANDRILL WITH PYROMANIA OF MELANCHOLY. I IMPORTUNE APPROVAL.' For a moment I toyed with the idea of a big blue-faced mandrill (a type of baboon) which, to the despair of his analyst, had taken to playing with matches after a fit of depression. But why was his owner so keen that I

443

should give my blessing to the fire-raising ape? It took several hours of head-scratching and a final telephone call to Naples to discover that the request for assistance was meant to be 'HELP PLEASE. HAVE MANDRILL WITH INFLAMED SPLEEN. REQUEST RECOMMENDATION.'

Many of the people contacting me from abroad spoke some English and, with the shreds of my School Certificate French and German, we got by. Even so, it could not have sounded very elegant to my foreign clients when in a serious medical discussion I had to use Rabelaisian synonyms—the sort which in a dictionary are followed by the severe epithet, '(vulg.)'—for key anatomical or physiological terms because of my poor command of the language. It just would not do; I had to achieve a basic working knowledge of French, German and Spanish together with all the most useful veterinary phrases. I got down to it seriously after a memorable visit to Duisberg Zoo in Germany, where I lectured to a group of keepers on the breathing system of whales and dolphins. In my mixture of English and German I talked about the amazing sensitivity of the blow-hole that lets air in and keeps water out, even in stormy seas, and about how the organ opens and closes apparently automatically when the animals sleep. It was the raised eyebrows of the zoo director and the helpless mirth of his staff as I repeatedly referred to the animals' blow-holes that eventually made me twig. I thought I had used the correct word for the hole in the creatures' heads—*blassloch*—whereas in fact I had consistently referred to the *assloch*, a more lowly orifice elsewhere in the anatomy.

The most illuminating demonstration of the value of even a limited knowledge of languages occurred later that year, when I went to the first conference of the newly formed European Association for Aquatic Mammals which was being held at the Dutch seaside resort of Harderwijk, a little town that boasts one of the finest Marinelands outside the United States. When the first day's papers had been deli-

444

vered and discussed, I repaired along with a group of other veterinarians, zoo directors, dolphin trainers and marine scientists to a local hostelry for the most important function of any conference: swapping gossip and talking 'shop' over a few litres of Amstel beer. In our corner of the bar were the director of Whipsnade Zoo, Victor Manton; a veterinarian from the US Navy Undersea Warfare research division, John Allen; the professor of anatomy at Cambridge, Richard Harrison; and Peter Grayson, later to succeed Raymond Legge as director of Belle Vue Zoo.

We had been jawing away for an hour or so when Peter whispered something in my ear. 'Have you got any drugs with you?' he asked.

Normally I never travel abroad to see a case without making sure that certain important anaesthetics, tranquillisers and other drugs which might be impossible to locate outside Britain are with me. So, should I or some other specimen of homo sapiens develop a headache, get bitten or suffer, say, the Kurdistan Collywobbles, I can usually root about under my socks and find a pill or a potion labelled 'For Treatment of Rhinoceros' or 'Gorilla: 3 drops daily in fruit juice', which makes life bearable again. On this occasion, however, I was not carrying even so much as an aspirin.

'Sorry, old boy,' I replied as our beer mugs were refilled again. 'Why, what's wrong?' It was difficult making myself heard above the jolly din.

'Got a pain, really bad,' Peter answered with a grimace.

'Where?'

'In my . . . in my urethra.'

The others noticed Peter's anguished features and asked what was up. He repeated his trouble and naturally everybody fell about laughing. Ribald remarks were made as to possible diagnoses and causes and no-one seemed inclined to treat the poor fellow's complaint as being in any way serious.

'But it's awful, bloody awful,' shouted Peter, clutching his groin. 'I'm not joking. If you haven't got any drugs, could

445

you give me a prescription or something then, David? I'll see if I can find a chemist. I must do something!'

Still loath to take Peter seriously, I agreed to write a note for some Penbritin capsules on the back of a beer mat, but warned him that it might not be acceptable in Holland. To the cheers of the rest of us, Peter dashed out clutching the prescription.

It was over an hour later that he re-appeared, relaxed and no longer wearing an agonised expression.

'You look better,' I said. 'Did you get the Penbritin?'

'No,' Peter replied, 'but I nearly got arrested!'

He went on to tell us what had happened as he hurried through the twilight-dim streets of Harderwijk, looking for a chemist to fill his prescription. With the pain in his water-works almost unbearable, he had at last spotted a shop with bottles in the window and a sign over the door that read 'Droguerie'. Dashing in, he thrust the prescription into the hands of a young lady in a white coat standing behind the counter. She turned the beer mat over, muttered in Dutch and looked distinctly nonplussed.

'Penbritin. Pen-bri-tin cap-sules,' groaned Peter. It was plain that the girl spoke no English. He tried another tack. 'Pain. Got pain down here. Bad.' He gesticulated towards his groin.

The girl was getting a trifle agitated, Peter noticed. She called out and was presently joined by another white-coated female who, equally puzzled, looked at the paper mat and then at the Englishman pointing miserably towards his trousers. Peter was at the end of his tether. He felt that at any moment his bladder would burst. Why didn't they do some-thing? There was no doubt in his mind: 'droguerie' sounded so like 'druggery', it must be the Dutch for 'pharmacy' to anyone with a glimmer of intelligence but no working Dutch.

Then he had an idea. Producing a pencil and taking the beer mat back from the shop assistant, he hurriedly drew the outlines of the human male genito-urinary organs and added a large arrow pointing to the source of the agony. He handed the beer mat back and said with great feeling, 'Pain. Have you got anything to take away pain?'

The girls' eyes bulged as they stared at the masterpiece. They began to fidget and talk rapidly to each other.

Perhaps, Peter thought, there was some confusion about the subject of his diagram and the girls had interpreted his squiggle wrongly: it did look rather like a plan of the motor-racing circuit at Zandvoort. Impatiently, he grabbed the beer mat, slapped it once again on the counter and pulled out his pencil. This time there would be no doubt. He carefully sketched in some anatomical details, shaded the thing to give it perspective and then thrust the paper under the girls' noses and waved it about. 'There,' he shouted, and jabbed with a finger at the spot where the figleaf should have been.

This latest effort produced an unmistakable reaction. With shrill squeaks the two girls lurched back from the counter, grabbed at one another for support and bundled themselves through a door leading into a back office. Moments later a man in a white coat appeared, red-faced and angry. He leaned over the counter and grabbed Peter tightly by the lapels of his jacket.

'Now, mister,' he said, 'English, eh? What the hell do you think you're doing? Looking for a burlesque show?'

Still holding firmly on to Peter's lapels, the man rattled on about how his shop was not a house of ill repute, his two assistants were good-living, God-fearing provincial girls, and how beery foreign day-trippers should confine themselves to the red-light district of Amsterdam. When Peter at last got an indignant word in, the truth on both sides came out: drogueries in Holland are cosmetics shops that do not deal in any medicines whatsoever, and the maidens recovering in the back room were beauticians.

The shop-owner was soon reassured that Peter really was in pain and in search of help. 'Go down the street and look for the sign "Apoteek"—apothecary—and good luck,' he said, smoothing my friend's creased jacket and leading him to the door.

The pain was now almost unbearable and to cap it all, when Peter eventually found the chemist's shop, it was closed. The poor chap dragged himself back to the bar where we sat, but before joining us staggered into the men's room to see if he could spot anything visibly wrong with his nether parts. Suddenly there was a 'ping' and the fierce pain literally vanished. He had passed a tiny bladder stone which had lodged in his urethra, causing obstruction and intense agony.

'I'd have given my eye teeth to be able to speak a word or two of Dutch,' said Peter as we listened to his story between further litres of beer and fits of helpless hysterics. 'Damned useful things, foreign languages.'

Five

I missed the end of that Harderwijk conference, because Shelagh phoned my hotel the next evening with news of an accident at Belle Vue. Pedro, the smallest of the zoo's bull giraffes, had been wounded in the neck. He was eating and drinking all right, but dribbles of food and water were running out of the wound when he did so. I took a taxi to Schiphol airport and caught the next plane back to Manchester.

It was past midnight when I met Matt Kelly, the stocky little Irish head keeper, outside the darkened giraffe house. 'Looks nasty to me,' he said, clicking his teeth. 'We'll have to be careful goin' in and puttin' the loights on.'

When zoo animals are put down for the night, they expect to be left undisturbed. Suddenly breaking the routine by switching on lights and making a noise can startle the resting or often snoring inhabitants, with disastrous results in that confined space both to panicking animals and to any humans who happen to be in their way. After 'lights out' you go back into an animal house very carefully.

We went up to the door. Before opening it, Matt began to talk just loud enough to be heard inside. Gradually he increased the volume, whistled a bit, tapped on the woodwork and finally turned the knob. Very slowly pushing the door open a crack, he addressed the animals pulling themselves to their feet and flaring their nostrils in the blackness. 'There, there. How're ye doin', me beauties? Oi'm sorry to be disturbin' ye.' He moved a hand to the light switches, put on one bulb, paused, then lit another, paused and lit a third.

We moved unhurriedly into the house, both billing and cooing softly towards the knots of zebra, giraffe and wildebeest that stood alertly, all with eyes upon us and ears pricked, ready to panic. After a few moments inspecting us, the animals relaxed: there was no mistaking the familiar, friendly tones of the head keeper.

Pedro, the giraffe, was standing in a corner. He seemed unconcerned about the ugly, six-inch long tear, caked with blood, in the left side of his neck.

'How did it happen, Matt?' I asked, as Pedro wandered over to the railings, craned over and curled a rough grey tongue round a twist of my hair to give my scalp a painful tug.

'We're not too sure, but it looks as if he got his muzzle jammed in one of them water bowls up high on the wall, panicked and threw himself about and crashed against the iron hay-rack. It came away from the wall and a bracket went through his throat.'

Matt pulled an apple out of his coat pocket and offered it to the giraffe, who took it willingly. Pedro chewed it, drooling saliva down onto us, and swallowed. We watched the sinuous waves of the gullet muscles carrying the mashed-up apple towards the stomach. As the waves reached the neck wound, a pink finger of foam welled out of the bloody hole and then, to my horror, soggy white pieces of apple pulp flecked with pale green slivers of peel emerged from the wound and dropped onto the straw-covered floor.

'Bejasus!' exclaimed Matt.

There was no doubt about it. Pedro had punctured his gullet, a rare and serious injury, particularly in an animal like a giraffe.

There was nothing to be done that night apart from shooting a couple of dart-syringes containing penicillin into his buttocks. The formidable prospect of trying to close the wound would have to wait until daylight. I drove home to Rochdale with my head full of questions. How to lay hands on the big beast in a place that was smooth walls on three sides and iron bars on the fourth? What type of anaesthetic to use on the most notoriously unpredictable of zoological patients? The operation itself: how badly damaged was the gullet? Repairing such a wound might present problems never encountered in the day-to-day cobbling together of skin and muscle injuries. Giraffe again, I thought. One of the most difficult of all zoo species to treat, and one which seemed lately to be needing a lot of my help—such help as I could give. At least things were busy, but the cases were rough.

'Well, you can always go back to speying cats and vaccinating poodles,' Shelagh said provocatively next morning as I worried over the turn of events.

'Don't be daft,' I retorted, stabbing at a fried egg that was not looking for trouble.

As I arrived at Belle Vue I was no nearer finding the answers which had haunted me all night. Matt was already in the giraffe house, looking worriedly at Pedro, whose appearance had altered distinctly in the past six hours.

'Would ye look at that, Doctor,' said the head keeper, pointing. 'He's gettin' fatter somehow.'

Sure enough, Pedro did look plumper. It was not that he was bloated with air or excess food in his belly, but he seemed simply to have enlarged. There was no question that his neck, chest and forelegs were fatter. Ominously, the giraffe had stopped eating and was looking depressed and miserable. Sticky froth had made a trail down his neck from the puncture wound.

'I'll need to examine him, Matt,' I said, 'but how?' There was at that time no proven reliable anaesthetic for giraffes, no swinging gate or funnel-shaped 'crush'.

'What d'ye want to do exactly?' Matt asked.

'First, I'd like to feel him to see why he's so much bigger than last night, then if possible get a finger into that neck wound.'

'It's goin' to be tricky. Let's try a door and some straw

451

bales.' He shouted to a bunch of keepers, 'Lift the elephant house door off its hinges, and look sharp about it!' The elephants were already outside for the day and had no need of their night-house door.

After a few minutes the keepers tottered into the giraffe house, straining and sweating under the weight of the massive, iron-studded door which must have weighed five or six hundredweight. The idea now was to take it into the giraffes' quarters, having moved out all the animals except Pedro, and then gradually press him against a wall by using the door as a portable barrier.

All went well at first. The door was introduced quietly and slowly. Pedro began to pace about nervously as the men under Matt's command advanced cautiously, carrying the door in an upright position. At least if the giraffe lashed out with one of his feet to deliver the powerful blows that can brain a charging lion, the solid wood should afford the keepers some protection. Gently cornered at last and unable to turn round, Pedro began to 'stargaze'—holding his head up so that his chin pointed directly at the ceiling—a sign of profound mental agitation. I told the men not to press the door actually onto the animal, for under such circumstances anything could happen. Pedro might try to climb the wall, jump amazingly upwards on four legs like a spring lamb, throw a limb over the door or even, seemingly, try to fly. Such remarkable displays always ended in torn muscles, fractures or even worse.

Matt piled up some bales of straw on our side of the door and I gingerly climbed up them. Now I was high enough to put my arm over the top of the door and do a bit of prodding around. 'Coosh now, coosh,' I murmured, the words that Pennine farmers would use when approaching a prickly-tempered cow. I lightly stroked Pedro's neck. Niggled, he swung his head to and fro and then lunged down awkwardly, trying to butt me with the hard pegs on his head. 'Coosh, coosh, boy.'

Pedro became accustomed to my touch on his skin, which flickered and jumped beneath my fingers. I prodded carefully. Scrunch! Scrunch! It was just like pressing shredded cellophane—I could hear as well as feel the crackling beneath the skin. This was not fat, nor was it the soggy fluid of dropsy. It was gas, gas collecting in thousands of bubbles under the animal's hide and puffing him up like the Michelin man. If the gas was being produced by bacteria that had entered through the wound, Pedro really was in trouble. Gas gangrene is usually lethal and runs a quick course, but somehow he did not look poorly enough for that. I looked at the neck wound from a few inches away and listened intently. As Pedro moved his head about I could hear the faintest sucking sound. A bubble of serum would appear at the hole, swell, shrink and vanish. That was it: movement of the neck was drawing air in through the wound, which acted as a valve. Once inside, the air was gradually working its way through the subcutaneous tissue. Another day or two of this and Pedro could be like a zeppelin right down to his hind feet.

The operation to repair the gullet and close the overlying tissues would put a stop to all that. As long as I continued to provide an antibiotic 'umbrella', the air under the skin would be absorbed by the blood capillaries and harmlessly dispersed. Ready for trouble, I moved my fingers up towards the wound. I touched the crusted blood, then, ever so delicately, pushed my index finger into the ragged hole. Pedro swayed about. I swayed with him, letting my hand ride with his neck. I felt my finger pass through a thin layer of split muscle and slip on the smooth lining of the gullet. The gap in its wall was as big as a plum.

I turned my head to look at Matt. 'There's a bloody great...' I began but then all hell let loose. Pedro had had enough. Kicking mightily sideways with a fore leg and a hind leg in concert, he connected with the door with a crash that shook the building. The heavy slab of wood fell away from him,

453

taking me and my pile of straw bales with it. The men buckled under the tumbling mass and collapsed to the ground. A yelling, struggling heap of keepers, plus one startled veterinarian, saw the great door come toppling down onto them. Only Matt Kelly had managed to skip out of the way. Luckily the straw bales in which we were tangled took much of the impact and saved us from being utterly flattened.

Unconfined once more, Pedro stalked haughtily from his corner and actually walked over the door beneath which we were sandwiched. The momentary addition of his weight resulted in a broken collar bone and a bloody nose for one of the keepers, and made my ear swell up like a tomato. When we emerged from our press we found Matt hopping about in a mixture of amusement and agitation like a red-faced leprechaun.

As our wounded were borne off I explained the situation and told Matt to prepare for an operation. At that time few attempts had been made to anaesthetise giraffe, and those who had tried it had found grave difficulties in coping with the tall beast: its peculiar circulation system seemed to distribute anaesthetics in an unpredictable way. Slowly induced anaesthesia resulted in dizziness, panic and awful accidents, while fast knock-out shots were dangerous, tricky to administer and brought the animal crashing straight down from its height of seventeen or eighteen feet. In the rare cases where the operation was completed satisfactorily, a giraffe might well refuse to get up on its feet ever again and there was the strange business of individuals which developed grotesquely twisted necks for some reason. Zoo vets had one recurring nightmare: that a giraffe might need surgery.

Even chiropody was a headache. In captivity giraffe hoofs sometimes grow long and curl upwards, but the difficulty was doing anything to remedy the situation. I had had some success putting the patient into a specially built travelling

454

box, removing the bottom plank on one side and working through the slot, but it was a dangerous technique. The horn, particularly in dry weather, can be hard as iron. A hoof-knife as used on sheep or cattle was useless, and there was not room to apply a blacksmith's hoof-clippers with the foot planted firmly on the ground and maybe a ton or more of weight resting on it. It was a painless operation but the giraffe usually resented his tootsies being fiddled about with, so it was difficult to decide which was best: to sweat away with a saw, waiting for the inevitable, lightning-fast kick to shatter the metal blade; to chip with a chisel and mallet and risk a broken arm or the chisel smashed into one's teeth; or to use a fast, electric portable saw and maybe amputate the giraffe's ankle when it suddenly struck. Just before leaving my old practice, though, I had used an injection of ace-promazine, a sedative made for farm and domestic animals, on an old bull giraffe at Dudley Zoo that had had terribly overgrown feet for years. It had worked well. The drug had left the animal standing but droopy-eyed, relaxed and uncaring. There had been no problems in darting the bull or cutting the horn and there seemed to be no after-effects to the acepromazine.

I had not wanted to use the drug just to examine Pedro, but for the operation on his throat I reckoned that the best and safest thing to do was to use acepromazine, put the patient behind the door again and then numb the operation site with plenty of local anaesthetic.

Even with the decision about the anaesthetic resolved, there were still the surgical problems. Left untreated or simply dressed with ointments or plasters, the hole would never heal as saliva and food passing through the orifice would encourage the formation of a permanent link, a fistula, between the gullet and the outside of the neck. I would have to close the gullet with special stitches that rolled the wound edges inwards, so that the mucous membrane lining the tube could knit together, and I must not cause an

455

obstruction to swallowing by narrowing the tube too much. I had opened ostrich gullets in the past in search of metal foreign bodies which they had swallowed and which we had located with army-issue mine detectors, but I had never had to operate on a mammal's gullet. Even in dogs it is rarely necessary—gullets get blocked sometimes, but they normally emerge from accidents unscathed. The rest, closing the muscle and skin, and thus putting an end to the air-sucking, would be simple.

The first step was to give the sedative. As usual, I worked out the dose by taking the average of three estimates of his weight, mine, Matt's and the senior giraffe keeper's. Then I assembled one of the aluminium flying darts with its ingenious, explosive-activated plunger and selected a needle appropriate for the buttocks of an adult giraffe. Finally I charged the dart with the calculated volume of ace-promazine, a beautiful golden-coloured liquid. There should be just enough to make this giraffe as peaceable and amenable as the one at Dudley.

With a soft 'phut', hardly loud enough to startle the animal, the dart flew from my gas pistol and homed perfectly into the giraffe's rump. So fast and surely do these devices travel that there is far less sensation for the recipient than there would be if a hypodermic needle were punched in manually. Pedro seemed unaware that he had been slipped a Mickey Finn.

I looked at my watch. Usually the first signs of drowsiness appear after five minutes or so. We all waited.

Six minutes went by. The giraffe started to droop his upper eyelids, instead of his normal alert expression he looked rather dumb, and his muscles visibly relaxed.

'Get the door, lads,' I said, 'and approach him nice and easy.'

As I spoke, Pedro gave a great sigh, keeled over as if struck by invisible lightning, and crashed onto the thick straw. I was stunned. The giraffe lay flat out, legs flailing and eyes rolling wildly.

Matt and I dashed over, and I put my ear to his chest, listening to the slow thud of the mighty heart.

'Get up, Pedro, get up!' yelled Matt, slapping the animal ineffectually on the flanks, his teeth grinding with tension.

I felt the pulse in the giraffe's femoral artery. It was soft and weakening.

'Come on, everyone. Prop him up on his brisket. Two of you hold his head up!' I shouted, and the keepers crowded round. 'Head up at all costs,' I repeated, and rummaged in my bag for syringes and needles.

Thoughts whirled through my mind. Certainly I had taken the correct drug from the correct bottle. Dose? We had all agreed that he weighed around sixteen hundredweight, and I had given 5 cc, a low to moderate amount. I looked at the dart to check. Yes, it was a 5-cc dart and could not have held more. It could only be a side-effect of the acepromazine: heart failure had been reported occasionally in domestic animals, and it was recognised that one effect of the chemical was to lower the blood pressure.

As Matt and his men pushed the now unconscious giraffe into some semblance of a normal sitting position, with the head propped on one fellow's shoulders, I drew a quantity of noradrenaline into my syringe, fast. I bent to pick up a skin swab and heard Matt's words as if in a dream.

'He's gone, Doctor. He's gone,' he said quietly.

I went over to the giraffe, cold sweat breaking out under my shirt. I gently touched the cornea of one eye. I jammed my head against the warm chest and listened. Matt was right. Pedro had died. Just like that. The acepromazine had over-expanded the blood vessels, Pedro's blood pressure had plummeted and his vital brain cells had been starved of circulating oxygen. 'Damnation,' muttered Matt. The men all stood back and let the giraffe's body slip onto its side.

'Unpredictable things, giraffes. Bloody terrible to treat,' I said. It sounded like an apology.

No-one said anything further as we collected our gear. Matt left silently to phone the knackerman.

I drove home in despair. Only a fool would take on the agony of zoo medicine, I thought. Pigs, cats, cows we understand; giraffes can only bring heartache.

Shelagh knew what had happened with one look at my face when I entered the house. She also knew that it was best to stick the lunch in the oven; I would not be eating. I went to my office to sit and think, go over all the possibilities, to try to get an inkling of what had gone wrong. The thought that one day there might, there would, be another giraffe was like iced water in my brain.

Shelagh brought me a cup of tea. 'Come on,' she said. 'The cup that cheers. By the way, there's been a veterinary student on the phone a couple of times. He wants to know something about lobsters. His name's Greenwood, Andrew Greenwood.'

'You can tell him what he can do with his lobsters, love,' I replied, and stared unseeing out of the window. The gangling, long-necked creature that the ancients had called a camel-leopard, *Giraffa camelopardalis*, was becoming my jinx.

On the way to Harderwijk for the conference which Pedro's accident interrupted, my old friend Mr van den Baars had invited me to Rotterdam to look over a mixed bunch of animals belonging to him which had just arrived from East Africa. One of his keepers took me round the live cargo: giraffes, antelopes, a hippo and zebras.

'You should be interested in this one,' the keeper said, pointing to one slatted crate. 'It's a young zebra.'

My heart leapt as I put my face to a slot in the woodwork and looked inside. A beautiful, nine-month-old zebra colt was looking directly towards me with his ears pricked forwards and his eyes glistening like cobs of coal. There were three spots on his forehead. It was Tatu!

I was ecstatic. Tatu had survived. Blind and concussed in

the heat of the bush eight months before, he was now a stroppy individual with glancing, arrogant eyes on his way to a zoo in Poland.

'Spirited little devil,' said the attendant. 'He kicks and bites as soon as look at you.'

'But does he look?' I asked. 'You've not seen him bump into things or miss objects, have you?'

'Definitely not,' came the emphatic reply. 'See this blue dent in my wrist? That's where he grabbed me a couple of weeks ago when I was mucking out. He saw all right.'

I was content. No doubt Tatu could have done better with a pair of bifocals or even contact lenses if such things had existed for wild animals, but he was biting folk accurately enough. That was just what I wanted to hear.

Pedro's death drove all thoughts of Tatu from my mind, and it was only some days later that I remembered to tell Shelagh about my reunion with the young zebra. She was thrilled.

'What's for dinner?' I asked when I had finished my tale.

'Can't you smell it?' Shelagh replied.

It was true there was a strong fishy smell about. 'Herrings!' I said, my mouth beginning to water in anticipation of baked rollmops with mashed potato and mustard sauce.

Shelagh shook her head. 'Wrong. It's mackerel today'.

'Fine by me.'

'And it's mackerel tomorrow, and the day after and Friday, Saturday, Sunday . . .'

'Whoa! Hold on!' I interrupted. 'What are you going on about?'

'Mackerel—twenty stone of it. It arrived on the front doorstep this morning, sent by Pentland Hick of Flamingo Park. He wants you to check its quality. He's bought a killer whale in Seattle and hopes to fly it over in two or three weeks, so he's been talking to merchants at Billingsgate about fish supplies. Oh, and that student, Andrew Greenwood, has been on about his lobsters again.'

Never mind lobsters—a killer whale! Determined to make his Flamingo Park Zoo in Yorkshire the finest in England, Hick had built one of the country's first dolphinaria and had become fascinated by the potentialities of the cetaceans——whales, dolphins, porpoises and the like. Harderwijk in Holland had had the first European killer a few months previously, but it had not survived long before dying, it was said, of a brain haemorrhage. Now with any luck I was actually going to touch one of the most awesome marine mammals, probably handle its medical problems.

A frisson of excitement ran down my spine as I thought about it. Since my first contact with Flamingo Park, capturing an escaped nilgai antelope for them, I had gradually seen more and more of Hick's growing empire of animals. I telephoned him immediately.

'Yes,' he said in his deceptively soft and sleepy voice, 'I'd like you to go to Seattle next month. Bring back a killer whale. Think about it. Check everything. Talk to the Americans by phone. But remember'—his voice took on the menacing tones of the Godfather—'nothing, but nothing, must go wrong, David.'

My contemplation of this momentous news was interrupted by Shelagh's more mundane but highly pressing problems as owner of 280 pounds of mackerel, a fish renowned for its lack of keeping quality. It was all over the kitchen, ousting my beer bottles from the refrigerator and filling the sinks. My daughters, Stephanie and Lindsey, peered somewhat mournfully from behind a stack of fish boxes which we had to climb over to get out of the kitchen.

'Lancastrians don't seem to eat mackerel,' Shelagh complained. 'I've managed to give away about ten pounds to the Schofields, old Fred the other side and even a pair to the postman, but look at the rest! I'm not going to waste them by dumping them in the dustbin, but what are we going to do with them before the house stinks of rotting fish?'

For the moment, though, they were beautiful fresh fish,

youngsters about seven inches long. I inspected a selection, checking gills, eyes, skin, oil content, smell, parasite load, muscle firmness; they were perfect. It seemed safe to order this for the new whale, but just in case there were invisible bugs in the fish I took samples from half a dozen for bacteriological culture and for analysis for heavy metals, an increasing worry as the seas become polluted by man and his industries.

That evening I was to be found bearing unsolicited fishy gifts wrapped in newspaper to friends and even mere nodding acquaintances all over Rochdale, and for the next week my enthusiasm for the hobby of cooking was put to the test as I experimented with the mackerel.

On the Sunday night, as I called the family to the supper table, Stephanie asked apprehensively, 'It's not mackerel again, is it, Dad? How have you done it this time? We've had it boiled, with white wine sauce, barbecued, as kedgeree.'

'And don't forget when we had it in cider, and with cucumber, and with tomato,' chimed in Lindsey, who was also approaching the table with less than her usual enthusiasm.

Shelagh pointed at the cat. 'Even poor old Lupin doesn't look like he could face a mackerel again for ten years.'

I knew I had plumbed the depths for this evening's meal but put a brave face on it. 'Tonight,' I declared gaily, 'my pièce de résistance—curried mackerel.'

With the groans of the family in my ears as I retreated to the kitchen to bring in the dishes, I began to doubt a killer whale's famed intelligence; after all, he would swallow a hundredweight of this stuff, day in and day out for years—and raw, without benefit of my sauces!

Before I had time to make serious preparations for my visit to America, I was summoned by the manager of the Garden of Eden, a sleazy night-club in Manchester, to sort out one of the alligators which had a 'funny tail'. My only previous contact with the establishment had been to treat an eye condition in the phython who was the working partner of Miss Seksi, the striptease dancer there:* I had never actually set foot inside the place and could not imagine what alligators were doing in such surroundings. Props in some exotic, erotic burlesque sketch—Tarzan and nude Jane, maybe? Perhaps they made alligator steak flambé out of them. After all, people rave over the rather indifferent soup made from that other enchanting reptile, the turtle—a dish which Shelagh insisted we never ate because of the cruel way the gentle animals are killed to titillate the palates of gourmets far away.

Reptiles form one of the most difficult and neglected areas of zoo medicine, and there are not the funds or the scientific facilities available for much research into the special problems of a group of animals that are rarely worth more than a few pounds apiece. So the more reptile practice I got, the better: as a student I had watched Matt Kelly first slip a leather or rope noose round an alligator's jaws, thus putting the more lethal end out of action, then jump boldly onto the thrashing muscular tail and eventually force the reptile over onto its back. With the beast in that position Matt had begun to stroke it gently and repeatedly in a straight line down the middle of its body, beginning at the point of the jaw and going right down the underbelly to the vent. After six or seven passes of this kind, the animal had become immobile and perfectly relaxed in a hypnotic trance. As a mere nuisance of a student I had not been allowed to participate in or get too close to these mysteries, but this Garden of Eden case might be my big chance. I had seen it all and was sure I was up to it, even if my alligator patient was a fine nine-footer like the ones at Belle Vue which had laid eggs in captivity—the first to do so in any European zoo. Noose, jump onto the tail, whip over and begin the Svengali bit.

*See *Doctor in the Zoo*

462

Taylor the Zoovet will emerge with flying colours this morning, I thought, as I pulled up outside the night-club.

There was no mention of alligators among the collection of curling photographs of fishnet-covered flesh on the billboard by the entrance, a small black door set in a grimy wall in a back street, but I could not help musing on the cosmopolitan spice in a zoo vet's life that is rare in the general-practice world of say, a James Herriot.

Nothing inside the dimly lit basement room recalled in the slightest the first Garden of Eden, unless it was a reek of original sin. There was not even a plastic apple tree. The place was tatty, smelling sourly of stale beer, yesterday's cigars and cheap perfume. Groups of small tables, with crumb-dusty, wine-stained covers and guttered candles stuck in empty Sauternes bottles, surrounded a minute dance floor. The whole garden of delights was illuminated coldly by blue fluorescent strip-lights which made the dandruff on the manager's jacket sparkle like snowflakes as he led me to my patient. Around the edge of the dance floor there was a narrow, water-filled channel perhaps twelve inches wide and six inches deep. The water was turbid and oily. Floating on the surface were cigarette butts, bits of cork and other scraps of debris.

'He's in there,' said the manager. 'There's three of 'em altogether. Quite a gimmick, don't you think?'

I scanned the grey water. Sure enough, three pairs of green-gold eyes just broke the surface. Yes, the Garden of Eden had alligators, each about one foot long and as lean as hazel twigs—not quite the monsters I had hoped for.

'That's the one, I think,' said the manager, pointing towards one of the three. 'They don't have names. There's something wrong with his tail. I wouldn't have troubled you myself but one of those bloody Eytie waiters seems to have got attached to the little perishers and said he'd report us if we didn't do something. I mean, I could understand if it was a dog or something, but well . . .' He sniffed disdainfully.

I plunged my hand into the channel and brought out the small alligator by the base of his tail. Four inches of his length was tail and half of that was brown, lifeless and rotting. It had obviously been gangrenous for weeks.

'What do you feed the alligators on?' I asked. Not only was the creature rather small, but the death of tissue without sign of infection, particularly on an extremity such as a tail, might well suggest something lacking in the diet. And the creature was rather small.

'What do you mean, feed them?' replied the manager.

I thought back. Perhaps I had phrased my question awkwardly. No, it seemed to make reasonable sense. 'What do you feed the alligators on?' I repeated. 'What food do you give them?'

The manager seemed perplexed. 'Food?' he mumbled. 'We don't exactly feed them at all. That's up to our customers.'

'What do you mean by that?' I felt the first stirrings of understanding and anger.

'Well, you know. The customers, the punters. They feed the little fellows. That's part of the gimmick—dancing with crocs all round you, throwing 'em bits to eat. Thrills the ladies no end. We're the only club in the North with the idea.' He smirked proudly.

'But what do the customers give the alligators?' I persisted. 'And how much?'

'Well, that'd be difficult to say. Prawns from the prawn cocktails, bits of steak, cheese of course, bits of melon—we do have quite a name for our Ogen melons filled with port wine you know, you ought to come some time and bring the missus—oh, and of course they get potato crisps and peas and scraps of lettuce.'

'Is that all they get in the way of food?' I asked, tight-lipped.

'Well, yes. But the people at the tables closest to the dance floor throw plenty in. They like to move 'em round a bit.

Trouble is, they do throw fag ends in as well. Never seen 'em eat those, though.'

'Have you ever seen them eat anything that's thrown in?' I looked at the carpet of decaying food remains and filth that lay on the bottom of the channel.

The manager reflected for a moment or two. 'Can't say I ever have, to be honest. Being so near the band puts 'em off, I suppose. Maybe they eat after closing. That's it—they're nocturnal, aren't they?'

'What do you think they normally eat in the wild?'

The manager frowned, then sniggered. 'Wogs, I imagine, natives, black boys, eh?' He gave me a jolly poke in the ribs. 'No, seriously, I reckon when they can't get human flesh they, well, they, er, graze on weed or chew reeds or something. Anyway, our food's very mixed, and the vegetables are good. They must get better fed here than up some mud creek among the fuzzy-wuzzies.'

Despite having to keep myself from punching this unlikely paradigm of zoological erudition in the eye, I was eager to hear more. 'How long have the alligators been here?' I inquired, gritting my teeth.

'Three years, about. They've grown a bit.'

'How big were they when you bought them, then?'

'Oh, about nine or ten inches, I'd say.'

It was appalling. The little reptiles had grown only two or three inches in three years. The reason was plain: eating little and very rarely, in cool water and a confined space, cold-blooded creatures like alligators grow barely at all. These should have been eight times their actual size. The wonder was that they were alive at all.

I inspected the tail of the little alligator closely. It was my first such case but I felt sure that the basic cause of the disease was vitamin B_6 deficiency. What was more, the bones of all three reptiles seemed unusually soft and pliable, so there was the complication of rickets too. The whole mess was one of gross neglect and malnutrition.

465

The manager paled when I asked him to hold the alligator while I amputated the gangrenous portion of its tail. 'Oooh! I couldn't possibly,' he said. 'Can't bear to touch the slimy beasts. Can't stand blood, really I can't. So sorry.' He edged away, muttering something about accounts to attend to and wine to order.

As it was the middle of the morning there was no-one else around. I took off my jacket and slipped the alligator inside head first, leaving just the tail protruding. Holding the wriggling reptile through the sleeve with one hand, I managed to inject a ring of local anaesthetic around its tail. Giving time for the anaesthetic to act, I prepared scalpel, suture needles and nylon thread. Meanwhile the alligator, alarmed at the prospect of imminent surgery, disappeared completely down my jacket sleeve. When I was ready, I pushed my hand down to feel for my little patient. As my fingers reached him, he bit down hard and painfully, seizing two of my fingers in a miniature gin-trap of spiky teeth. In agony, I withdrew my hand, bringing with it the tenaciously engaged alligator. I did not want to break the little fellow's teeth so I slowly used the blunt end of a scalpel in my other hand to prise open his mouth and release my punctured digits. That done, I wired his jaws securely together with an encircling strand or two of nylon.

At last the operation could begin, but without any helper I had to hold the animal, cut and stitch. The problem began when the tail had been amputated, a fraction closer to the body than the line where the rotting tissue ended, and I was attempting to suture the wound neatly. How was I to tie knots in the nylon? The slightest relaxation of my grip on the alligator's body and he prepared to scuttle off. I turned him upside down on the nearest table and stroked his tummy in the style of Kelly, the croc mesmerist. He seemed to like the tickling sensation and lay still. When I thought he had gone properly into a trance, I released my hold on him. Quick as a flash, he flipped onto his feet and fled over the dirty tablecloth. I cursed the Garden of Eden and its fallen angels. Retrieving my bolting patient, I held him up to my mouth with one hand. I would have to use my teeth. I passed the needle and nylon thread through the edges of the scaly skin with my other hand, caught and held them between my teeth while I slipped a knot round with my bleeding fingers. Right under my nose, the soggy rear end of the alligator smelt distinctly unpleasant. Slowly, one by one, I 'toothed' surgical knots across the tail stump until it was completely sealed. Then I gave all three alligators stiff shots of vitamins and liquid minerals.

My final job was to deal with the manager and I went to his office.

'I've operated on the alligator,' I told him, 'but the Garden of Eden is a bloody disgrace. You've kept those animals for three years in abominable conditions and with no provision for proper diet or care.'

The manager stood up abruptly from behind his desk with a look I imagine he normally reserved for clients requiring the attentions of his bouncer. There was no bouncer at hand.

I continued, 'You know nothing at all about these creatures, you've been neglectful and cruel and you're not fit to keep tame bluebottles!'

'Now look here, young fellow, I don't know who you think you are, but . . .'

'I give you one week to donate those alligators to the zoo, otherwise I blow the whistle. *Manchester Evening News*, police, Cruelty to Animals Act, the lot—you get my point?'

The word 'police' seemed to quieten the manager down immediately. 'Yes, er, quite, quite,' he said. 'Now how about a drop of short stuff before you go?'

'Thank you, no. But please remember my advice about your donation to the zoo.' I had made him make an offer he could not refuse.

Sure enough, the manager did remember, for three days later the local newspaper carried a publicity shot of Miss

Seksi, she of the python and the striptease, presenting Belle Vue with the trio.

'"Do take care of them, we're so fond of them," said Miss Seksi,' read the blurb beneath the photograph.

The three alligators from the Garden of Eden were named Adam, Eve and Abel by Clive, Belle Vue's reptile keeper, and under his care they began to grow long and fat. When Belle Vue closed in 1977 they were all around eight feet long and they went off to sunnier climes in the new Zoo de la Casa de Campo, Madrid, where I still see them.

Six

There were only three more days before I was due to fly out to Seattle to see how the Americans went about shipping the killer whale. It was breakfast-time again when Shelagh answered the phone and said it was Matt from Belle Vue. My appetite vanished as I pushed back my chair to take the receiver.

'What now?' I asked tersely, steeling myself for further catastrophes. Not more giraffe problems, I prayed.

'A woipe out. Not a survoivor,' came the Irishman's voice. Yet he sounded remarkably cheerful for a bearer of sad tidings.

'How many of what?' I barked.

'Oh, the lot. Around three dozen, they say.'

The man must have cracked under the shock, I thought. He was quite clearly chuckling.

'Three dozen dead what?' I bellowed.

Matt paused for maximum dramatic effect and then said quietly, 'Fleas, Doctor, the whole bally lot of 'em, the performin' fleas.'

Belle Vue possessed the last surviving example of that Victorian curiosity, the flea circus. In a small round kiosk in the centre of the zoo, the flea trainer would crouch over a miniature ring set on a table-top and put a troupe of shiny brown fleas through their repertoire. The circle of paying customers huddled round him would see two of the minute creatures fence with swords made out of fuse-wire, another couple pull Lilliputian chariots and a supposedly female star do a high-wire act along a filament of cotton whilst clasping a diminutive parasol. The fleas worked well. They submitted gamely to being harnessed with the aid of a magnifying glass and tweezers, they pushed and pulled and lifted in demonstrations of their relatively enormous strength, and the show went on. It was not actually true to say that the fleas were trained; they did what they were supposed to do quite naturally. Put a well-fed flea on a thread and he (or she) will walk along it. Give him a little parasol to grab and he will grab it for sure in one pair of legs and still walk happily along on the remaining two pairs. Place two fleas face to face, give them each a bit of fuse-wire and they will wave the useless things in front of them (what else should a flea find to do with fuse-wire?), looking for all the world like a pair of miniature Errol Flynns.

If that makes it sound too simple, let me hasten to point out the pitfalls before you tell your boss what he can do with his job, shake the cat in search of an off-the-peg and out-of-work company of artistes and take a one-way ticket to Broadway. First, there are fleas and fleas. To put it another way, there are Thespian fleas, fleas that have greasepaint and the roar of the crowd in their yellow blood, that are invigorated by the limelight, that dream dreams of playing Hamlet or Macbeth, and then there are the common herd, the fleas lacking in pizzazz. It goes without saying that flea circuses depend on a plentiful supply of the former variety, plentiful because of the brevity, if brilliance, of their lives and because of the tendency, so well known among flighty show-biz types, to be unreliable, miss rehearsals, elope. Experience has shown that only *Pulex irritans,* the human flea, has got what it takes to make the grade in flea circuses.

The second necessity, common to all performers whether they be Laurence Olivier or a six-legged blood-sucker one-eighth of an inch long, is nourishment, and where Lord O. might make do with a cold cutlet or fish and chips, fleas demand meals of blood. Human fleas prefer human blood and take other brews with reluctance. The provider of the meals, usually by baring his forearm, is the long-suffering trainer who owns the flea circus.

Now I come to the bit that will bring tears to the eyes of every dedicated animal conservationist: along with the blue whale, the Javan rhinoceros and the okapi, the human flea faces the sombre possibility of extinction, at least in the West. The plain fact that the species is becoming increasingly difficult to find is no doubt the principal reason why flea circuses, those bizarre backwaters of show business, are no longer around. The decline of *Pulex irritans* was brought on by increased standards of hygiene in the human population and especially by the universal use of DDT and other pesticides and fly-sprays around the house. What applies to the human flea, however, does not seem to have worried unduly the hundred or more other species of flea that make their homes on almost all kinds of mammals and birds throughout the world. They thrive, but the trouble is that their histrionic abilities are said to be abysmal.

'The feller runnin' the flea circus is as sick as a parrot,' Matt was saying. 'Some joker squirted Flit in the room where he keeps his insects. He thinks it was his woife after they'd had a bit of a barney. Anyway, he comes in this morning and foinds the lot with their legs in the air, croaked.' He chuckled louder than ever.

'Can't he get replacements easily enough?' I asked. My knowledge of the flea business at that time was zero. I assumed that a quick dash down to the nearest Salvation Army doss-house would have a full complement of performers on cue for the afternoon performance.

'No chance,' said Matt. 'Human fleas are loike gold nowadays. His last batch he had sent in from a scientist in Wales at two pounds apiece. But apparently that source has petered out.'

'And they must be human fleas?'

'So he says. It's traditional. Apparently if they're content and well fed they'll march about and not indulge in too much jumpin'. Other fleas object to marchin'.'

'Surely some other species of animal flea would do as a substitute, at least temporarily?'

'Well, that's whoiy oi'm ringin' you. The flea circus man doubts it'll work but he thinks it's worth a go. Perhaps some of the zoo animals have their own fleas on them, fleas mebbe with a little bit of talent. Dog and cat fleas he says are an absolute dead loss. They clear off before you can say Finn McCool.'

'So?' I queried.

'Well, if you could spare half an hour, he'd be most obloiged if we could look through some of our animals.'

'To round up candidates for audition?'

'Correct, Doctor.'

I went to the zoo. Apart from the reptile house, where blood-sucking ticks on snakes and lizards were carefully controlled, our defence against external parasites was simply to powder, bath or spray any bird or mammal on which ticks or mites had begun to cause skin disease or itching. Newly arrived animals were inspected for fellow-travellers and dealt with as necessary. Fleas, of all the various types of creature that pass their days browsing beneath the fur or feathers of their hosts, are rarely seen.

Matt and the mournful flea trainer, whose name was Alf, met me and we set off round the gardens, carrying with us a handful of small, waxed pill-boxes. There was no question of picking over some of our beasts, and we passed by the big cats, the wolves, the gorillas and such. A selection of monkeys was clean as a whistle. (People often think that these creatures can be seen picking fleas from one another's coats but it is not so: what they see is mutual grooming, with the groomer taking skin scales and grains of salt from the other animal's body.) We parted the lush wool of the llamas and alpacas, grabbed a Barbary sheep or two and frisked an amazed group of kangaroos. They had not got a single flea among them. On we went, like the School Inspectors who came once a year and scratched around our heads in search of 'nits' when I was a little boy.

Then we made our first capture. A little black fellow fumbled his take-off leap from the belly fur of an Arctic fox and was collared by Matt. Soon we bagged a rather somnolent brace of bigger reddish ones which were napping on a parrot. Within a couple of hours we had almost twenty fleas of various sorts safely incarcerated in our pill-boxes. We went back to the flea circus kiosk to see them auditioned. When we were inside and securely battened down, Alf illuminated the table-top where all the action took place, set up his props and laid out the pill-boxes in front of him. Each box had been labelled with the name of the host species. If by any chance there was a minuscule Richard Burton waiting to be discovered in one of the containers, we needed to know where more like him might be obtained.

One by one the pill-boxes were opened and the inmates removed with tweezers. Alf first examined them through the magnifying glass. Some he thought were far too small, as apart from the difficulty of putting on the cotton harnesses, the audience would have difficulty seeing them. He tried the bigger ones in the ring. The first three of these, from a coatimundi, took one look at the Big Top and vanished, never to be seen again. The next, a solitary, mahogany-coloured individual plucked whilst still sucking brunch from the neck of an ostrich, was found to have expired in the pill-box. So it went on. Some jumped straight out of the ring, others keeled over, legs bicycling furiously in the air, when urged to walk. The few that Alf actually managed to encumber with parasol, fuse-wire or harness seemed to be struck with instant stage fright and froze up, feigning death.

'Just like I thought,' muttered Alf. 'We've always said in the profession that there's no substitute for yer grand old 'uman variety.' He shook his head sadly, recalling the gracious, flea-ridden days gone by.

My part in the attempt to save the death of another little bit of theatre ended there, and although Alf eventually obtained a small troupe from somewhere, the growing difficulties of supply did finally bring down the curtain on Britain's last flea circus.

The news of Alf's misfortune had got into the early edition of the evening paper, I found later that day, and before I had finished reading my copy, there was a phone call.

'My name's Andrew Greenwood,' said the voice. 'I'm a veterinary student at Cambridge. I live over the hills from you and read in the paper about the flea circus at Belle Vue. I wondered if I could be of any help.'

It was the chap who had been chasing me up about lobsters, I suddenly remembered.

'I've collected some of the biggest fleas in Britain, if you'd like them,' continued the voice earnestly. 'They're mole fleas, a quarter of an inch long. I'd be delighted to bring them along.'

The mole flea certainly is a giant of its kind, though still not as enormous as the pea-sized monster of a flea once seen in the nest of an American beaver.

'Thanks anyway,' I said, 'but I don't think we're in the market for any more fleas today.'

Less than a week later, I was sitting in a restaurant on the Seattle seafront, chewing whopping great pieces of broiled lobster and outsize oysters. Like so much American seafood, they looked delicious and were temptingly served, but had somehow outgrown their subtle, flavourful birthright, sacrificing delicacy and taste for sheer size. Oh for a Cornish lobster or a dozen Whitstable natives, I thought, as my jaws began to ache with the effort and I washed the rubbery chunks down with a dispiriting beverage that claimed to be wine and went under the enigmatic name of 'Cold Duck'.

Through the window I could see below me the round

metal pools of the Seattle Aquarium. Floating motionless in the one nearest to me, like an inflated plastic bath toy, eleven feet long with oil-smooth, jet-black skin and crisp, snow-white markings, was the young killer whale I had come for. He was a perfect specimen, about two-and-a-half years old, with the teeth at the front of his jaws only just beginning to push through the gums. I was stoking up for the two-day journey to Flamingo Park. He was fasting; whales and dolphins never travel on full stomachs.

Don Goldsberry and Ted Griffin, the two owners of the Aquarium, were the pioneers of killer whale catching. Using a mile of immensely heavy and unwieldy stainless steel netting, they trapped the powerful and sharp-witted whales in Puget Sound. Goldsberry, Griffin and their veterinarian, Bill Klontz, were the experts at what was a fairly new game. All I was supposed to do was watch and listen and learn.

The first of their killers had been given the Eskimo name of 'Namu'. Later animals were christened 'Shamu', 'Ramu' and so on. They had a few appropriate, noble-sounding suggestions for my little fellow.

'Sorry,' I said, 'Pentland Hick has already decided what he is to be called. His name is Cuddles.'

The Americans did not like it. I hated it. But Hick was a shrewd entrepreneur with an eye to publicity: 'A fierce hunter of the oceans with a soft and winsome name. It's a good gimmick that will catch the imagination of the media men,' he reasoned. He was right.

Goldsberry and Griffin gave me a long list of do's and don'ts concerning the whale, all of which I meticulously noted down. This was the gospel to be followed—any infringement and Cuddles would undoubtedly run into trouble. 'If his dorsal fin flops over he's short of sweet water'; 'Use a three-inch needle if you have to inject him'; 'The only safe vaccine is 5 cc of such and such'; 'A shot of penicillin before he travels is all he needs'; 'Eggs are bad for him'; 'Sugar and glucose aren't absorbed by his gut and may do him harm'; 'If he falls ill give him a quart of Maalox and fly us over'.

It sounded daunting, but who was I to judge? The practical study of larger cetaceans in captivity may have been in its infancy in the United States, but it had not even been born in Britain. It was prudent to go along with the instructions that accompanied the goods, not least because Pentland Hick had paid fifteen thousand dollars for Cuddles and was in no mood to quibble. It would be two years or more before we realised that the Seattle team knew little more about the care and treatment of these complicated marine animals than we did.

Next day Cuddles' long journey began. A padded hammock with holes for his eyes, flippers and vent was slipped under him as he floated in three feet of water. He did not fight or complain as a crane picked him, dripping, out of the pool and lowered him gently into a framework of tubular steel in which the hammock was to be slung. At last I got a chance to touch him. It was a wonderful experience. As I leaned over the placid beast after clambering up the bars surrounding him, he exhaled with a soft roar. A blast of hot air, carrying a not unpleasant, cow-like smell, hit me in the face. I revelled in the sensuous delight of passing my fingers over the skin. It was polished, very finely grooved and had the consistency of hard india rubber. It was soft and cool under his axillas, like sheet-steel across the blade of his tail fluke and warm as toast on his forehead, or melon. I climbed down and looked through the holes in the hammock. I waggled the paddle-like flippers and tried to trace the outlines of the bones within, bones that are identical to those in the fingers of human beings. Then I peered close to one large round brown eye. It was streaming with transparent tears as thick as syrup. The eye with its pleated, chocolate-coloured iris rolled slightly and fixed on me. He was looking at me. I stroked the nearby flipper and whistled.

To my utter delight, the eye remained gazing at me and a

squeaky, high-pitched chirruping was squeezed out of the blow-hole on top of Cuddles' head. I whistled again. The whale chirp-chirped in turn. He was answering me. Cats answer back, Henry, my goat, willingly exchanges bleats, dogs do it and tigers have a lovely habit of replying to a low 'prrh-prrh' with a similar welcoming sound that never fails to excite me, but this was something unique and it touched me deeply. It was to become a regular feature of my relationship with Cuddles, but that first moment when I came eyeball to eyeball and conversed with a Lord of the Sea, as the Eskimos call these magnificent beasts, was one of the most moving of my life, a vivid instant of sentiment, not sentimentality. Quite inexplicably, a bond had been forged between the whale and me. Whales, and particularly this one, were going to be something extra-special from now on.

As a greenhorn with whales, I was allowed to help in coating every inch of Cuddles' body with thick lanolin grease. This would stop the delicate skin drying out and cracking. Next, towels were spread along his back and smoothed to get rid of air-bubbles that could 'burn' the skin during the long journey. After that, hundredweights of crushed ice were sprinkled on and around the whale. The entire framework was shrouded in plastic sheeting and a water-spraying system of pipes, pumps and electric batteries was set up. The animal would go all the way sticky, wet and cold to avoid the killer's principal enemy, the risk of internal overheating.

We set out for the airport by road, on the back of a long low-loader. In the freight hold of the TWA jet freighter purposely kept at 1°C to help keep the whale cool, it was no fun clambering over his framework for a solid twelve hours. Don Goldsberry, Ted Griffin and I had to keep a constant watch for 'bed-sores' that can end weeks later in death from toxic gangrene, for blobs of lanolin melting and running into the blow-hole, for shifting towels that could be sucked in by one powerful inhalation of the whale's breath. The water sprays had to be kept going, batteries replaced, the system cleared of blocking particles of faecal matter re-circulated with the water. Most important of all, the whale must be constantly reassured. Stroking his forehead, whistling to him or just talking nonsense into his pinhead-sized but highly sensitive ear—it did not matter what, as long as we kept doing it, hour after hour. I had brought my *Collected Poems* of John Betjeman with me, a constant companion on my travels, and I passed the time on my spells of duty at the head end by reading aloud from the book. Apart from the comforting murmur of my voice, I wonder if Cuddles got anything more from such Betjemania as the delightful, awful Miss Joan Hunter Dunn.

Arriving at London Airport, we passed smoothly through Customs, then came the inspection by the Government vet. He had never even seen a whale before and would not have been any the wiser if our boy had been lying there in the terminal stages of rabies complicated by bubonic plague. His main function, he said, was to count incoming animals. To my amazement, he climbed up onto the whale container, looked down and said, 'One'. This he wrote in his notebook before jumping down and bidding us good evening.

After a six-hour road journey up into the north-east of England, where Flamingo Park lies in the sleepy village of Kirkby Misperton, the whale was unloaded from his truck and hoisted above the floodlit figure-of-eight pool that was to be his new home. Gently he was lowered into the icy cold water where several of us were waiting in wet-suits to release him from his hammock. The cold water and my tiredness were forgotten as the canvas fell away. Heart in mouth I waited, bobbing by Cuddles' side. If he had become stiff and could not flex his tail flukes, if he sank out of control, or if he listed because of a congested lung, we would have little chance of manhandling his great bulk in the deep pool. I saw that the two Americans who were conducting the releasing operation were looking tense, too.

For a second Cuddles hung in the water. Lazily he raised his great tail. Its deceptively powerful upbeat thrust the water into foaming furrows and his torpedo body glided gently forwards into the centre of the pool. We paddled after him—not that he needed us, but with all the photographer's flash-bulbs popping we wanted to look useful. Goldsberry called for a mackerel and threw it a couple of yards ahead of the whale. It sank in a flickering spiral through the blue water. Instantly Cuddles saw it, blew out a broad plume of water droplets and dived. Half-turning gracefully ten feet down, he opened his mouth a mere inch or two, sucked and the mackerel shot in. To the cheers of the crowd Cuddles rose to the surface, floated vertically with his head well clear of the water and opened his jaws wide. For the first time I saw the salmon-pink expanse of Cuddles' unmistakable grin.

Half an hour later this untrained animal that had roamed the north Pacific only one month before, that had raided fishing nets, murdered great whales, out-run and out-thought sharks and sealions and dolphins, this grinning, cuddly Cuddles with the appealing chirrup, was seen to begin playing with a floating beach-ball.

During the following weeks the killer whale settled down admirably in his new home. Every few days I made the 200-mile round trip over the hills, through the cities of Leeds and York and across the fertile farmland of the vale of Pickering that stretches east to the coast, to see that all was going well. This usually entailed swimming with Cuddles in his pool of artificial sea water. In a wet-suit and face mask I inspected his ventral surface under water; it would be several months before he was trained to roll over on command so that his tummy could be viewed and prodded from dry land. Underwater, too, I had a chance of catching for parasite analysis a sample of his elusive, near-liquid faecal matter before it dispersed irretrievably in his wake. Even so humble a task as collecting droppings from these remarkable creatures presented quite special complications, as the whale, ever curious about the submarine antics of this ungainly caricature of a drunken walrus, buffeted me with his rounded nose.

Giving injections was another poser. Asian 'flu swept through the human population of Britain shortly after Cuddles' arrival and, on learning that Sea World in San Diego had evidence that the influenza virus could attack cetaceans, I had to think of some way of jabbing Cuddles with the current strains of 'flu vaccine. In the early days we had no special slinging device for 'dry-docking' the whale, and emptying the 300,000-gallon pool except for serious emergencies just was not on. For one thing, artificial sea water is expensive to make up. For another, the local river authority did not take kindly to so vast a quantity of brine passing via the drains into their waterways. The salt injured freshwater river life and could poison vegetation along the banks. I had already seen the effect of brine discharge into a stream near the Marineland on the Côte d'Azur: every one of the three dozen majestic palm trees in the gardens of villas running down to the stream was dead as a dodo in a couple of weeks and had to be given fake crowns of branches cut from other trees. The villa owners played hell. On top of these problems, pools like the one at Flamingo Park, built in sandy soil with a high water table, often object to being emptied by collapsing inwards when the enormous outward pressure of their contents is removed.

Cuddles had behaved like a playful, amenable child so far. He doted on humans, craved their attention and was impeccably well-mannered. Pondering the problem of the 'flu vaccination, I decided to try simply swimming up to him in the water and slapping a needle in. I was a dab hand at doing this sort of thing with large land animals. Take an elephant: thump his buttocks hard with your clenched fist one, two, three times so that he knows you are there and is accustomed to what is, to him, a friendly pat on his inch-

480

thick skin. Then, O wily elephant doctor, still keeping up the regular rhythm, with the fourth thump flick forward the wide-bore hypodermic needle that you have concealed in the palm of your hand. Slap goes your fist for the fifth time and the needle zooms to the hilt right through the tough grey leather. The elephant does not feel a thing and consequently has no nasty memories to never forget. This technique is used on horses, cattle and pigs by James Herriots all over the world.

I looked at the whale contentedly basking on the surface after a snack of twenty pounds of mackerel and I reckoned there was a good chance of doing it the same way with him. The press were going to take pictures of the novel inoculation, and I came forth from the dressing room looking like Dustin Hoffman in *The Graduate*. Apart from the frogman outfit I carried a disinfectant aerosol in one hand and a syringe fitted with a ten-inch needle in the other. With the panache of a commando off to plant limpet mines on the *Tirpitz*, I somersaulted backwards into the pool. This flashy entrance was then followed by a more feeble dog-paddle towards my prey. As I arrived at Cuddles' glistening hull, steam was rising from his forehead where it was drying while he basked. He tolerantly rolled a liquid brown eye at me and gave me the salmon-pink grin. The sloping rows of conical white teeth sparkled.

I selected a spot on the top of the killer's back at the base of the dorsal fin. Supporting myself by throwing one arm over his loins, I sprayed the area with disinfectant and then threw the can away from me. Cuddles was most intrigued. Only his big eye moved, following my every movement.

I balanced myself in the water and raised the syringe and needle high in the air. Cuddles watched it go. Then with my free hand I slapped at the disinfected spot. One, two, three. 'What *is* the lad up to?' I could imagine the whale musing good-humouredly. Four, five—down came the syringe, straight as an arrow, and at exactly the same instant I had

481

the impression that someone had dropped an atom bomb on the *Tirpitz*, prematurely aborting my mission. The pool water beneath me seemed to levitate itself. I was in no doubt that the entire three million pounds of liquid was unexpectedly on its way up towards the ceiling. Certainly I was proceeding in the opposite direction. Somehow I had been transported into a giant washing machine. Arms and legs flailing, I was sucked down, tumbled, rolled, swept and swirled in a maelstrom of foaming water. What looked like a nuclear submarine with a full-open throttle was tearing round me. My lungs were bursting. I had swallowed what felt like a hogshead of salt water du maison. My syringe and needle had vanished, and my shins had received an excruciating blow from something that could only have been Neptune's iron trident.

A half-drowned veterinarian was hauled miserably over the edge of the pool and lay, puking salt water, in a very un-commando-like fashion at the feet of the pressmen, who found it all very interesting.

Apparently, as soon as the needle had touched the whale. he had launched himself forward with full, fast beats of his flukes. The entire muscle strength of a cetacean's body is concentrated on the focal point at the hinge of the tail. The energy contained in this highly efficient propeller is enough to storm-toss incredible volumes of water in the twinkling of an eye. I had been the centre of such an instant storm and the painful bruising of my shins had been caused by the tip of a flipper grazing by.

Half an hour and a stiff shot of brandy later, I felt ready to try again. I was loath to use the dart-gun, since its longest needle measured only three inches and anyway I was afraid that the wide bore might carry unsterile water into the tissues. I would not have been able to disinfect the skin and there was the problem of retrieving the spent flying syringe.

The question of needle length interested me. It was generally assumed that a long one that could reach beyond the thick blubber layer was essential: everyone talked as if the blubber was inert stuff, without blood vessels that could pick up and circulate drugs and vaccines. But even fatty tissue must have blood to remain alive, and I decided to try a foolproof but shallow injection method on Cuddles. I telephoned a friend at a Leeds University dental clinic, and a car was sent over with what I wanted: the needle-less gun that fires liquids at high velocity into human gums or skin. It was the instrument being developed for mass vaccination against cholera, typhoid, polio and so on.

The dose of vaccine for a killer whale was my next problem. With most vaccines it is by no means true or safe to give, say, six times the amount of vaccine to an individual who weighs six times the average for any particular dosage. Vaccines do not work like that. Nevertheless it was possible to use too small a dose—in Seattle Cuddles had been given what was thought to be an adequate shot of a vaccine against germs of the lockjaw family, but tests I had done on his blood when he first arrived showed virtually no antibodies to lockjaw circulating in his system. He was not protected as everyone thought. In the end, I decided to give Cuddles three times the human dose of 'flu vaccine and then take blood after a couple of weeks, by when, I hoped, a dry dock would be ready. I would check the level of 'flu antibodies and give bigger booster shots if necessary.

The intrepid frogman re-entered the water carrying the vaccine-gun. Once more Cuddles was resting and gave no sign as I approached that only a couple of hours before I had tried to harpoon him and had been summarily demolished. Again he grinned disarmingly. A trainer on the pool-side threw a mackerel into the gaping jaw. Cuddles sucked it down with smooth ease and ogled me. I raised the gun and drew in a big breath. If the typhoon struck, I was determined to keep my mouth shut this time, no matter what.

I pulled the trigger. There was a sharp crack. I got ready for drowning.

Cuddles grinned benevolently again and did not move an inch. He was vaccinated and had not felt a thing. Now all I had to do was wait and hope that the inoculation was effective.

I was quite pleased as I struggled out of the pool for the second time that day. One way or another, I had injected my first real live killer. By the time I had showered, admired the blue and red protuberances on my shins and got into warm clothing once more, everyone had gone from the dolphinarium except one fellow. He stood at the water's edge, looking down intently at the whale, a camera slung from his neck and his pockets bristling with notebooks. I took him to be the last of the press, or possibly the usual late arriver from the local rag who always gets upset when you politely explain, 'No, it isn't possible to do it all again just for you. No, not even mocking it up. No, even though I appreciate how bloody-minded your editor's going to be if you return without the hoped for pictures of Dr Taylor being eaten by a killer whale or stomped by a rhinoceros.'

'Get what you want?' I asked the mousey-haired young man with the faintest resemblance to Robert Redford.

'Oh yes, very much so,' came the reply. 'By the way, I'm Andrew Greenwood. I spoke to you a few months back. Lobsters, fleas—remember?'

'Come and have a spot of lunch and tell me all about your lobsters,' I said.

Andrew barely touched the meal, he spent so much time enthusing over his determination to practise with zoo animals once he had qualified from Cambridge.

'How did you know I was working on the whale today?' I asked.

He grinned. 'I drop a keeper in the bird section a packet of fags every week or two to keep me informed.'

His chutzpah appealed to me. 'And the lobsters?'

Earnestly, he explained. 'You may well know of the significance of lobster blood serum in identifying a certain

484

type of haemophilia in humans. It's a very rare condition, and only about eight cases have been reported so far, but Manchester Royal Infirmary are working on a test for the disease. That test relies on a supply of lobster serum.'

'Quite. To detect the missing clotting factor in the human blood,' I said, nodding sagely but not knowing the faintest thing about the rôle in such obscure areas of medicine of a crustacean that until then had been useful to me only when coated with a mixture of cream, parmesan cheese, white wine and garlic, and lightly broiled.

The intent young student appeared to think that I knew all about the matter. 'So I've been asked to supply the laboratory at Manchester with lobster serum and I came to you, Dr Taylor, for advice on taking blood from lobsters.'

It was flattering, of course, but I had no idea where to begin finding veins on such an armour-plated creature.

'I'm afraid I can't help you,' I confessed. 'Lobsters don't fall sick very often these days.' (In fact, within a couple of years Reg Bloom, a zoologist friend, started flying plane-loads of Canadian lobsters over the Atlantic to stock his 'lobster farm' at Clacton, and I discovered then that the species can be expected to feel poorly with monotonous regularity.)

Andrew Greenwood seemed disappointed that I could not shed any light on how to persuade the shellfish to enrol as blood donors, but I had the feeling that he was not the type to let it rest at that. When we parted he asked if he could contact me and keep me informed of his progress.

'There must be a way of sampling a lobster without doing it like the Dutch scientists do—simply chopping off a claw and letting the poor thing bleed into a jar,' he said.

I liked that. Andrew seemed a promising sort of bloke.

I was further impressed when, three or four weeks later, he proudly appeared at my home in Rochdale carrying a little tube of pale blue liquid. He had studied the architecture of the crusty old lobster and had found a particular soft spot

485

where a needle can be inserted and blood drawn off easily without hurting or damaging the lowly creature in any way. It was his unusual début in the world of wild animal surgery.

Seven

From the vast room's high ceiling, tattered strips of red velvet wallpaper hung down in rows like Tibetan prayer flags. In the centre of the floor stood a full-length billiard table lit by hooded lights and with a small Capuchin monkey curled up asleep on the green baize over the spot reserved for the blue ball. The air was heavy with an aroma of mothballs, Cologne water, Capuchin monkey and sheer age. A velvet-covered sofa was drawn up before the deep, broad hearth where a cheap electric fire's single bar glowed dully amid gently waving cobwebs.

On the sofa reclined Mrs Crabbe. A Singer sewing machine and a large pile of Tetley teabags were on a card table nearby. She had been neatly stitching two lines across the middle of each teabag and then separating the halves with a snip of her scissors when we arrived. Renowned in the town for 'having nowt to learn about making brass go a long way', Mrs Crabbe was worth half a million and found it easy to stay that way. Two stools, low and wooden like milking stools, were placed before her and slightly to one side to avoid blocking the feeble heat from the fire. On one sat Dr Aspinall, Doctor of Medicine, humans for the treatment of, and on the other sat I, Doctor of Veterinary Medicine, physician to the countless other living things on this planet that Dr Aspinall was not concerned with. Dr Aspinall and I both held a liqueur glass brimming with a thick yellow liquid. Mrs Crabbe had a firm grasp on a tumbler filled with the same stuff. Dr Aspinall and I sat in silence, glumly sipping the sickly Advocaat from time to time. Mrs Crabbe gulped large mouthfuls at frequent intervals while giving us an imperious dressing-down.

Over eighty, small and wiry, with hennaed hair and a face thickly powdered with what looked like flour, the old lady was not having any nonsense. It was the first time Aspinall or I had met her, but like every Rochdalian we had heard much about the history of this remarkable woman. Widow of the Crabbe who expanded the Crabbe cotton textile mills into the largest family concern west of the Pennines, she had chased over the moors on foot, following the Rochdale Hunt, until well into her seventies; with one swipe of a lacrosse stick she had broken the arm of a canvasser who had imprudently distributed Labour Party leaflets to her gardeners; and she had literally closed down a Methodist chapel of which she was the patroness and main financial support when the new young minister had professed a belief in evolution. Since her spouse had abruptly expired while doing the hokey-kokey at a Masonic function twenty years before, Mrs Crabbe had soldiered on in the great black stone house, served faithfully by a small staff, the youngest of whom, referred to as 't' gardener's lad', could not have been more than ten years younger than his mistress. Time creaked along in the house set on the moor edge above the chimneys of the family mills that filled the narrow valley below with smoke. House and inhabitants were slowly grinding to a halt. Essentials were attended to. Non-essentials were not. The brass knobs and knockers bearing the ornate 'C' were crusty with verdigris, the Victorian wood and ironwork were dull. The kitchen, which six nights a week had handled the victualling of a gaggle of mill owners, Conservative Party notables, parsons and their wives, lay cold and dank, its shelves empty but for Weetabix and Ovaltine. The garden, once trim and spruce, was regaining a wild beauty and making for the moorland. The cellar, though, was full—not, as in years gone by, with crusted port and well-bred clarets but with rack upon rack of Advocaat. Mrs Crabbe doted, depended, survived upon

488

egg-flip. Therein lay the problem, for both Dr Aspinall and myself.

It was actually by pure coincidence that the doctor and I had driven up to the house at precisely the same moment. We had parked our cars on the circle of cobbles through which a forest of vigorous weeds was thrusting six inches high, greeted one another—Aspinall had stitched me up once and I had treated some of his sheep-farmer patients who had picked up orf virus from their flocks—and knocked on the imposing front door.

'D'ye think we've been called to see the same patient?' Aspinall chuckled as we waited.

'Hope not,' I said. 'Apparently the old lady's got a monkey. What are you here for?'

'Mrs Crabbe herself.' He sighed heavily. 'This is my first visit. She's a private patient, just switched to us from Landau's practice. I can't say I'm over-enthusiastic. She's a bit of a tartar by all accounts. She led Dr Landau a hell of a dance and would never take his advice.'

The door opened at last with much groaning of hinges to reveal a bad-tempered crone in high button-boots. She showed us into the room where Mrs Crabbe was treadling furiously away at the suturing of teabags. The whirring of the machine continued until the old lady had bisected several rows of bags to her satisfaction, then she stretched out on the sofa, protectively nestling two bottles of Advocaat in the crook of one arm and surveying us unblinkingly over the tilted brim of her glass. Breaking the ice, I suggested that I wait outside while Dr Aspinall did his stuff. I had already spotted my patient slumbering soundly on the billiard table.

Mrs Crabbe emptied the glass, looked from one to the other of us dolefully, slowly passed a furry tongue across thin lips and then reached for one of her bottles. Without speaking she leaned sideways, felt under the sofa and produced two liqueur glasses. These she filled before replenishing her own glass. Eventually she addressed us in loud and plummy tones.

'Sit down there, both of you. Take a glass. And listen.'

We did as we were told.

'Let me make myself clear,' she continued. 'Ethel, my housekeeper, let you in at the front door. You came to the *front door*.' She uttered the words 'front door' like Edith Evans as Lady Bracknell referring to 'a *handbag*' in *The Importance of Being Earnest*. 'The front door is never opened. I want that clearly understood. In future please remember to use the tradesmen's entrance.'

Dr Aspinall and I cowered on our stools. Mrs Crabbe downed half her tumbler and made a gargling noise.

'Now then.' The old lady's plumminess was sounding distinctly over-ripe. 'I take it you are the two doctors. Are you going to look first at Thoth?' She turned her head briefly towards the sleeping monkey.

'I'm here to see you, Mrs Crabbe,' said Aspinall bravely. 'I'm Dr Aspinall, your new doctor. I've come to give you a check-up and . . .'

'Who's that, then?' interrupted Mrs Crabbe, pointing accusingly towards me and snatching a deep swig that emptied the tumbler.

'Er—I'm the vet. To see the monkey. You rang, I believe.' I smiled reassuringly.

She kept her pointing finger firmly in position and frowned intently. Her dark, deep-sunken eyes bored into me. 'You're Dr Aspinall then. What do you know about monkeys?'

Aspinall groaned and put down his glass. 'Mrs Crabbe, if I might explain, Dr Taylor is here to see your monkey and I'm here to . . .'

Mrs Crabbe's imperious finger swung instantly round, aiming at the unfortunate Aspinall. 'Ah, I see,' she interrupted effortlessly. 'You're his assistant. Quite right. Good. Must have the best for poor Thoth there. Now you may examine him. But don't hurt him, mind. You, Dr

Taylor'—she was speaking to my companion—'hold him gently. Watch what Dr Aspinall does. I've heard he's got quite a way with monkeys.'

I looked at the doctor and he stared helplessly at me. It was perfectly plain that the old battleaxe was suffering from a combination of the passage of time and a surfeit of egg-flip. I raised my eyebrows and bit on the edge of my liqueur glass. With a sharp crack a crescent of glass broke off the rim and dropped from my lips onto the carpet.

'Really, Dr Landau!' barked Mrs Crabbe. 'That's Waterford. Fifteen and sixpence if I'm not mistaken. I shall deduct it from your bill at the end of the quarter.'

Dear God, I thought as I dabbed my bleeding lip with my handkerchief, quarters! What I needed was clients who paid cash or at least promptly after receiving one of Shelagh's monthly accounts.

Aspinall shrugged and rolled his eyes. I tried once more. 'But you sent for the doctor yourself,' I explained. 'Wouldn't it be better if Dr Aspinall—he—your own human doctor examined you elsewhere while I attended to the monkey, to Thoth?'

The old lady grunted indignantly. 'Certainly not. Examined by your assistant, Doctor? What are things coming to? No, sir. You must see to my poor Thoth first, then you can take a look at me and see about my little problem.'

'But, Mrs Crabbe, he is your doctor.'

'Doctor? Doctor? Is he or isn't he a veterinarian, qualified to work with monkeys?'

'No, madam, he isn't, but . . .'

'Quite so.' She squeezed out a stern smile. 'I don't mind him assisting you, Dr Aspinall, while he learns, but I couldn't possibly allow him to treat Thoth alone.'

'I'm the veterinarian, Dr Taylor,' I half-shouted in exasperation.

'Of course you are, Doctor,' she said quietly. 'That's why I called you. And I've every faith in you.'

'Tell you what—why don't you look at the monkey and get that part over with?' Aspinall sounded strangely faint. He stood up and stared intently at the peeling ceiling.

I walked over to the billiard table and looked down at the monkey. 'What's been worrying you about Thoth, Mrs Crabbe?' I asked.

'It's his teeth, Doctor. They seem to be giving him a bit of trouble. He drools and holds his face and is easily offended.'

'Offended?'

'Yes. For example, old Fairbanks, my solicitor, looked at Thoth in a wrong sort of way the other day and Thoth bit his ear.'

'How long have you had him, Mrs Crabbe?'

'Oh, at least forty-five years.'

I gasped. Forty-five years was a sensationally long life-span for a Capuchin monkey.

'Forty-five years for sure?' I asked.

'At least. Possibly longer. He was ever such a smart young fellow when my late husband was in short trousers. I remember his father before him.'

'He was bred round here, you mean?'

Mrs Crabbe slopped a thick stream of Advocaat into the tumbler again. Taking a mouthful, she closed her eyes and seemed to be thinking deeply. 'I think not, Doctor,' she said eventually. 'His family originated in Rhodesia or Nyasaland or somewhere like that.'

'Thoth? He's a South American species, not African, Mrs Crabbe.'

'What are you talking about, Doctor? Old Fairbanks' parents lived in Bulawayo as near as I can recall. Fine stock.'

A muffled choking noise came from the direction of my medical colleague. I dared not look round at him.

'How long have you had Thoth, Mrs Crabbe?' I persevered.

'Nearly ten years now. He's never had a day's illness. You may wake him up if you like.'

I tickled the little creature at the back of his head and, remembering Fairbanks' luck, put on an expression of which the monkey would approve when he opened his eyes. He awoke immediately and glared at me. Then, baring his teeth, he crawled off awkwardly and stuck both legs in a corner pocket. I looked at him carefully. He was an ugly specimen, with a swollen, punch-drunk boxer's face and lips bulging over an upper jaw that seemed too big for his mouth. No, ugly was not a fair word to use. His whole face was deformed. There was no symmetry to it and all the features were askew. Its bones were lumpy and seemed to be trying to press out through the skin.

I approached the Capuchin warily and put out a hand. He pulled himself out of the pocket and shuffled on his knees across the green surface of the table. Now I could see that not only his face but the whole of his puny body was totally deformed. With grotesquely bowed limbs and sunken ribs, this monkey was a hunchback, a miniature Quasimodo. I went after him, grabbed him swiftly behind the neck and with one hand swept his arms behind him into a full nelson. He gibbered infuriatedly but was not able to reach me with his teeth. Gently I put him down onto the floor and released him. The distorted little body dragged itself like a wounded beetle across the dusty carpet. It was not walking. Its feet were redundant. It was crawling, slithering, hauling itself along on elbows and knees.

'Has he always moved like this?' I asked, dismayed.

'Always,' came the reply. 'Why? Capuchin monkeys always walk like that, as you should know, Doctor. Have you ever seen a nicer specimen? It's just those teeth, those naughty peggy-wegs that bother him.'

Quite often I had come across owners, pet-shop dealers, folk who claimed to know a bit about monkeys, who really believed that Capuchins and other New World species such as woolly and spider monkeys naturally haul themselves about in this bizarre and pitiable manner. As a student I had heard zoo men declare that such a way of moving was a classic characteristic of a group of primates who spent their entire lives high in the forest canopy and whose legs as a result were as obsolescent as the human appendix.

I picked the monkey up again, immobilised him in the full nelson and lifted his upper lip. Mrs Crabbe was quite right: Thoth had a mouthful of tooth problems. Looking in, I saw a scene of utter shambles as if a miniature grenade had exploded between the jaws and blasted every tooth out of its foundations. The teeth were there OK but apart from that everything was most definitely not OK. There were teeth growing down from the middle of the roof of the mouth, under the tongue, in clusters one on top of another, three or four abreast struggling to occupy a socket meant for a single one. There were teeth doing their own thing—growing upside down with their roots just visible and their crowns buried deep in the gum, some pointing in towards the tongue, others taking the opposite direction and burrowing into the cheeks.

'Look at this, Doctor,' I said. Aspinall was still studying the ceiling.

'Yes, young man,' said Mrs Crabbe. 'Go and give Dr Taylor a hand and learn something. You'll never be much of a monkey vet if you moon about like that.'

As if in a trance the doctor quietly obeyed.

'SAPD—South American Primate Disease, worst case I've ever seen,' I whispered. 'Malnutrition essentially. Head bones soften while the teeth are developing, letting them drift off into any old place. Ribs cave in. I'm surprised he's not dead long ago with pneumonia. I'll probably find half a dozen pathological fractures in his limbs if I X-ray him.'

The doctor nodded. A more complex and dramatic disease, it nevertheless has some of the features of human rickets.

'What does Thoth eat?' I asked, although I had a pretty

494

shrewd idea—sugary junk with minimum protein and hardly a vitamin.

Mrs Crabbe was silent.

Right, I thought. 'Grapes, bananas, chocolates, sweeties, cakes, biscuits, apples, oranges, sugar lumps, tea, fruit drinks—that's the sort of thing he has, isn't it, Mrs Crabbe?' I inquired confidently.

'No, Dr Aspinall. Definitely not.' Mrs Crabbe's voice was distinctly plummier. 'Thoth has what I have. None of that rubbish you mention. He's got a very sweet tooth and I see he gets plenty of nourishment.'

'What exactly, Mrs Crabbe?' There seemed to be a bleat of desperation in my voice.

'Good wholesome food.'

'Yes, but what exactly? In the wild these monkeys get very high levels of protein including animal protein, minerals and a massive daily intake of vitamin D_3. Does he get meat, chicken, vitamins, cereals as well as vegetables?'

'He gets eggs.'

'That's good. What else?'

'Eggs.'

'And?'

'Eggs in the most nourishing form.'

Light dawned. Of course—the Advocaat.

'Does he drink the egg-flip, Mrs Crabbe?' I asked.

'Of course. I do. It's what keeps me as fit as I am. So does Thoth. It has eggs—there's a whole meal in eggs, Doctor—sugar for energy and grape spirit. It's first-rate stuff.'

'What else does he get, Mrs Crabbe?'

'What else? Nothing else. What else would one need, sir? Advocaat's a perfect diet. Tell me any other monkey you know that's so well cared for. Advocaat's not cheap, you know.'

I lifted Thoth back onto the billiard table and returned to my stool. 'Mrs Crabbe,' I said, picking my words carefully, 'you're killing Thoth. Advocaat is an atrocious diet. He's a cripple because of it. He's deformed because of it. His chest is collapsing because of it.'

The old lady stared at me in stunned amazement.

I went on, 'I can't undo all the damage you've done, but with a little luck I can help him. Maybe he'll walk again for the first time in years. But no more Advocaat for him, ever again. From now it's going to be meat, chicken, milk, nuts, cereals, fruit and daily vitamins and calcium. I want you to have a run built for him outside so that he can get direct sunlight with its ultra-violet light. As for medicine, I'm going to give him some stuff called Sterogyl—an ampoule now and another in three weeks. You understand?'

Mrs Crabbe poured herself another tumbler of the yellow cream and glowered at me. Then she muttered acidly, 'Very well, Dr Aspinall, but I hope you know what you're doing. However, I have decided that I do not need you to examine me. I'll do very well, thank you.' She fussed pettishly with the hem of her dress.

'But there's your doctor.' I pointed at Aspinall. It was starting again.

'I will certainly not be handled by your assistant, Doctor.'

Admitting defeat in the battle of words, I took an ampoule of Sterogyl out of my bag, broke it and poured the alcoholic solution of vitamin D down Thoth's mouth. A connoisseur of booze, he seemed to relish the change of liquor.

'That's me done,' I said. 'Now I'll leave you with Dr Aspinall. I can assure you he's an excellent doctor.' I made for the door.

'Come back,' boomed the plummy voice as I put my hand on the knob. 'Very well then, have your way with a poor old lady. Get on with your examination. After all, Thoth seemed to like you. But please ask this animal doctor friend of yours to leave the room while I undress.'

I turned the door-knob and kept going.

Three weeks later I revisited the black stone house. There

was no sign of Dr Aspinall this time. Again I banged on the front door. After four or five minutes I heard someone come to the door, the letter box was flapped open and the house-keeper's tetchy voice told me to find the tradesmen's entrance. It was a sunny day and I was in a good mood so I walked round to the back of the house.

In the billiard room something dark brown and chirruping darted about the floor. It was Thoth. Mrs Crabbe, reclining on the sofa, greeted me with a charming smile and asked me to sit next to her. There was no sign of Advocaat bottles anywhere.

'Dr Landau, how nice to see you,' she murmured, taking me by the hand. 'Now do please have a little of this.' She reached under the sofa as before and pulled out a bottle of dark red liquid. Two glasses followed, a sherry size for me and the tumbler for her. She poured out the Buckfast Tonic Wine.

'Not drinking Advocaat, I see,' I said, toasting her.

'Oh dear me no, not since that nice Dr Taylor was here the other week. He gave me a thorough examination and said that I was short of protein, vitamins, roughage and heaven knows what else in my diet. He made me have steak and fish every day. Vitamin pills, too. I feel marvellous. I might even consider getting married again.' She gave me a roguish wink. 'Yes, Dr Taylor said that having the Advocaat and not much else to eat was giving me these dizzy spells and cracked lips. Anyway, I mustn't go on about me. You've come to see Thoth, haven't you, Dr Landau?'

Though still grossly mis-shapen, Thoth was indeed a different monkey. He was using his legs, walking and even running for short distances. He looked happier and more energetic. His pugilist's face had softened, the lumpy bones were not as prominent. The progressive collapse of his skeleton had been halted, though he would be scarred for life. It was a dramatic change that I had seen many times before in such cases. Now, with the jaws firmer and less likely to shatter as I pulled with my tooth forceps, I could begin sorting out the jumble of teeth in his mouth. Thoth was going to need at least three sessions of dental surgery under general anaesthetic.

'Isn't it absolutely wonderful, Doctor? said Mrs Crabbe. 'A miracle in three weeks. I'd never have believed it. But what about the toothache?'

I explained the next stages of treatment, gave the monkey another ampoule of Sterogyl and inquired how well Thoth had taken to his proper, teetotal diet.

'Have a close look at the billiard table, Dr Aspinall,' commanded Mrs Crabbe.

I looked. The six net pockets had been lined with pieces of newspaper. One had been filled with chopped hard-boiled egg, another with peanuts, a third with dates and raisins and so on. Each pocket contained some item of suitable food. One was even brimming with shiny, writhing mealworms, a fine Capuchin delicacy. A crystal bowl of milk stood on the pink spot and a matching piece containing vitaminised water was on the yellow spot.

'First-rate,' I said.

'Now before you go, Dr Taylor,' beamed Mrs Crabbe, 'just have a little drop more of this most wholesome wine and tell me what you think about this rheumatic joint of mine.'

She began unbuttoning her dress before I could say a word.

The balanced diet and the Sterogyl continued to transform Thoth. Under anaesthetic I extracted all the rogue teeth and left him with a small but adequate set. At last the time came for my final visit. Thoth now had his outside run built onto the billiard room. As far as I could see he was on the wagon, and seemed to relish his mixed diet and his new-found ability to exercise with gusto. He did not drool, showed no sign of pain in his mouth and was altogether more amiable. He had not drawn another drop of human blood and did not seem to

498

care how you looked at him. Apart from his physical improvement, I assumed that his mind was enjoying a certain clarity of thought after ten years of toping; Thoth the easily offended had probably been the equivalent of the bellicose bar-fly.

Mrs Crabbe, on the other hand, had quickly dispensed with Dr Aspinall's diet and was subsisting on voluminous quantities of the tonic wine which, as she said, had the added spiritual dimension to its nutritive qualities of 'having the church behind it'. Naturally her dizzy spells had re-appeared.

'Thank you for everything, dear Dr Aspinall,' she said thickly when I told her that Thoth, though hardly a show specimen, should get along fine if she stuck to the diet. 'Now before you go, there's something I want you to have. Follow me.'

I followed her uncertain path through the corridors of the old house, up a wide staircase of orange marble where our steps raised puffs of dust and sent balls of fluff rolling like tumbleweed, and through rooms smelling like mushroom farms. Eventually we came to a small boxroom that was empty save for an enormous, rust-encrusted safe.

Rocking slightly on her heels, Mrs Crabbe brought forth a large key from her décolletage and with much difficulty found the keyhole.

'Now, Dr Landau,' she puffed. 'Please turn the handle for me and pull open the door.'

I twisted the heavy brass lever and heaved against the protesting stiffness of the old hinges. The door gradually yielded and came open.

Mrs Crabbe stepped forward and started sorting through a heap of trays and boxes. It was a stupendous sight: dull gold rings by the score; old-fashioned pendants and earrings heavy with succulent emeralds and rubies as big as damsons; dusty tiaras which burst into diamond flame as the old lady blew winey breath over them; the baubles of Freemasonry, the tie-pins, signet rings, seals, swizzle-sticks, cuff-links, loving cups, heirlooms of the Crabbes; silver presentation salvers from the mills; gold fobs from Victorian Crabbes; sapphire souvenirs from Edwardian cruises long forgotten.

'In here I have something specially for you, my dear Doctor,' she whispered as she rooted about.

It was as exciting as Christmas morning. What was she going to bestow on me? Some nugget, some pea-sized diamond of the first water that had belonged to old Crabbe? I could not see anything that was not worthy a tidy sum. How very unprofessional, a little voice chivvied inside me. How bloody marvellous, breathed another.

At last Mrs Crabbe appeared to have found what she was looking for. She withdrew a lumpy, brown paper bag, about the size of two clenched fists. 'There,' she said, giving me the bag, 'and thank you so much, Dr Landau. Please also thank your assistant, Dr Taylor.'

We retraced our steps with me clutching my present and my mind whirling. The bag weighed about one pound, I guessed, but its lumpy shape mystified me. Precious stones, gold dust, an assortment of jewellery, watches? I could hardly wait to get outside to my car and look inside. Anyway, I thought, as I shook hands at the door (tradesmen's entrance), from what I've seen of the safe's treasures, whatever it is it's bound to be fabulous.

Jumping into the car, I opened the bag and looked inside. Beneath a scrap of paper, on which was scribbled in pencil 'To Doctor Aspinall, the best vet in the world, with grateful thanks from Thoth', lay seven or eight plump, fresh tomatoes, undoubtedly not long picked from the greenhouses behind the big black stone house.

'Where did you get these from?' asked Shelagh, as she sliced the tomatoes that evening and mixed them with slivers of raw mushrooms and onion to make my favourite salad.

'Well, love, in a nutshell,' I explained, 'from treating the monkey of an old lady who thinks I do wonders for her rheumatism and whose doctor is a dab hand at . . . oh, forget it—it's so confusing that I'm not quite sure who I am anyway.'

My wife gave me a curious look and kept on slicing. Stephanie and Lindsey, drawing at the kitchen table, looked at each other then raised their eyes to the heavens at this further evidence of the mysterious behaviour of grown-ups.

Dotty and befuddled Mrs Crabbe may have been, but she justified the townsfolk's opinion of her canny attention to all matters financial. Months later, when my bill was settled, she faithfully deducted exactly fifteen shillings and sixpence.

In those early months of 1970, I was happy to realise that my practice was becoming busier and busier. I had been on my own now for eighteen months, and it seemed that the venture might have turned the corner. Cuddles, the killer whale at Flamingo Park, occupied a good deal of my time and attention, of course: like any infant, he had teething pain as more of his ivory fangs came through his gums, but I soothed his mouth with vast quantities of babies' teething jelly held on by water-resistant denture paste. That winter was becoming quite eventful elsewhere, too, which was why I came to be sitting on a Derbyshire hillside one freezing afternoon, cradling my dart-rifle.

Whereas America has its Big-foot and the Himalayas their Yeti, not forgetting Scotland's own *Nessiteras rhombopteryx* as Sir Peter Scott so precipitately named her, the English have to make do with the more mundane monsters which are reported every six months or so in the newspapers and are usually identified as pumas or, less frequently, lions. Regularly these large felines are spotted by ostensibly sober members of the community in the suburbs of Birmingham or on the village green at Wormwood Magna. 'I was hoeing the radishes one evening when this mountain lion walked out of the privet hedge and jumped over the fence into next door's garden,' affirms a worthy citizen, or 'I glanced out of the loo window of the bingo hall and there was this puma mooching round the dustbins.' Occasionally in mud or snow, Foot-prints are Found, which the 'local naturalist' pronounces as those of no animal known to science. The constabulary wearily assure the townsfolk that they are checking all zoos and circuses in the vicinity just in case no-one noticed that one of the big cats had not shown up at roll call. The story hangs around in the papers for up to a week and then, no doubt tiring of the humdrum series of brief encounters with postmen, gardeners, schoolboys and late-night strollers, the beast clears off and lies low for a few months, to re-appear as sure as fate miles away.

I often marvel at the certainty with which folk whose knowledge of the jungle is limited to admiring the Town Hall palms will cry wolf (or tiger, or puma) when a twitching brown tail is spied vanishing into a thicket three hundred yards away. Sadly, lions no longer roam wild in England, bears and wolves became extinct more recently and, unlike the Scots, we cannot boast even one wild cat in our forests. The mystery pumas are almost invariably big dogs enhanced by the unreliability of the human eye, a fertile imagination, alcohol or fabrication.

The 'puma' which surfaced that January in Derbyshire, fifty miles south of Rochdale, was bothering the inhabitants of a little town set on a hillside criss-crossed with limestone walls. The beast had been seen by the schoolmaster, several farmers and various other people. It was exactly three feet to eight feet long, a minimum of four feet to six feet high at the shoulder and was variously black, dark brown, gingery and light yellow. It was known to have a long tail or none at all, showed no signs of timidity or shot off at the slightest sound, and ate remarkable quantities of other people's chickens, cats, pet rabbits, dustbin waste and garden-pond goldfish. I was asked to go over with a dart-rifle and join in a concerted hunt by police, RSPCA men, journalists and small boys.

Apart from the cold, the weather was good for puma

502

hunting. I was being paid well for a leisurely stroll over fine countryside, and was confident that I would end up by tea-time, when the exercise was due to end, feeling as fit as a fiddle and without having seen anything more wild than a hare. There are wild wallabies living and breeding success-fully in the Derbyshire heather; they are rarely spotted but I reckoned that the 'puma', if it existed at all, was probably one of them.

The local village constable organised the sweep of the countryside very efficiently. He had plotted the most recent sightings on a map and when I arrived was distributing walkie-talkies, maps and thermos flasks of tea. He lined us up and announced the Orders of the Day as if he was sending us in after Bonnie and Clyde. Off we set, and I soon found myself alone on the hillside, pushing through beds of drip-ping bracken with the wind making my cheeks tingle. When I was almost at the top of the main ridge and could look down at the streets of glistening grey slate roofs, I was told over the walkie-talkie to find a sheltered spot by one of the moorland walls and wait. The constable had deployed his posse in a circle enclosing hundreds of acres. I was the centre point of that circle and the order to beat inwards would now be given.

Squatting on a dry stone out of the wind, I passed the time outstaring the curious sheep that had gathered to inspect me. The object of our game was to see who blinked first. I could not see any of the other searchers although I could hear the constable chivvying his right flank, his left flank and his centre with the authority of Rommel making a dash for Tobruk. There was no doubt, I thought, that before long the complete bunch of hunters would find themselves on top of me, puma-less.

The sheep got bored with me and resumed grazing. Suddenly I heard my name called urgently over the walkie-talkie. I took in the astounding message that came crackling over the air in the excited voice of the village constable: 'Dr

Taylor, Dr Taylor, hold your position. Animal sighted coming in your direction.'

I looked hurriedly around and pressed in against the dry-stone wall. My heart began to beat rapidly with excitement. The beast existed and was on its way! I still could not see any of the men and there was no sign of the monster. I carefully checked that the safety catch on the dart-gun was securely in the 'off' position. When the man-eating minotaur or whatever it was breathed fire down my earhole I did not want a repetition of what had happened once when I was called to recapture an escaped axis deer in Sussex. After hours of painstaking stalking, its keepers had driven it so that it stood, a perfect target, only a few feet away from a special camouflaged hide in which I lurked, peering out through a tiny hole. I had aimed, pulled the trigger of the dart-gun and heard that depressing 'clunk' which means that the safety catch is on. Like lightning the deer had leapt off, startled by the 'clunk' and far too rapidly to let me put my mistake right by flicking the dratted catch. No axis deer had been retrieved that embarrassing day.

Now I was certain my gun was in fighting condition. There was a new compressed-air cylinder in the chamber, a syringe loaded with enough phencyclidine to clobber a grizzly bear was up the spout and the safety catch was most definitely off.

The walkie-talkie crackled again. 'Dr Taylor, Dr Taylor, keep down, keep down. Animal seen still coming your way, approximately quarter of a mile from you. Other side of your wall. Running at present time parallel to wall.'

If they had been able to identify the creature, no-one had bothered to tell me. I decided not to talk back in case it was frightened off. At this point, quite honestly, I felt a trifle apprehensive. I had tangled with big cats many times in zoos and in Africa, but under controlled conditions. Still, I thought, the poor whatever-it-was was probably scared to death. Escaped zoo big cats never enjoy life on the run and appear positively relieved once they are back in their own territory, among sights and sounds they know, with warm beds and regular meals.

The difficulty I faced now was knowing when to stand up and look over the wall. Too soon or too late could obviously be disastrous. The wall was too well built to have any chinks in it. The trusty constable solved the problem almost at once. 'Dr Taylor, Dr Taylor, animal now one hundred yards approximately to your left. Still running parallel to wall.'

He said nothing about speed or range from the wall. My mind raced. I would have only a few seconds in which to stand up, aim and fire after taking into account the wind, which might deflect the bulky dart, and the low temperature, which affected the gas pressure and consequently the maximum range of my weapon. Whatever it was, I would aim for the middle of the target. That would give me some latitude for error. I had fitted my shortest barbed needle, so that no matter what the creature or virtually where I hit it, there was the smallest risk of the needle entering a major body cavity. I would swing the gun round with the movement of the animal, assuming it was still running. I do not like using the dart-gun on moving targets, but that way I might have least risk of a bounce-off.

The nettle must be grasped at once. I stood up and rammed my rifle over the wall. Twenty feet away, slightly to my left and going at a steady pace, loped a tawny creature which at first sight looked dramatically like the Hound of the Baskervilles.

The beast that had been blamed in the locality for every sort of misdeed, with the possible exception of the spate of obscene phone calls that was also occupying the constable's busy life, was a long lanky Great Dane. Looking closer, I saw it was in terrible shape. Scurfy skin was stretched tight over its prominent skeleton, its sides were disfigured with numerous red scars and L-shaped wounds where wire and thorns had left their marks, the eyes were sunk and desperate and ropes of glutinous saliva speckled with soil hung from the slack lips. It was an animal that must have been out on the run for weeks if not months, and it was easy to see from the slight sway of its hindquarters that it was coming to the end of the road.

All the same, my sudden emergence like a jack-in-the-box produced a surge of alarm and determination in the dog. Its eyes bulged with the effort as it strained for more speed and veered away from me. I looked down the gun barrel, made my split-second assessment of wind and likely trajectory and fired. The dart flew strong and straight—straight over the back of the Great Dane. It thwacked impotently into a tussock fifteen yards away, the dog vanished over a rise in the ground and I shouted unrepeatable epithets at the re-gathering sheep. You never get a second chance in such cases.

It was a very subdued marksman who shortly afterwards explained to the constable and his troops what had happened. They took it very politely and we started another, rather half-hearted hunt. By late afternoon there had not even been another sighting of the dog and we were about to call it a day when an amazing piece of good news came up from the town: the Great Dane had dashed into a timber yard and someone had had the good sense to close the yard gates. It was holed up behind a pile of wood and was in a mean mood.

Somewhat cheered by this turn of events, I went down to the yard with the constable and some of his men. Distressed and terrified, the animal crouched behind a pile of wood, obviously prepared to go down fighting. It was snarling and snapping in earnest, and no-one dared go near it. There was no way I could find to get a shot at the dog other than from directly in front, but with the way it was barking and moving its head, and with its emaciated frame presenting no expanses of muscle from that angle, I was afraid that the dart might hit the head. Even hungry animals like this one are not always easy to knock out by drugging meat, but I sent a boy to the nearest butcher's shop for a pound of pork sausages. When he came back with them I threw a couple to the dog, which swallowed them ravenously. Next I took a third sausage and carefully pressed it in the middle. The meat within the sausage skin compacted towards each end, leaving an inch of empty skin in the middle. Now, with a fine hypodermic needle passed through the sausage meat and into the empty space, I slowly injected a quantity of powerful narcotic. The sausage was now fixed and ready, with no smell and no taste. I tossed the Trojan Horse morsel to the wild-eyed dog. One gulp and it was gone. In eight minutes the poor creature was sound asleep and I could approach him to make a thorough examination which confirmed my earlier opinion. He must have been straying for a very long time and was suffering from malnutrition, multiple wounds, a grass awn embedded in the cornea of one eye and a tumour on the breast.

The owner was never traced but the story ended happily. Now no longer equipped with an operating room for domestic animals, I arranged with a colleague to hospitalise the wanderer, operate on his eye, remove the breast growth and generally tack him together. A good home was found for him by the RSPCA, and when I saw him a month later he had become plump, glossy and relaxed on an intensive diet of steak, eggs, fish and milk—but no more sausages. And the would-be 'puma' nearly licked my hand off.

Eight

The family sat at breakfast. I had just taken the first call of the day and it had produced an instant cloud over the grilled kippers and marmalade toast. 'Doesn't Daddy look grumpy all of a sudden?' piped Stephanie as I pushed away my plate.

'Grumpy as Rump . . . Rumpul . . . Rump . . .' Lindsey agreed, fumbling for the word.

'Rumpelstiltskin.' Stephanie's dark eyes bored into me as she leaned over and reached up to pat my head. 'What's up, Doc?' The girls chuckled happily.

Shelagh knew instinctively what was likely to have made my face so bleak. She frowned at the children and shook her head. 'What was it, love?' she asked quietly. 'Giraffe trouble?'

I nodded as I put on my coat and picked up the instrument bag from the cloakroom. 'Yes,' I said, 'at Flamingo Park. A young giraffe's been beaten up by an ostrich. It might be a broken leg.'

Shelagh knew what that meant. I raised my eyebrows and tried a smile. It felt an effort.

Giraffe surgery was really beginning to prey on my mind. Since the death of Pedro, I had noticed the quickening of my pulse when the phone rang and a voice brought tidings of sickness or accident in some member of this particular species. If the complaint seemed to be essentially a medical one—upset bowels after a Bank Holiday's over-indulgence in visitors' titbits, or skin disease—my heart rate returned quickly to normal and the knot in my stomach would melt away. It was the surgical side of this beast, the prospect of

508

having to knock out any more of these jinxes that was, I realised, making me lose my nerve. Sometimes I would wake in the small hours when nightmares crowd in the coiling dark, and sweat over the difficulties of struggling to be a giraffe-doctor. An animal half camel, half leopard? It almost seemed true—such freaks of nature could hardly be other than doom-laden.

I had seen the results of a furious attack by red-neck ostriches on zebras and giraffes before. Flailing their powerful legs, beaks agape and stubby wings jutting out like ragged flags, they had snapped limbs, broken skulls and staved in chests. This time the curator had talked of a six-month-old giraffe with a hind leg that dangled and would not bear weight. Dear God, let it be severe muscle bruising! If it was a femur broken, there was just a simple choice—surgery or death. I would not contemplate euthanasing the animal, so then there would be no choice. Please let it be bruising and crushing of muscles. I had some marvellous drugs in my bag for such conditions: cortisone, Novalgin, trypsin. They were all first-class, and could be administered without anaesthetic. By the time I turned into the gates of the park I had quite convinced myself that I was going to face a simple case of severe bruising.

One glance at the giraffe with its swinging hind leg quickly put me straight. I felt slightly sea-sick as I stood and watched the calf, a male, lurch gracefully on three legs. The femur—the thigh-bone—was broken, although the blow from the ostrich's horny foot had not left so much as a scratch on the skin surface.

Frank, the curator, was impatient for my decision. He had hand-reared the youngster himself when its mother had refused to stand for her offspring to suckle. 'What about it, then, Doctor?' he asked. 'Plaster of Paris?'

I shook my head slowly. 'No chance. If the break had been lower down the leg, maybe. That or fibreglass. But with high fractures in the femur there's too much ham muscle round the site. The plaster can't hold the bone pieces firmly.'

'What then?' Frank sounded a fraction aggressive. He would not have agreed to euthanasia even if I had suggested it.

I took a deep breath; it seemed to ease the queasiness in my guts. 'I'll have to pin the leg with a vitallium spike. Maybe screw a plate on as well. I can't say more for sure till I open up the leg to look.'

Frank's tense body sagged in relief. He managed a tight smile. 'Great, Doctor.'

While Frank and his keepers prepared ropes, straw, water and all the other things necessary for surgery al fresco (it was a warm sunny day and I prefer to operate outside in the cleaner air whenever possible), I turned my attention to the old bugbear of anaesthetic. Should I pre-medicate with valium instead of acepromazine to avoid the blood pressure effects which had killed poor Pedro? Then what? A touch of xylazine as a tranquilliser with a final knock-out shot of etorphine, or etorphine alone? There was no chance of using tubocurarine or succinylcholine to relax the muscles completely; either would be too risky without gas and giraffes are terribly difficult to put onto a closed-circuit gas machine. I pondered. If the broken ends of bone had overlapped I would have to use brute force to re-position them. I settled for the valium, xylazine and etorphine cocktail.

When all was ready the giraffe, calm as a child's pony, was coaxed into a narrow, high-sided box. Before starting, I listened to its heart through my stethoscope. It was bounding but I could not detect any abnormalities. The animal accepted slivers of apple from Frank while I began the injections into its neck muscles. I worked like a zombie. There was just me and the giraffe and the box in the whole universe. I could hear nothing but the breathing of the animal, the tap of its hooves from time to time against the woodwork, the dull rush of blood in the centre of my head. I could see nothing but the long camouflaged neck and the

510

dark rivulet of blood that lay on the skin like a twist of thread where my needle had been.

After the valium the calf soon became droopy with half-closed eyes. The xylazine settled it down gently onto its knees in the straw. I still felt queasy, but the giraffe showed no sign of the fainting that had finished Pedro. Now to bring oblivion down onto the gentle creature and to begin the surgical equivalent of the furniture repairer's craft. The door of the box was lifted and I squeezed inside. The giraffe's colour was good. It was drooling saliva, I noticed, but there was no sign of the dangerous regurgitation of stomach contents that can sometimes drown an unconscious animal. I felt the pulse. It was reasonably regular and the volume was good. Quickly I injected a small dose of etorphine into the neck. Once flat out, the giraffe would be hauled out of the box by Frank's keepers and I could work in the open.

Again I put my stethoscope to the rib-cage. 'Lub-dup, lub-dup, lub-dup.' All sounded well. 'Lup-dup, lub-dup, lub-lub-dup.'

My hand clenched over the diaphragm head of the stetho-scope. What was that again?

'Lub-dup, lub-lub-dup,' then 'Lub-lub-lub-lub-dup.' Pause. 'Lub-lub-dup.' I instantly began to pour out tacky sweat. One hand still on the stethoscope, I groped with the other beneath the animal's groin to take the pulse in the femoral artery. It was hard to find. The sound coming through my ivory ear-pieces seemed softer now. I pushed the diaphragm hard onto the animal's chest and checked its position over the heart. 'Lub-dup, lub-dup, lub-lub-lub-dup.' Pause. 'Lub-lub-lub-lub-dup.' Long pause. 'Lub-lub . . .'

Wildly I looked at the breathing. It was barely detectable. I took a deep breath, fought down the panic. 'My bag—quick,' I hissed to the curator who crouched behind me. 'He's collapsing.'

The words echoed round my head. All else was silence.

The keepers were hushed. It took me a few seconds to load a syringe with theophylline, a circulation booster, and another with cyprenorphine, the antidote to the etorphine. Thank God giraffes have jugulars like drainpipes, I thought, as the drugs shot into the bloodstream. Then I thought, why did I ever dabble in giraffes and such? The old times at the Rochdale surgery with a bitch for hysterectomy on the table—predictable, my assistant to help, my partner coming in to have a chat whilst we stitched up—oh, the fond remembrance of times past. 'Lub-dup, lub-lub . . . lub . . . lub . . . lu-u-b . . .'

I could not believe it. There was no more sound, at least no more heart sound. Just the distant squeak of the bowels, contracting after life had slipped away.

'I'm afraid he's dead,' I said bluntly. 'And I haven't got a bloody clue why.'

It would be nice in some ways to be able to run away from such disasters, to jump in the car and get the hell out of it, shake the dust off one's feet, have a whisky and talk tough about 'c'est la vie', 'you win some and you lose some', and 'when they gotta go, they gotta go'. But it can't be done. The indefinable sense of guilt must be expiated in the rites: the explaining, the analysing, the agonising, the excusing, first in public to the keepers, curators and directors then, more importantly, to oneself in bed at night. An autopsy forms part of the ritual and sometimes yields valuable information that might save future lives. I decided to do an immediate post-mortem on the young giraffe. The scalpel revealed white, dry areas of tissue scattered throughout many of the muscles of the body and most significantly in the thick muscular wall of the heart. It was quite unmistakable, but the first time I had come across it in a giraffe: 'white muscle disease', which I had often seen in calves and even wallabies and pelicans. The diseased heart had simply failed when the added stress of anaesthesia had been loaded onto it.

512

It was little consolation for Frank as I explained the cause and gave my opinion that the animal's days had been numbered anyway. 'Irreversible change caused by a deficiency of a chemical called selenium in the fodder and herbage,' I said. 'I'll take some samples of soil and hay for analysis.'

So it turned out: there were barely two parts in ten million of selenium in the soil and even less in the fodder. Selenium is a rare element, named after the Greek word for 'moon' and of little interest to anyone except the occasional scientist. It is a by-product of copper refining, is used in the manufacture of photo-electric cells and is invariably ignored completely by schoolboys swotting for chemistry examinations. Selenium means as little to them as it does to, say, chimpanzees or giraffes. The difference is that to giraffes the presence or absence of the invisible element in the soil and herbage of their environment can be literally a matter of life or death. A mere five parts in ten million of the strange 'moonstone' would have been enough and perhaps there would be a giraffe walking around Flamingo Park today with a shiny pin in his mended leg.

That evening Shelagh listened as I fumed over this latest giraffe débâcle. The girls kept tactfully out of the way while I cursed the day I had ever decided to specialise in exotic animals.

'Not only do I feel I'm wasting my time, but I'm beginning to think that I'm a positive menace where giraffes are concerned. Cats and dogs, pigs and ponies—that's where I should be. They're more my measure. Bring back the budgies and the moggies.' My bitterness was without humour and almost the real thing.

'Do you really mean that?' Shelagh asked quietly after a moment's silence. She smiled gently and fixed me with unblinking green eyes.

'Er, no,' I said. 'No.' I tried in vain to adopt the air of a martyr.

'I'll get you a cup of tea while you work out a dose for supplementing the other giraffes with selenium,' said Shelagh, rising to her feet.

There was trouble back at Belle Vue that winter, too. It came not from the giraffes but from homo sapiens: Belle Vue's director, Ray Legge, was up to his neck with complaints from bothered visitors. The female chimpanzees were a perennial source of trouble, as they are at many zoos. When these animals are mature and come into season, the skin round the vulva becomes remarkably red and swollen. Biologically this phenomenon is a visual sexual signal to what must be rather slow-witted males, but you can be sure that it also triggers off a response from some animal-lover who visits the great ape house and decides to tackle the authorities about the matter.

On this occasion a worthy middle-aged lady teacher—of biology!—had stormed into the director's office demanding to know why something was not being done about the chimpanzee with the prolapse. The animal must have been in terrible pain, she declared in high dudgeon, and she as a woman as well as a teacher knew about such things. What was more, she was not leaving the office until the veterinarian appeared and did something. She then grabbed the office phone to put a call through to the RSPCA and was about to do likewise to the police, press and BBC until physically restrained from doing do by the director's secretary. A conversation was eventually arranged with me by telephone. It got rid of the good lady, but despite my lengthy explanations as to the nature of the swellings I got the impression that I had not calmed her down much.

'I cannot believe,' she said huffily at the end of our conversation, 'that so alarming, so . . . so . . . blatant a display could be part of the Creator's design. I warn you I shall take the matter up with my gynaecologist, Doctor.'

Well, I thought, even the Creator himself would have

514

difficulty persuading such folk that chimpanzees and their ways were made for chimpanzees, not for lady teachers and their gynaecologists.

Hot on the heels of that little fracas came a similar incident involving a camel that had calved happily enough and immediately after the birth could be seen in the paddock with the placenta still hanging from its behind. That really stirred up one old lady, who complained that it was utterly disgusting that children might witness such scenes of gory intimacy. I am afraid I give such people short shrift—no doubt they mean well, and I entirely accept that the visiting public has a duty to ensure that zoos maintain a good standard in the care of their animals, but I do not believe that animals mating, giving or having just given birth should necessarily be kept off exhibition. If seclusion would be good for the mother or baby, fine, but otherwise I am strongly for folk being able to watch such miraculous goings-on. The true appreciation of living things must involve real life in all its facets. It is rarely ugly, except where homo sapiens is involved; indeed it is generally beautiful and always edifying. Zoos particularly have a lot to gain by presenting animals as they really are, warts and all. Thank God animals are not intricate toys made of icing sugar or ormulu. Elephants smell, camels burp, predators kill, scavengers rake muck. The blood, the guts, the excrement, the new life and the old death all knit together into a flawless, balanced unity.

More trouble came when a Belle Vue keeper let an animal which should not have been on display out into its paddock and could not get it back again. It did no harm to the creature, in fact the fresh air and sunshine did it all the good in the world. The trouble, once again, was with the paying public. This time the outraged visitor went straight to the nearest telephone kiosk and rang the police. Before long the police called Ray Legge, the zoo director.

'We've had a complaint from a visitor to your zoo,' said

the constable. 'Sounds bloody horrific if it's true. They say you've got a young lion with shirt buttons stitched all over his ears. Is this right?'

'Yes, it is,' replied Ray.

'And could you explain what a lion is doing decorated with pearl buttons, sir? Have the vandals been at it again?'

Ray roared with laughter, as I did when he told me later. Both of us tried to imagine a couple of typical louts, the sort that cause such annoying trouble at city zoos all over the world, climbing over the wall one night after an energetic pub crawl. Full of Dutch courage and bravado, one suggests to the other that they indulge in a merry prank. Whereas normally this involves harassing, chasing or simply killing any animal they can find, preferably one of the gentler species such as wallabies or penguins, this time they decide to try something more spicy.

' 'Ere, Bert,' says one. 'Wot abaht givin' that lion over there a bit of the old 'ow's yer father?'

'Wotcha mean, 'Arry?' says the other.

'Well, you grab 'old of 'im, see, an' then I'll stitch some o' me shirt buttons on 'is lug'ole.'

'No sooner said than done, me old son,' says Bert, catching the snoozing lion by the tail and holding its jaws closed with finger and thumb.

Harry meanwhile snaps the pearl buttons off his beer-stained shirt front. Producing in a trice the needle and thread that Saturday night revellers always have to hand, he proceeds to attach the buttons deftly to the astonished lion's ear flap. Harry and Bert then stagger off home, leaving the button-bedecked lion to resume his rudely disturbed slumbers.

Happily, this dramatic fantasy of drunken prowess was not quite the explanation of why the lion was indeed sporting a number of ordinary pearly buttons stitched to one ear as he yawned in the pale winter twilight. Jambo, the lion in question, had been playing with his companions and the fun

516

had involved rolling, tumbling and cuffing one another, claws retracted, about the head. One over-boisterous right hook had burst a blood vessel beneath the skin of Jambo's ear, and within minutes a giant blood-blister had developed, puffing out the curved leaf of the ear into something more like an outsize piece of ravioli. It was the first stage of the process which in humans leads to the formation of a 'cauliflower ear': left alone the blood would clot, the clot would gradually be converted into scar tissue and shrink, and the ear would be crumpled up like a ball of waste paper. It was not painful or dangerous, but I had to do something about it for the sake of Jambo's looks, if only to keep the little old ladies at bay.

With Jambo dreaming happily under phencyclidine anaesthesia, topped up with drops of barbiturate from time to time, I made an S-shaped incision in the ear flap and removed all the clot lying between the skin and the central plate of cartilage. To avoid the ear simply filling up once more with blood, I needed to pin the skin down to the cartilage long enough for adhesions to fill any space where blood might accumulate. I therefore put in stitches all over the surface of the ear, but to avoid the risk of cutting and to distribute pressure efficiently, I incorporated a flat, sterilised button, supplied by Shelagh from her sewing box, with each stitch. It worked perfectly: Jambo's ear would be uncrumpled and as good as new when I removed the buttons and stitches after ten days. Meanwhile I had suggested that he be kept in the big cat house to avoid the incredulous stares of the public and possible re-matches with his playful mates. My prediction about the visitors' reaction was proved right when a keeper lifted Jambo's slide door by mistake.

Of course, the matter ended with Ray Legge explaining all this to the police, but I suggested that in future the enclosures or houses of any animals under treatment and on show should carry notices explaining the position. I believe it is

517

good that the public should be able to see that most zoo inmates receive medical care at least as good as that given to pet poodles and racehorses.

As for Jambo, who soon regained a matching set of respectable lion lugs, he would have been amazed at all the fuss.

I had a chance to get away from such bothersome incidents for a few days when February came round. The Association of Marine Mammal Veterinarians, of which I was a founder member, was holding its annual symposium in Miami. Off I went for the anticipated binge of scientific shop-talk and gossip from the close world of dolphin doctors. One of the snags of living in a cotton town in north-west England was always that there was no-one within hundreds of miles with whom I could indulge in an occasional talk-fest on exotic beasts of the oceans. The symposiums were, and still are, a chance to wallow with others who shared a passion for walruses and whales and a deep curiosity as to what makes them tick.

If California, with its Sea World, Marineland of the Pacific and US Navy research units, is the Mecca of cetacean buffs, then Florida, home of Seaquarium and the major catching grounds for dolphins, is the Medina—and it is now only a hop away from London by non-stop jet. All the same, I was delayed checking in to the symposium by bad weather over the Atlantic. Lightning struck the 707 with a fearful bang, sending a blue ball of light straight down the centre aisle, and the plane had to land at Nassau for inspection. I felt like a limp lettuce when eventually I set thankful feet on US soil. I knew that by arriving late I would find that the best hotel rooms at the conference centre had already been allocated, that the restricted list of delegates wishing to visit some particularly interesting laboratory had been closed and that copies of papers to be given had been snaffled by folk who wanted multiple sets. As I walked into the hotel lobby, my only thought was for a large Jack Daniels to restore my confidence in aeroplanes.

Someone touched my arm. 'Dr Taylor, you're here at last.'

I turned round. It was the lobster-sampling student again, Andrew Greenwood.

'What on earth are you doing here?' I asked, astounded. Students are chronically impecunious by tradition, and Cambridge to Florida and back by air ain't potatoes.

'I leaned on my father,' he replied cheerfully. 'It seemed too important a programme to miss.'

I marvelled at this further evidence of the chap's tenacity.

He went on, 'I've organised everything for you—got you a super room overloooking the sea, collected a full set of papers plus some new microfilms that were in short supply, put your name down for the trip to the shark research place and made sure you're one of only six delegates invited to join a dive on a new sea-lab mini-sub.'

I was speechless. Not only did this young man pop out of the woodwork with surprising regularity, but he was beginning to act like a first-class, unpaid personal private secretary!

'How very kind of you,' I said faintly.

He beamed happily and picked up my bag. 'Oh, by the way, Dr Taylor, when you've had a shower, I've got a large bourbon and dry ginger waiting for you in the lounge.'

That conference went like clockwork. My batman, advisor, aide-de-camp and new-found apprentice did everything except fan me with a palm frond when the lecture hall got stuffy. Andrew and I became firm friends and I grew increasingly aware of his powerful intellectual approach to the wide world of animal medicine.

Back from Florida, I found a message waiting. It was my jinx again—giraffes. A fine female at Rio Leon Safari Park in Spain had suddenly dropped dead and I was wanted to fly out to do a post-mortem examination. I was beginning to get a complex about giraffes, although this one had at least had the grace to give up the ghost without me being anywhere within a thousand miles.

Rio Leon is delightfully set in a valley by the sea about fifty miles west of Barcelona. Its slopes were terraced centuries ago and are covered with olive, cherry and almond trees. On the ridge tops above the valley the wind murmurs unceasingly through conifer groves where occasional escaped baboons can be glimpsed, sleek and rounded as they gather cones and berries. On the valley floor, zebras, elands, elephants, rare lechwe antelopes and ostriches mingle amicably on sandy flats. The little village of Albiñana nearby has barely changed in nine centuries. It has narrow streets of earth and boulders, Roman wells in overgrown orangeries, and old ladies in black who serve you peppery snails and succulent roast hare and press olive oil as thick as treacle. The village grows juicy, pale green clumps of garlic that are the most heavenly and unsociable in the whole of Spain. Visits to the park are delights, marred by the fact that my purpose is always one concerned with disease or death.

The autopsy on the giraffe was quite straightforward. The cause of death was almost identical to that in the case of the Flamingo Park giraffe: heart attack brought on by a deficiency of selenium in the soil and vegetation. I ordered the immediate addition of tiny percentages of selenium to the food of all the creatures in the safari park.

The director, my good friend Rolf Rohwer, was now faced with the problem of replacing the female giraffe. There was one available, a young beauty, so they said, but it was some four hundred miles away at a safari park which was closing down west of Madrid.

'I want you to come and look at it with me,' said Rolf. 'If you give it a clean bill of health, we'll bring it back together with a couple of African elephants they're selling as well. I suppose you'll want to tranquillise the giraffe for loading.'

I bit my tongue, thinking of Pedro and of Flamingo Park, but said nothing.

Next day we set off for the park that had the animals for sale, about forty miles from Madrid. It was set in a sleepy, unremarkable region of peasant farms and silent forests, and was approached by a narrow road that seemed to wind forever through the hills. It was not difficult to imagine why it was folding up: it was way off the tourist beat and could not have been easy for day-tripping Madrilenos to find. Rolf and I found a handful of peasants looking after the stock that remained in the crumbling clusters of buildings and fenced reserves where wind and weeds were waging a war of attrition on the entrepreneur's faded dreams.

The visit began badly. On hearing I was el veterinario inglés, the caretakers asked us to look at a fox they had locked up in a wooden box, an adolescent with all the signs of canine distemper. Looking into the box through a grille in the lid, I gave that as my diagnosis and offered to leave them some drugs and hypodermics. It is always inexcusably slipshod to make glib, split-second diagnoses, for when one of the men lifted the box lid and brought out the fox by the scruff of its neck, I saw to my horror that the sad-faced animal he held aloft had only three and a half legs. The fox had lost part of a fore leg in a gin-trap, and the fly-covered stump was a mess.

'Que pena terrible!' I said. 'I am sorry, Señores, there is nothing to be done. I will kill the animal painlessly. I have an injection in my bag.'

I was turning to go to the car when the man holding the fox shook his head and walked, still carrying it, towards a low, lean-to shed. His companions gathered round. A piece of cord was produced from somewhere. Incredulously, I watched as one of the Spaniards fashioned a noose in the cord and slipped it over the fox's mask. Transfixed with thunderous anger, the blood leaving my face icy cold as it drained rapidly away, I saw the other end of the length of cord thrown over a beam. They were going to hang the suffering beast!

With real effort, for all my powers seemed to have been turned to frozen clay, I managed to force out the biggest shout I have ever shouted. 'Stop at once, you!' I screamed, with plenty of volume but weak content: in my anger I forgot even the simplest words of Spanish.

The men ignored me and strung the fox up. I found I could still not move my legs.

'Rolf!' I shouted. 'Tell the bastards to stop or I'll kill one. I mean it!'

Rolf, grim-faced, was already running across the sandy yard towards the lynching party. My legs began to work. I remembered at last how to speak and be understood, and remembered too that Rolf had once told me the most obscene word in the Castilian tongue. I bellowed it out repeatedly as I ran. 'Cut that———rope, you———!' The fox was twisting in choking agony as the men, scowling, took the weight of the creature and let it down.

I pushed in among them, white-faced and trembling. They stood silently and still as I cradled the semi-conscious animal in my arms and went into careful detail about their parents, their mothers' gynaecological histories and how the descendants of Philip II and El Cid had, by some process of reversed evolution, descended into two-legged piojos—lice. Instead of sticking a blade between my ribs, the rough countrymen dispersed, snarling incomprehensibly and spitting onto the sand. I injected the fox with a massive overdose of xylazine anaesthetic, the stuff I normally use for quietening bison and buffalo, and it died peacefully in my arms.

Not surprisingly, Rolf and I were unaccompanied as we set off to inspect the animals. There were lions, including the uncommon Atlas Mountain variety, living in a compound littered with heaps of stinking bones; Imperial Spanish eagles, a protected species that should not have been there at all; and, in a large, undulating reserve, the most dangerous and unlikely animal I have ever met.

Before going into the reserve we scanned the terrain thoroughly with field-glasses. It was a tranquil place of pale sand slopes dotted with small clumps of locust trees. A trio of ostriches pecked about in the dust two hundred yards away, a Watusi cow was daydreaming in a shallow mud hole, and in the far distance a couple of wild horses of some sort, impossible to identify accurately, were standing nibbling one another's manes. With such creatures around there could not be a bunch of grizzly bears or tigers lurking in the bushes and we carried wooden sticks for use against animals such as male red-neck ostriches, which are more of a nuisance than a danger but get a kick out of stomping on you. As we walked into the reserve, a blackbuck darted up from behind a boulder and sprang silently away.

'We should have brought a bucket of corn,' Rolf murmured. 'Those fellows think it's feeding time.' He pointed towards the two horsey creatures, which were now staring at us. One began to move slowly towards us. At that distance it looked as big as a mouse.

I lifted the field-glasses as the approaching animal broke into a gentle trot. No, it was not a Przevalski's horse, it was a species of wild ass that I had chased over the water meadows of Holland, an onager. A pair of such beasts, barely twelve hands high and nervous as Derby winners, had arranged a smelly dunking in a Dutch canal for me.*

Rolf took the glasses and squinted through them. 'He must be hungry,' he said. 'He's coming in at a fair old canter now.'

The onager was now growing much bigger and was more easily recognised. It had covered half the distance between us. I could see puffs of dust rising from its hooves as it came straight as an arrow over the rolling land.

*See *Doctor in the Zoo*

'It certainly is keen to meet us,' I said, uneasily noticing that the canter was now more of a full gallop. It was absolutely head-on towards us. We had stopped walking and were standing, watching.

'Look at those legs go,' Rolf drawled easily. A tanned, lean Coloradan who had been a professional hunter in East Africa, he had been charged by more tough customers—elephant, lion, buffalo—than I had had hot dinners. He watched the approach of the harmless little pony, as unflappable as if he had been back in Zambia at the right end of a Winchester Express. 'Darn me—see how he's got his ears back,' Rolf chuckled.

It was true, they were so flat as to be invisible. What was more, the onager's lips were drawn back. Its beeline course was unwavering. It was a hundred yards away, still in top gear, and the sun glinted off a perfect set of upper and lower incisor teeth. Forty yards to go. Both of us could see, and hear, those incisors gnashing. Now the onager began to make an ugly, pig-like, squealing noise. My uneasiness became plain, naked fear. Rolf suddenly swore: he had not tangled with wild asses before, but his hunter's instincts had seen enough of this jet-propelled little pony. 'For Chrissake jump!' he yelled.

I had never considered myself to be much of an athlete, yet a moment later I found myself in the narrow fork of a locust tree. The ground was ten feet below, and I was tangled in an undignified embrace with Rolf who had taken wing simultaneously and lighted on the same cramped refuge.

The onager had screeched to a halt. It stood on its hind legs at the base of our tree, pawing and biting furiously at the bark. There was no doubt about it, the maniacal creature that was baying like a demented banshee a few inches beneath our trouser bottoms was trying to climb up and join us. Hatred blazed in its face.

'Don't that beat all?' said Rolf, as we hugged one another for support. 'Tree'd by a doggone ass!'

524

In the distance I could see a knot of Spaniards, the would-be fox-lynchers, watching the drama with expressions of rapt delight: 'Estupendo, the loud-mouthed veterinario and the Americano with the Corona Corona between his teeth are about to be torn to pieces. Que maravilloso!'

'Clear off! Vaya!' I shouted at the onager.

In reply it strained up the trunk and whinnied with such venom that I was surprised not to see sparks amongst the steam belching from its gaping, red nostrils.

Rolf broke off a twig and threw it down at our attacker. It bounced off the onager's muzzle. This really provoked the beast. It did a remarkable standing leap with its hind feet, such as only a few highly trained circus horses can do, or so I thought. Not only did it rise bodily a further six inches up the tree, but its teeth actually glanced off my shoe heel.

Pulling my knees up to my chin and clinging on to Rolf for dear life, I tried to think things out reasonably. 'Ever read the book by that woman who thinks you can communicate with animals by breathing at them nose to nose?' I asked.

'You ain't gonna use my nose with that bastard,' Rolf replied, trying to keep hold of me while extricating his buttocks from spiky branches that had pierced his jeans and embedded themselves securely in his flesh. 'I'll get those goddammed Spaniards to come down and chase it away.' At the top of his voice he shouted in Spanish towards our distant audience. 'Venga! Get down here and get rid of this blasted horse!'

The men heard him, I am sure, but stayed where they were, sitting on a fence, slapping their thighs, scratching and grinning like monkeys.

I tried a stern look at the onager, right in the eyes, no blinking. It looked sternly back and bit off another apple-sized chunk of tree. 'Animals don't like to be stared at usually,' I said.

'Well for Chrissake stop staring at the critter then,'

groaned Rolf. 'Mebbe you're provoking the son of a bitch.'

'He'll get tired and go back to his mate in a minute if we're patient,' I said confidently.

Half an hour later, 'He still ain't tired,' replied my companion.

The onager was on patrol, circling the trunk of our tree. It marched steadily, never stopping, never more than a couple of feet away from our precarious perch. From time to time it would look up at its prey, give that horrible, frustrated squeal and lunge up at a juicy portion of one of us in the hopes that it might get just one little taste.

'I don't understand it,' I told Rolf. 'We haven't tried to get between him and his food or a mare in season. We haven't said any rude words in onagerese. We're just innocent passers by!'

'It ain't no use analysing,' growled Rolf. 'This bastard's just a man-hater, that's all.'

That seemed the only logical explanation. This was not the aggression even of a creature that has been cruelly treated in the past by humans. It had the chilling appearance of irrational, intrinsic hatred, the blind rage of a rabid animal that has turned into a deadly robot obeying the virus infesting its brain cells.

Rolf had the same thought simultaneously. 'Couldn't be rabies, could it?' he asked.

I went through the cobwebbed mental pigeonholes containing what I knew of rabies in equines. Rag-and-bone-men's ponies in Rochdale did not often chase folk up trees, and Britain has been effectively free of rabies since 1921. I had never seen rabies in horses of any species, but those who had wrote of it taking the 'furious' rather than the 'dumb', paralytic form. They had, I dimly recalled from lectures long ago at Glasgow University, spoken of excitement, mania, uncontrolled actions that were violent and dangerous, including blind charges, and frequently chewing of the animal's own skin. Rabies was reported from time to time in Spain.

The onager, rabid or not, was still as determined as ever to destroy us. Detestation of us fuelled every straining sinew and corded vein in its body. All the symptoms of rabies taught me as a student seemed to fit the beast below me, except the bit about uncontrolled actions. Rolf agreed that this demon pony seemed highly controlled and calculating. It knew what it was after and was trying damned hard to get it. The absence of robot-like movement gave me just enough confidence tentatively to rule out rabies.

'The one driving force in the animal seems to be that it wants to eat us,' I pointed out when another hour had passed without the slightest change in the situation. 'I wonder if it'd be happy with a limb as a diversion while we escape.'

Rolf laughed bitterly. 'What do you want me to do? Amputate one of your arms with my penknife and throw it down like a spare rib to a hound-dawg?'

I looked at Rolf's natty suède jacket and then at my old denim one. I made the choice. 'Try to break off that thick branch above your head,' I said.

With great difficulty, while I hugged his waist, he tugged and pulled and went red in the face. Suddenly the branch broke with a crack and we both rocked violently. Only just did we avoid toppling straight down into the gnashing fangs below.

I took my jacket off and stuffed the branch down one sleeve, then I slowly proffered the bit of 'me' down to the onager. I saw delight and triumph sparkle in its bloodshot eyes. The one in blue was coming down like a lamb to the slaughter! With a great lunge the wild ass seized the 'arm' in the jacket, tore it away from me and flung it with immense force to the ground. It then began to stamp, rip and gnaw at it with terifying ferocity. It was utterly absorbed in reducing the 'arm' to pulp. Postage-stamp-sized pieces of denim began to flutter around. Rolf whispered just the one word, 'Go!' We dropped down from the tree and somehow ran like the wind on aching, numbed legs for the gate in the fencing. I was scared as hell, more scared than any escaped circus lion, elephant with raging toothache or tiger coming round prematurely from an anaesthetic had ever made me feel.

Miraculously we made the gate, crashed through and collapsed on the ground as it slammed behind us. At that instant, five hundred pounds of squealing, thwarted onager hurtled into the wire mesh beside us. The fence bulged alarmingly, some metal strands 'pinged' as they parted but mercifully held. After a valiant attempt to leap over the top at us, the onager returned to the remains of my jacket and its wooden arm and took up the furious attack again. We picked ourselves up and limped stiffly away. As we passed the grinning group of Spaniards, Rolf said something terse and explicit that wiped the grins from their faces.

We decided to buy the two elephants and the giraffe; when the weather was warmer we would move them by road to Rio Leon. We also made some enquiries about the onager, which turned out to be well-known as a fearsome scourge of homo sapiens, with two near-kills to its credit among the park workers. There was no chance of its being sold and we were told that it would have to be put down.

'When they do euthanase it, ask them to use a heart shot,' I said to Rolf. 'I'd very much like a look at its brain if that could be arranged.'

Weeks later Rolf took the trouble to acquire the brain of the dead onager and put it into a tub of formaldehyde for my next visit. When I eventually had a chance of examining it, I found a tapeworm cyst as big as, and bearing a close resemblance to, a table-tennis ball embedded in one side of the brain's frontal lobes. The onager had been a sort of robot after all—tragically controlled by a parasite picked up maybe years before when grazing. A blade of grass must have borne a tiny beetle which contained within its minuscule muscles the microscopic larva that would one day drive a wild ass mad and give a friend and me a very rough couple of hours.

Nine

Cuddles the killer whale had by this time settled down wonderfully at Flamingo Park. The 'flu vaccine worked and no booster shots were needed. He was devoted to the American girl whale-trainer, Jerry Watmore, who had come over from the USA to school him, and he was eating like a horse. A whale sling that could be run over the pool on massive steel beams had proved a success, and Cuddles had swum into it at our first attempt. Blood sampling and health inspections were easy and quick, and the only problem was to persuade the whale to back off out of the sling when the examination or whatever was over. He loved this giant doctor's couch, and never showed any of the 'once jabbed, twice shy' wariness of chimpanzees, who remember always their first encounter with nefarious individuals like me who chuckle heartily, bear gifts of grapes and then treacherously produce the syringe that had been hidden behind their backs. Cuddles was the perfect patient, provided you did not try to stick needles into him while he was swimming free in his own environment. Killer whales I have met since have behaved quite differently when faced with their medical advisor.

I fussed over every little ailment, real or imagined, that beset Cuddles. Slight cracking of the skin in the corners of his mouth? I had read of scurvy, the disease that was once the bane of mariners, cropping up in whales, so I trebled his daily dose of vitamin C. A small spongy wart on his dorsal fin? Into the sling, a shot of local anaesthetic and off it came. A slight iron-deficiency anaemia appeared a few weeks after his arrival, caused by some of the natural blood in mackerel being lost as we thawed out the whale's meals of deep-frozen fish. I boosted his iron pill supplement and the anaemia cleared; I was beginning to get the 'feel' of this animal. Every time I visited I swam with him for a few minutes. He adored having his tummy scratched and lightly kicked by my flippered feet as he hugged me between his flippers.

One day, Cuddles' keeper noticed that the whale's dorsal fin was bleeding. It had been unblemished the night before, but now, at 8.30 in the morning, it was oozing blood from a small group of what looked like ulcers. I was soon on my way over the hills in response to yet another breakfast-time phone call.

Once at the park, I arranged for the whale sling to be run out and Cuddles slipped in without a murmur. A few cranks on the winch handles and he was clear of the water. I walked out along the catwalk and inspected the skin disease. They were not strictly ulcers, more like ragged little wounds on the leading edge of the triangular black sail that is so characteristic of male killer whales. They did not seem to be infected and I had no idea what they were. I smeared them with neomycin ointment, plastered thick lanolin and denture-fixing paste on top, and coaxed him back into the pool.

Next day, more of the skin damage had appeared. It was all in roughly the same place, and the base of the dorsal fin was beginning to look rather ugly. Under a magnifying glass, the splits in the skin could be seen to be quite deep. Their ragged appearance was vaguely familiar, but I could not place exactly what they reminded me of. Over the next few days the skin disease worsened. One curious fact was that the bleeding area did not expand at all by day, but extended noticeably during each night.

'Any chance of vandals, or keepers with a grudge of some sort doing him mischief?' Pentland Hick asked me.

Mutilation of animals, sometimes by outwardly normal keepers, was not unknown to us, but the dolphinarium was securely locked up at night and it had high walls. Nevertheless, I asked for a dolphin trainer to sleep in a hammock slung near the whale pool for a few nights to see whether that might help. It did not. The damage to Cuddles' dorsal fin progressed steadily and the dolphin trainer was adamant that no-one had entered the dolphinarium.

My concern over what had begun as a relatively small if mysterious skin problem was by now considerable. Phone calls to the marinelands of America produced no concrete suggestions from their veterinarians and I simply kept on applying my antibiotic ointment and hoping that something would turn up. Laboratory tests had revealed nothing significant.

Andrew Greenwood's bush telegraph, fuelled by packets of cigarettes, had once again worked perfectly. Whenever I drove into the park to review the latest developments in the mysterious Case of the Bleeding Dorsal, a puzzle that was proving anything but elementary, there would be Andrew already at the pool-side, eager to play the role of Dr Watson.

We talked about the puzzle one day over tea in the cafeteria. 'I'm intrigued by the nocturnal aspects of the darned thing,' I said. 'It extends when he's floating and dozing during the wee small hours, but never in broad daylight.'

'What about setting up a surveillance system?' Andrew suggested.

'To survey what? Microbes dancing about in the moonlight? Little water sprites paddling out to the whale in fairy canoes and hacking at his fin with elfin axes?'

We both smiled. Suddenly I had an idea—maybe surveillance was not such a bad idea. 'We'll try it, Andrew,' I said. 'I'm going to phone the Green Howards.'

This reference to one of Yorkshire's most famous army regiments mystified the student. 'To do what? Hire a howitzer to blow up the water sprites with?'

It took several phone calls before the Army public relations people oiled the wheels and arranged what I wanted. A squad of soldiers would come out that evening with infra-red searchlights of the type being fitted at that time to some battle tanks, and some sets of night binoculars. I was going to light up the dreaming Cuddles in his pool with 'black' light and observe him through the hours of darkness. Maybe he was doing something odd like rubbing the fin against the piping or pool edge. With this system and warm clothing, plus flasks of strong coffee laced with rum, we might get a clue to the cause of the trouble.

The soldiers and their officer duly arrived and set up the equipment. As darkness fell, we took our places high in the rows of seating around the pool. Besides the military contingent and me, there was the ubiquitous Andrew, who seemed to carry in his little sports car clothing, equipment, victuals and all sorts of paraphernalia for impromptu exploits such as this.

It was a dark, moonless night. After the novelty of looking through the night-glasses and seeing the pool and its inmate sharply displayed in ghostly, lime-green light, the vigil became a cold and cheerless affair. No talking was allowed. We passed the night-glasses silently from one to another, took gulps of the coffee when the cold began to bite and cursed that no-one had thought to bring cushions for the hard wooden seating that was numbing our bottoms.

At 2 am, just when I was regretting having thought of so daft a piece of time-wasting, I was hit hard in the ribs by the army officer, who was holding the glasses at the time. He thrust them into my hands. I lifted them and looked.

Cuddles was where he had been since early evening, and at first I could see nothing that I had not seen before. Water, pool-side, whale—the usual lime-green scene. But wait! There was something new. Two luminous blobs had appeared on the pool-side, small, green like all the rest, but moving. They stopped briefly, changed places, merged into

533

one, separated and then moved slowly on. It was like something out of a badly out-of-focus horror movie. Fascinated, I watched the little ghostly forms go down onto the platform, approach the water's edge and stop. Then the blobs moved again: with graceful hops they sprang onto the whale's forehead and began to move up past his blow-hole. Cuddles gave no sign of movement.

When the blobs reached the dorsal I had had enough. 'House lights on!' I shouted. Andrew flicked a switch and the pool was flooded in powerful visible light.

'Good God,' Andrew muttered.

Two startled brown rats turned their heads towards us as they crouched on the broad expanse of the whale's back. In a twinkling they had scurried back to shore and disappeared down a floor drain.

I had heard of other zoo animals being chewed alive by rats, but usually they were sick or dying creatures. An amphibious assault on a fit and floating whale by such bold buccaneers was something else. Whether their vampire-like visits had irritated Cuddles or whether he had been as unconcerned about them as he was about needle pricks, I will never know.

The blobs had been unmasked. The next day we called in the vermin-control people, Cuddles' skin wounds healed and there were no further attacks from the drains.

For once, an early-morning telephone call brought glad tidings—my first hippopotamus birth. Fifi, the bucolic old female at Belle Vue had sprung a surprise and borne a lusty little 'horse of the Nile' during the night. I forgot utterly the planned luxury of a morning spent pottering in the garden and snatched a handful of buttered toast to munch as I drove down to the zoo. All new-born animals give me a marvellous thrill, and I wanted to see my first brand new hippo before he or she had a chance to become blasé with this sad old world of ours, while it still blinked brightly in the

534

artificial Africa that men had built for it to end its days in, in the middle of a smoky, grey city.

The baby was a beauty. Only fools compare the physical features of animals and debate the relative charms of wombats and warthogs. The impala cannot be judged against the bullfrog, nor the sloth against the lyre bird. Apart from man, who sorts out the minority of his kind that can be expected to pass muster at beauty contests and similar sad gatherings, it is a universal truth that there are no ugly animals. The Vietnamese pot-bellied pig produces piglets that I consider utterly charming and close behind, for my money, come baby hippos. This one was plump and in showroom condition. The mother looked watchfully proud and had an udder whose teats bore globules of colostrum. Matt Kelly and I agreed: everything seemed absolutely OK. I arranged for Mum to get extra rations of food and half a cupful of cod-liver oil each day and told Matt to inform me if the complete afterbirth was not expelled within thirty-six hours.

Two days later Matt called me. 'Afterbirth came away OK,' he said. 'Mother seems foine. But oi'm not too sure about the little feller.'

I went to look. I agreed with Matt. The baby was not as perky and plump as it should have been at three days old. It looked listless and unhappy, though the keeper was adamant that it had been suckling vigorously on several occasions. Cautiously Matt and I tried to grab the baby for a thorough examination. Not a hope—the mother hippo was not having any such shenanigans and sent us hurriedly back over the barrier by charging with the speed and nimbleness of which these lumbering, tank-like creatures are capable.

'The best I can suggest is a dart injection of the baby,' I told Matt. 'I don't want to knock out Mum just to get at the little one.'

I do not like the old-fashioned guess-agnosis with zoo animals, but on this occasion I felt a flying syringe full of vitamins would be a good idea. It was easily done, though the mother indignantly pulled the emptied dart out of her baby's rump and chomped it up between her enormous teeth. I lose twenty-five pounds' worth of dart syringes every month that way.

The next day the baby was distinctly fading. Our initial exuberation had turned to despair. The baby was not feeding as frequently, although its mother was brimming with milk. It wobbled slightly on its feet. It slept more than I liked, and Matt noticed something else: the urine it passed was the colour of dark coffee. 'Looks like changed blood,' I said unhappily. 'My bet is a severe cystitis—inflammation of the bladder.'

While I went to fix another flying dart containing a dose of ampicillin, I asked Matt to try to dab up a spot or two of the baby hippo's urine, using a long pole with an absorbent tissue tied to the end. Despite defensive action by the mother, Matt got some of the brown liquid. To my surprise, tests showed no blood in it. But if the deep, murky colour was not caused by blood, what on earth could it be? I gave myself the benefit of the doubt and darted in the anti-cystitis antibiotic anyway.

'Ye know, Doctor,' Matt said, as we stared glumly into the pen, 'the little feller's not passed a motion yet.'

There was no simple way of administering a laxative, and surely the natural action of the mother's colostrom would produce droppings before long. Anyway, with a sickly baby hippo I would prefer constipation to debilitating, dehydrating diarrhoea.

The ampicillin had not the slightest effect. After a further three days, with the baby steadily deteriorating, I took more samples of the black and muddy urine. Still the blood tests read negative. I was puzzled but switched my antibiotic attack and brought in the expensive but powerful chemical called gentamycin. I might as well have been darting the baby with lemonade for all the good it did. It looked as if I would have to neutralise the mother with an anaesthetic and haul out the baby for a thorough going-over, but before I could go ahead with the plan, Matt phoned me with the worst possible news: the baby had died suddenly. It was heart-breaking.

'Get the little fellow's body out,' I instructed. 'I'll come over and do an autopsy.'

But when I arrived at Belle Vue no little corpse was lying ready in the post-mortem room. 'Can't get at it,' explained Matt dejectedly. 'She'll kill anyone who troies to go near it.'

I went to look. The bereaved female stood guard over the leathery little heap in the straw that was her first-born. Keepers with boards, brush handles or even thick doors lifted off their hinges were driven mercilessly back by the determined animal. No-one, but no-one, was going any-where near her baby. I threw her tranquilliser powder in hollowed-out loaves of bread; she would not eat. We tried raking the body out with hooked poles; she broke the poles effortlessly with great snaps of her jaws. I darted her with valium; she drooped her eyelids but remained on guard, wheeling her hind legs whenever one of us tried to creep up behind her. Matt tried to lure her into other quarters with fruit and fresh vegetables; she never even looked in his direction. The day came to a close with us defeated and the hippo still standing four-square over the lifeless infant.

'She's stood over the baby all noight,' Matt told me next day. 'She won't eat, drink or go into the pool. Oi've tried lettin' the bull in with her. She went for him like a mad thing, took a lump as big as yer fist out of his cheek and now he's sulkin' scared in the river house.'

It would have to be anaesthetic. But suppose as she went under the effects of the drug she staggered into the water? It would take all day to drain her pool. No, I was not justified in darting any one of my hippopotamus anaesthetics with deep water so close to where she stood.

The hippopotamus and elephant house at Belle Vue had an old gallery running along the back of the animal pens. I looked up at it. Suppose we went up there with a rope and fished for the corpse? We tried it. It was a long drop. Matt fashioned a lasso out of thick cord and, leaning over the edge of the gallery that was caked with almost a hundred years of bird droppings, slowly lowered the loop down towards the little hippo. The mother did not once look up, but as soon as the cord dangled close to her head, she snapped at it with loud clumping noises of her teeth. Each time Matt nearly had the cord in place round the baby's muzzle, the mother's jaws swept the lasso away. The head keeper was red in the face and grinding his teeth in frustration. Suddenly, as he lowered the cord yet again, the female actually caught hold of the loop in her mouth and gave a mighty, irritable yank. Matt was snatched violently forward and his chest came up hard against the low balustrade. A section of the old wood-work broke away before him and crashed down onto the hippo. Only the fact that I grabbed him by the back of his shirt and jammed my feet against the surviving bit of rail saved him from going down as well. The mother had not budged an inch under the surprise aerial bombard-ment. Splintered wood littered her back but she was intently nuzzling the cold, dark form lying between her fore legs.

'Sure, there's only one thing for it,' puffed Matt, getting over the shock of his narrow escape from death either by breaking his neck or by being chomped by the hippo. 'Lower me down on the rope, Doctor—ye'll need two or more fellers to help ye. Then oi'll grab the little 'un whoile she's dis-tracted somehow.'

It sounded perilous to me, not least because for over twenty-four hours now this animal had shown itself immune to every sort of distraction we had come up with. Matt would need at least five or six seconds to throw the rope round the baby and secure himself for the ascent. What could we do that would guarantee at least that much time? At the very best the mother would still be only a few feet from the head keeper, and hippos can turn their heads and the rest of their bodies like lightning.

'Oi've an oidea,' Matt continued. 'Jim!' he called to one of his keepers who was standing down below. 'Go to the souvenir shop and ask 'em to let you have three or four of those mechanical toys they're sellin'—the animals that move. The biggest they've got!'

Jim returned shortly with three brightly coloured plastic animals, a tiger, a pig and a dinosaur. Each had a clockwork motor that Matt wound up with a key. He put them on the floor, gave them a nudge and the three toys started to move round in loudly whirring circles. Matt seemed satisfied. We went down to the ground floor again and he cautiously opened the door of the pen containing our distressed mother. He wound up the mechanical pig, placed it on the floor just inside the door and set it off. Fizz-fizz-whirr went the toy, beginning to move in a wide circle. We watched the hippo. Her ears pricked, then she turned her head slowly towards the strange sound, fixed the mechanical intruder with a baleful gaze and advanced upon it, mouth agape. Stomp, stomp, crunch! The pig would never move or whirr again. Its clockwork spring remained impaled on one of her tusks.

'Foine! Foine!' crowed the head keeper. 'Oi reckon she was ten seconds away from the baby. We've two more of the same. We'll get into position and then when oi give the word, Jim can set both of 'em off in the same place.'

Reluctantly I went along with Matt's stratagem. I had nothing better to offer. With four keepers I accompanied him back to the gallery and we fixed a new length of one-inch rope to his waist, leaving a long piece free for him to attach to the corpse.

When all was ready and Jim had fully wound up the two toy animals, Matt gave a shout and the operation began. We took the strain and slowly lowered Matt from the gallery while Jim's animals did their bit like Trojans. The head keeper touched down gently as soon as the hippo was seen to be turning away and moving in to deal with this second wave of invaders. Crouching tensely, eyes fixed on the rear end of the hippo only a few feet from his face, Matt quietly fished in the straw for some extremity of the baby to pull on. Scrunch! One down—the mechanical tiger had bitten the dust. Matt had got hold of a leg and was hurriedly throwing a loop of rope round it. It was all up to the dinosaur now. Cra-ack, whirr—the hippo had lunged and split open its casing but the little hero was still going. The hippo was having difficulty biting satisfactorily at so small an object. Matt gave us the thumbs up and yelled 'Pull!' just as the dinosaur met a sticky end at last, stomped flat. The hippo whirled, we pulled like demons. Matt's broad head appeared over the edge of the gallery and the body of the little hippo bumped against the balustrade as the mother made her final charge. She missed Matt's boots by inches. It was done.

The autopsy showed the cause of the baby's death and of the dark-brown urine. It had been born without an anus, a congenital fault, and the large bowel ended instead in the bladder of all places. The deformity was too gross to have been curable, so there was some minute comfort in knowing that I could not have done anything for the little mite, but I was depressed by the evident psychological upset of the now lonely mother. Her milk would dry up without any need of drugs, but to ease her mind I put her on a course of euphoria-giving chemicals for a couple of weeks. She needed and deserved a bit of a 'high' for a while.

I congratulated Matt on his efforts. We had used toys in animal work before—for example cuddly ones for orphan monkeys and apes to cling to—but I had never thought of using clockwork animals as unmanned decoy missiles!

Any remaining worries I had about enough work coming my way vanished when Pentland Hick made me an offer. Frank, the curator of Flamingo Park, was leaving. Would I go to live at Flamingo Park and take the position of Curator and

Group Veterinary Officer? Hick said I could retain an essential degree of independence, visit Belle Vue regularly, go out to other exotic animal clients if they called, and use all the facilities of the operating room he was building for my use at Flamingo Park. More, he would pay for me to travel around the world, studying wild animals and visiting other zoos and animal dealers. I could keep the old farmhouse in Rochdale and would live a bachelor life in a caravan on the site set in a peaceful corner of the park. It would mean, too, that I could see even more of Cuddles, for whom I had developed something of an infatuation. The offer was a unique one and without hesitation I accepted: few zoo veterinarians have any experience of the other side of the fence, of general keeping, curating and management, yet they can never be fully efficient without it. It was to prove a watershed in my life.

Ten

Flamingo Park Zoo was built round an early Victorian manor house and occupied the house itself, the grounds and two or three outlying farms. The house and lake stood at the top of a rise, from which the ground sloped away to a stream and the caravan site. Across the Vale of Pickering, the hazy line of the North Yorkshire moors stretched across the horizon like a lilac-coloured rock garden. My first days as curator were highly discouraging. There was far more than I had ever imagined to running a zoo with a couple of dozen keepers and hundreds of assorted animals, not to mention the thousands of human varieties that arrived by car and coach each week. The veterinarian finds it salutary to see for himself that 99.9% of the important affairs in the life of the lions, camels, parrots and crocodiles, which he thinks he knows well, go on day after day in a subtly changing kaleidoscope while he is not normally there. Headline-grabbing, glamour bits of surgery on cute zoo inmates, the occasional dramatic intervention and the midnight emergency were not as central to my life from now on as keeping the drains unblocked and dealing with grumbles from visitors about catering, lost boys, too few lavatories, spectacles snatched by monkeys and coats ruined by wet paint.

I soon found caravan life too spartan for my more sybaritic tastes. Days that had started with one of Shelagh's fine breakfasts and time for a stab at the *Daily Telegraph* crossword in front of the log fire were replaced by the miseries of tea stewed over a calor-gas heater, cold baked beans and no morning paper.

An unusually depressing spring, with icy winds and snow right through till May, turned the land round the caravan into a gumboot-removing quagmire. The caravan-site manager was a cussed individual who took a malevolent delight in switching off the lights in the cold, brick lavatory block just after watching me wade there across the mud in pyjamas and oilskins late in the evening. I resorted to carrying a box of matches with me when attending to calls of nature. As soon as the lights went off I quickly unravelled several feet of toilet paper and set fire to it. The blazing roll gave enough light for me to complete the ceremonies with a measure of decorum.

Apart from the visitors, the zoo stock and lesser beasts like the caravan-site manager, I also had my hands full with staff problems. I had to maintain discipline, try in vain to get them to clean their rooms and show them the rudiments of good stockmanship. One guy always stole the pennies thrown by visitors into the pools of the park. His intelligence did not match his greed, however, since he had no more wit than to spend the piles of verdigris-coated pennies in the zoo cafeteria or bar. Despite being warned by me, he continued to retrieve the coins which brought good luck to the throwers and Christmas comforts to the local charity to whom the pools' monetary contents were donated once a year. I had to fire the fellow for his own good, when I discovered him paddling about early one morning in the bear-pit pool. Two sweet-faced but lethal adult polar bears were standing on the water's edge, watching his treasure hunt.

Another keeper was asked to carry the bags of a newly arrived girl trainee to the caravan she had been allocated half a mile from the zoo. Neither of them returned for three whole days. Such instant passion had to be rewarded by instant dismissal when the two dreamily put in an appearance on the fourth morning. Even among my patients, I had never come across such importunate mating behaviour.

But by and large, the staff I had at Flamingo Park at that

time were a talented if colourful bunch. One is now the director of a famous safari park, another looks after the menagerie of the ruler of Abu Dhabi, another is a distinguished fine arts dealer, and there is one boy, who helped me to deliver the first baby dolphin conceived and born in England, who is now serving a life sentence for fitting an acquaintance with a pair of concrete boots and dropping him alive into the sea. If only he had stuck to the less flamboyant aspects of marine mammal studies!

Despite the weather, the drains, the staff and the visitors, I soldiered on. I had the animals, and for the first time in my life they were all under my care and not just with respect to veterinary matters. Want to hire an elephant for a store opening in Leeds? I was the chap who said yea or nay and organised everything. The rewards for putting up with the mud and the baked beans and the toilet roll torches were the opportunities to touch, see, smell and just be with a whole variety of animals all day long.

Everyone taught me something. I was initiated into the highly complex business of water treatment and filtration by the dolphinarium staff. Violet, the head of the animal food kitchen, showed me how to present acceptable and appetising meals to some of the rare animals like lesser pandas, pangolins and Gambian pouched rats.

Most of all, the animals were always instructing me. Mangrove snakes went into convulsions when I experimented with what I had found to be a safe anti-tick aerosol on other sorts of serpent at Belle Vue. The great elephant seal demonstrated the uselessness of a dart-gun on him even at point-blank range; the near-liquid blubber in this species absorbs the shock of the syringe impact, and the charge that actually pushes the injection in does not detonate. Tigers, camels, elephants, cockatoos and kangaroos taught me respect—respect not of the kind I had always had for living things but for the way in which they insisted on certain standards of behaviour by human beings in the daily routines of cleaning, feeding, watering and general maintenance. Break the routine, disturb their ordered lives, be brusque, cocky or absent-minded and they meted out punishment by employing one of the vast range of physical weapons they are fitted with, by embarrassing you in front of the public through non-co-operation or, worse, by escaping or by falling ill and dying.

I was learning the hard way, but I was learning fast.

With the arrival of early summer, caravan life at Flamingo Park became less stark. Shelagh and the girls drove over at the weekends and we would all swim with the whale. He was as good-natured with them as he was with me, which gave Stephanie and Lindsey something of an unusual advantage when talk among their school friends turned to dogs, cats and other more mundane pets. The light evenings meant the end of the site manager's jape with the lavatory switches, and it was my turn to discomfit him. I was rearing a lion cub in the caravan. On warm days it would roam round in the grass and play cubbish games of hiding behind clumps of weeds and springing out gleefully to give the legs of passers by a left, right with its paws. The site manager did not like cats, small or large, and suffered continual harassment of this sort. Worse, he watched with impotent chagrin as the cub lay in my caravan doorway, gnawing at the surrounding woodwork; the slow demolition of one of his beautiful painted mobile homes sorely grieved him.

There was lots of animal training going on at the park. Sharp-eyed macaws played pontoon with members of the public and always won. Their opponents never realised that the crusty-natured birds had been trained to spot marked cards which bore minute black dots on their reverse side. I learned how easy it is to train dolphins and how much easier it is for dolphins literally to train and condition their trainers. I also spent long hours watching the American girl, Jerry Watmore, turning Cuddles into a star performer. When she

545

had given him a full repertoire of jumps, rolls, handshakes and tricks of all kinds, and every one produced by kindness and rewards of mackerel, she handed Cuddles' presentation over to a young English boy who had the makings of a marine mammal trainer. He did well. Cuddles liked him and appointed him one of the select coterie, which included myself, who were allowed to ride round the pool sitting on his back either in front of the dorsal fin or, should one prefer a more exciting, bumpy journey, perched directly behind it. The training programme continued smoothly until one day there was a misunderstanding. Perhaps there was a foul-up in the system of signalling, the language of precise movement by which the man communicates his commands to the whale; perhaps the trainer was momentarily sloppy in his gestures; perhaps Cuddles was doing a spot of daydreaming about fat salmon or shoals of mackerel.

Cuddles was being trained to play the trumpet. He was to hold the toy instrument between his teeth with his head out of the water. The fanfare would in fact come not by his blowing into the trumpet (whales cannot exhale air through their mouths) but from loud hootings from his pursed blow-hole. There were a series of distinct signals governing the various stages of this performance: one hand movement caused Cuddles to raise his head and take the trumpet gently between his lips, another started him hooting, and a third stopped the hooting and persuaded him to release his hold on the trumpet. When things began to go wrong on that fateful morning, the trainer had got Cuddles to hold the trumpet perfectly and produce hoots that would delight the audiences in future but make Louis Armstrong turn in his grave. With the trumpet between his teeth Cuddles suddenly opened his mouth, no doubt impatient to receive his reward of succulent mackerel. Whatever the reason, the great jaws gaped, and the shiny plastic instrument fell onto the back of his tongue.

The trainer immediately took sensible action by giving a

hand signal which Cuddles had already learnt, and which meant that he was to shake his head vigorously from side to side as if rinsing out his mouth. Somewhere between man and animal there was a break in transmission. Cuddles closed his mouth, gulped and the trumpet was gone. Killer whales have wide, dilatable gullets; adults can swallow big tuna and seals whole. Within seconds the trumpet must have splashed down into the cavern of the first of the whale's four stomachs. As if he had not noticed a thing, Cuddles at once opened his jaws again in anticipation of fish for a job well done. The horrified trainer gave him a handful of mackerel and then dashed to the phone.

I was at the pool-side within minutes and went into urgent conference with Martin Padley, the head of the dolphinarium. First we had to make sure that the trumpet really had been swallowed. We grilled the poor trainer and sent a couple of scuba divers down to scour the pool bottom. We had had false alarms in dolphinaria before where trainers swore blind that they had seen an object swallowed by a marine mammal. Dolphins and sealions had been stomach pumped, X-rayed and dosed with emetics and purgatives. Then the object had turned up, thrown out of the pool by the animal and lying hidden behind seating, in someone's pocket or on the shelf in a locker. The cardinal rule was to check the pool and its surrounds meticulously, no matter who said they had witnessed the actual swallowing, before pursuing the foreign body into the animal itself.

Usually we had been concerned with nuts and bolts, coins, torch batteries and the like, things that can be overlooked on a pool bottom or elsewhere. You can hardly miss trumpets that are sixteen inches long and canary yellow with bright red valves. There was no doubt, we concluded eventually—the trumpet was inside the whale. I was pretty certain that it must be in the first stomach, since foreign bodies in cetaceans very rarely get through the tight little valve that guards the entrance to stomach number two. Being plastic,

547

the thing would not dissolve although it might conceivably break. In one piece it could do damage as the lining of the stomach contracted down onto it. Broken, it might cause severe internal bleeding.

I considered the medical implications. I would not be able to use my ex-army mine detector in the way that I did on ostriches that gulped down bits of old iron; the machine could not pinpoint the position of non-metallic objects. X-ray was out, too; there was not a set in the country, even at the University large animal clinics, that could have shot a picture through Cuddles' girth. Fibre-optic gastroscopy, the technique that Andrew was later to pioneer in dolphins, could not be used; even the longest fibre-optic instrument, the colonoscope for peering up humans' lower bowels, was far too short to reach down the whale's throat and gullet. Laxatives would be useless; the damned thing was safer in the stomach than trying to slide through the hundreds of feet of narrow bowel. Emetics? I baulked at the dose of sodium carbonate or hydrogen peroxide that I would have to use to try to induce vomiting. As for apomorphine, an injectable drug that causes retching in some species, it had never been used on whales and I feared it might rupture his guts. Abdominal operation on a killer whale was, at that time, totally beyond our capabilities.

So what was I left with? Only two approaches. One was the oldest medical therapy in the world (and arguably the safest)—do nothing but wait. The other was to use the good old stomach pump and try to flood the trumpet out. After much thought I decided to begin by doing nothing since I was sure that the trumpet would soon be regurgitated. It was a tough decision and even tougher explaining to Martin and Pentland Hick why I chose masterly inactivity. I went back to my trailer, poured a Glenlivet and tried to unwind by losing myself in Gerard Manley Hopkins' poetry, a sure remedy for tensions of the day.

Next day Cuddles was still in fine fettle but there was no

sign of the trumpet. The scuba divers searched again and we opened the pre-filters to look for pieces of plastic. Nothing was found. Cuddles ate a hearty eighty pounds of fish and played gleefully. Tests showed no blood or other abnormalities in his excrement. To keep everyone on their toes in case of a regurgitation, I promised a bottle of champagne for whoever brought me the troublesome Jonah of an instrument. I decided to wait another day. When that passed uneventfully I waited yet another.

By the fourth day I had lost enough sleep agonising over the possible ulcerating effects of the trumpet's mouthpiece, bell or valves on the soft stomach lining. 'I'm going to pump out his stomach,' I announced.

Like a genie conjured up by my words, Andrew Greenwood drove up to the dolphinarium at that moment. He walked blandly in as we rolled out the whale sling. His timing, as usual, was perfect. The grapevine extended down to his college in Cambridge and was functioning well.

'It'll be a wet business,' I told him, 'and I'm afraid there aren't enough wet-suits for everybody. If you want to get in close, strip down to your underpants.'

'Don't worry about me,' he replied, slapping a grip he was carrying. 'I've got trunks and towel in here.'

Once the dry-dock was in position it did not take a minute for the whale to cruise happily into it. We wound him up and I gave one keeper the job of wetting down Cuddles' entire body surface with a hosepipe.

'Don't let one inch of him dry out for an instant,' I warned. 'When we start pumping, his temperature will go up with stress and excitement and he'll steam like a Christmas pudding. Keep spraying the water, don't worry about soaking the people round him.' Stomach-pumping whales is never fun.

I had the plastic stomach tube and pump ready. Stainless steel buckets of warm water were lined up by my side. All I had to do now was pass the tube down the mouth and into the stomach. In horses, stomach tubing can go wrong if you forget to check that the tube you have shoved gaily down the animal really is lying in the gullet. You begin pumping in the liquid, and may find you have a drowned nag on your hands; the tube has slipped down the windpipe. But any fool can stomach-tube a cetacean safely because there is no opening between the larynx and the back of the throat, so the tube cannot go wandering off towards the lungs. Whales and dolphins are vet-proof by design.

All the same, trumpet-chasing inside Cuddles was not going to be all that much of a piece of cake. Before I could pass the tube I naturally had to get Cuddles' mouth open, and whereas he would open it at the drop of a hat when floating in water, as soon as he was suspended in his hammock he resolutely clenched his teeth and refused to open them even a millimetre, not even for a mackerel dangled in front of his shiny eye. I tried prising them open with my fingers; I fancied he sniggered as he felt my puny hands working against jaw muscles that can wrench the entire giant tongue out of a blue whale at one bite. I had a tapered, four-inch-square piece of wood to use as a dental gag during the operation. I attempted to lever his mouth open gently by inserting the tapered end of the wedge between his lips. No go; Cuddles blew foamy bubbles through the fine spaces between his teeth. An onlooker suggested I might chisel out a tooth to provide a window for the tube. He quailed under the storm of ridicule and indignation. Multilate our Cuddles? The man must have been out of his mind!

The man with the hose was dutifully concentrating on his responsibilities and chilling us humans in the process. No-one complained. I noticed that when he sprayed his jet of water at Cuddles' lip, the whale would wriggle slightly and give some piggish squeaks. Taking the hosepipe, I rammed it hard up against the arcade of shining white teeth and told someone to turn the water pressure on full. Tickly jets of tap water squirted through the gaps in the whale's teeth and struck the tongue and roof of the mouth. It must have produced some sort of fizzy sensation. Whatever it did, Cuddles suddenly opened his jaws a fraction and then clamped them shut again, cleanly amputating three inches of hosepipe.

'That's it!' I exclaimed. 'Two of you get ready to push in the gag when I do it again. Remember, once the gag is in place he'll throw his head around. Ride with him!'

I repeated the squirting business. Again Cuddles momentarily opened his mouth and the men rammed in the gag. Surprised and insulted, the whale threw his head to left and right, trying to dislodge the offending piece of timber. The two men holding the gag were flung about but clung on desperately as Cuddles beat them against the hammock framework. Suddenly one lost his grip. The gag slewed across the whale's mouth. The other gag-holder was pitched headlong into the pool and, with a final mighty shake of his jaws, Cuddles hurled the block of wood from him. It hit the shins of the water-spraying keeper with terrible force. As the poor fellow was carried off in agony with what turned out to be a fractured tibia, Cuddles contentedly shut his empty mouth tight.

Beefier gag-holders were recruited and the whole rigmarole was repeated. This time the men managed to survive the whale's onslaught. The gag was well and truly jammed into the space between the back teeth. As it was made of soft, white wood, Cuddles' teeth sank into it slightly, which was just what I wanted; it could not skid away like one made of resistant hard wood.

Cuddles protested with hoots and querulous squeals. I greased the stomach tube with liquid paraffin and passed it quickly over the back of his tongue. It slid easily. I felt the slight resistance as it curved round the larynx, then a fast transit of the gullet and finally more resistance as the tip pressed through the weak valve at the entrance to the stomach. I was in.

'Right, Andrew,' I said, 'start pumping as fast as you like. Go!'

Andrew bent to the machine lying in the first bucket of warm water and started working the handle rapidly up and down. Within a minute the bucket was empty. Nothing had changed at Cuddles' end of the tube.

'Start on the next,' I ordered.

That bucket also was quickly empty. Cuddles blinked but that was all.

'Next! Fast as you can!'

Andrew puffed away with the effort. The third bucket was half empty when suddenly Cuddles' stomach responded at last to the involuntary expansion. There was a rumble and a retch and Cuddles opened his mouth. I was drenched in a tidal wave of warm, fishy-smelling water. Wiping partially digested fish bones from my eyes, I looked around. No trumpet.

We did it all again. Four buckets went in this time before the wall of water inundated me. Still no trumpet, but at least there were fewer fish remnants.

Andrew inspected the whale, feeling the flippers and tail-flukes to test the temperature reaction. 'He's heating up noticeably,' he reported.

I could not risk much more stress. 'Just one more try,' I said.

It was another failure. The water returned promptly and in full measure; of musical instruments there was not the slightest sign, not even a grand piano. Despondently, I ordered the whale to be lowered back into his pool. Now all I could do was return to the so-called Turkish treatment or, as we say in Lancashire, 'doing nowt'.

I 'did nowt' for the next two weeks. Cuddles remained outwardly hale and hearty and the daily searches for the trumpet continued. I began to wonder if the whale would carry the object for life. I had been slightly consoled by talking by phone to Dr Sam Ridgway of the US Navy marine

552

mammal research unit. He had told me of some of the large radio-telemetry packs which they were placing in the first stomachs of dolphins and which stayed in place for long periods without producing any signs of discomfort or disease. As the days went by we came to accept the fact that maybe Cuddles would have to live permanently with the trumpet.

I was surfacing from sleep one morning when there came a furious knocking on the caravan door. Half asleep, I tried to make sense of the noisy fool so rudely disturbing the delicate hour. Dammit, was this some keeper still drunk after an all-night binge? I pulled back the blankets and listened.

'Champagne, Dr Taylor, open the bottle of champagne!'

Suddenly, with crystal clarity, I knew what he was hollering about. Although it was raining hard outside, it was a wonderful, glorious, halcyon day.

I kicked open the caravan door. A dripping wet dolphin trainer stood on the steps with a grin like a slice of watermelon and a yellow and red trumpet held high above his head.

Cuddles had regurgitated the instrument without any fuss during the night and it had been found floating on the surface when the dolphinarium was opened up. I was overjoyed and immediately sent to the bar for half a dozen celebratory bottles. Forestalling the grapevine, I also telephoned Andrew to tell him the good news.

'Marvellous!' he replied. 'Like Benjamin Franklin wrote, "God heals and the Doctor takes the fee."'

I agreed, laughing, but reminded him in return of the Emperor Tiberius who claimed that every man at thirty is either a fool or a physician.

I could not have cared less into which category I fitted at that moment. All that mattered was that Cuddles was safe. There would be no more musical items in his repertoire.

Whitsuntide and its important bank holiday was approaching. There are three holy days in the year of a British zoo or safari park. These solemn festivals when the coffers are open and waiting to be filled to overflowing are the bank holidays at Easter, Whitsun and in the late summer. If the Gods smile and arrange for particularly favourable weather, these three days alone can put the zoo's accounts at the end of the year securely in the black. If it rains, or worse still snows or blows hard, these fateful few hours may well mean uncomfortable visits by the company accountants in October and bullets in the brain for a handful of lions.

Now you may well assume that the unwitting inmates of the zoo should be down on their paws, claws, fins and flippers praying to Pan for burning sun and bright blue skies on these three crucial days. Not so. Brilliant weather lures too many trippers to the beaches and swimming pools. Hot sun beating down on a car full of brats, with windows closed as per regulations while driving through lion and bear reserves, is a penance these weak souls cannot endure.

To be perfect, to lure human pilgrims to come and cough up their alms, to linger long at the hot dog stalls and treat the kids to elephant rides, these Holy Days must be warm enough to produce optimism and deter ladies in frocks from demanding an early return home, but cool enough to promote the sale of pies, jellied eels and hamburgers. The sun must be in evidence but without too much burning enthusiasm; as long as it nips unexpectedly in and out of small clouds, families considering a drive to the coast are uncertain, thrown off balance. As for rain, there is no harm at all in just a soupçon of the stuff around breakfast time. Not only does it put paid to the aspirations of would-be bathers and promenaders, it will without doubt prompt some member of the family to point out that zoos have shelters: you can always go to the monkey house if it pours down. Ah, you may say, but surely rain ruins the chances of an outing altogether? Might not the family opt en masse for television or the cinema? Not at all. At these great festivals, the British family Goes Out For The Day as Holy Writ commands. Obedience to these ancient traditions, together with faith that it might well clear up later, are all that it needs to get the family on the road. Once away, miles of traffic jams cannot stop these sturdy creatures from enjoying themselves—at the zoo, comes the chorus from the zoo directors.

Now you can understand why zoo directors can be seen actually going to church on the eve of the bank holidays, why some can be seen staring at the heavens, talking to old yokels wise in country weather-lore or scratching in the soil to see how deep the snails are burrowing, and why others take to drink, sorcery or self-flagellation.

These busy days are rough ones for zoo staff and animals alike. The latter engorge a surfeit of potato crisps, mouldy sandwiches, ice cream and foreign bodies that keep veterinarians in work for weeks afterwards. The staff sweat it out and wait for the blessed sight of the last human backside passing through the gates in the evening. As curator-cum-veterinary officer at Flamingo Park, I dashed at these times from drunkards throwing bottles at the bears to small boys locked in the lavatory to escaped monkeys causing havoc in the self-service cafeteria.

Pentland Hick always liked to have some special attraction for a bank holiday, something to get publicity in the press. That Whitsuntide it was a giant red Pacific octopus. We had had these monsters before and I had found them spectacular creatures but a bundle of trouble. The biggest problem was the shipping of them from the north Pacific. Although they were wonderfully packed in sea water and oxygen-filled plastic bags surrounded by ice and insulation and flown on non-stop jets, I was having great difficulty combating their tendency to poison themselves. On the journey they naturally emptied their bowels, and the nitrates which thus accumulated in the water made them mortally sick.

This latest octopus I met personally at London Airport. I gave him a fresh supply of sea water and ice, pumped pure oxygen into his bag and drove north like a madman with the fifty pounds of angry red mollusc slurping about on the back seat of my Citroën. A refrigerated tank was waiting for him at Flamingo Park. I had three days to get him fit before the bank holiday. After showing promise on the first day, he collapsed and finally expired on the morning of the second, thirty-six hours before the big crowds paid to see the only giant red Pacific octopus in Europe, whose pictures had been in all the papers. Now he lay in a motionless heap on the floor of his tank, although I was intrigued to see that the animal's skin retained its ability to change its colour shade and patterning according to the background on which it was placed.

Pentland Hick took the news of the octopus' demise very badly. He had spent a considerable sum bringing the red monster the best part of seven thousand miles. 'It can't be dead,' he said in that ultra-quiet voice which indicated that he was very angry.

It was time to switch my veterinarian's hat for my curatorial one. 'It can't be dead,' I said to Martin Padley some time later. 'At least, not till the end of the bank holiday.'

For an instant he looked puzzled. Then he grinned as he understood what we were going to do.

The great day dawned perfectly and the coaches and cars began to roll up for what promised to be a bumper bank holiday. Down in the aquarium below the whale and dolphin pools, the first visitors ambled around. The big refrigerated tank in one corner was the main attraction. There, nestling in some rocks and illuminated dramatically by a pale spotlight beam, was the famous new arrival. From the other side of the armour-plated glass, the holiday-makers watched the tentacles tremble as if itching to unleash their fury and saw distinctly the flapping of the mighty creature's crimson mantle. It was surely breathing. It was alive. It was fantastic!

Martin and I were rather pleased with the octopus' resurrection. It had been a simple matter of running one of the aeration pipes under the mollusc's body and adjusting the air flow so that the body vibrated just enough and the actual gas bubbles made their way to the surface through the rocks. The spotlight was a moment's work. In fact, terrible though it sounds, the dead monster presented a far grander spectacle than the live monster would have done. One thing live octopuses utterly detest is spotlighting, and it would have cleared out of the limelight in a cloud of black ink. Of course our deception was indefensible—except by the attention the beast received and by the shudders of delight from the onlookers, many of whom had come that day to see just such a sight and who went on their way none the wiser.

By noon things seemed to be going perfectly. The crowds were emerging from the aquarium and discussing enthusiastically their first face-to-face encounter with a real live Kraken. Then came the inevitable small boy, complete with small boy's earnest father. I was standing admiring our shameless bit of theatre when the pair came up to me.

'You the chap in charge?' began the father.

I nodded proudly. Now what have they lost, I thought, or have they dropped the lad's spending money into the dolphin pool?

'Clifford here, my boy, says that octopus is dead!' The words were uttered in a strident, Black Country voice. Nearby heads turned at the sound. The boy, around twelve years old, red-faced and weasel-eyed, looked up at me with a sly smirk as I registered what I hoped was incredulous horror at such sacrilege.

The father continued, 'See, Clifford knows about such things. Mad on animals, he is. Not much he doesn't know about 'em. And he says it's dead.'

I looked down at the horrid child and wondered whether I was looking at myself twenty-odd years before. I shivered at the thought.

'Why on earth should you think that?' I murmured with forced avuncularity.

557

More folk nearby were now paying attention to us. Were our sins about to find us out?

The boy spoke for the first time. 'Been down 'ere watching him for an hour. Been down as well before that. 'E don't move 'is tentacles one hinch.' He was speaking in confident triumph. 'No doubt about it, mister, that specimen of *Paroctopus apollyon* is gorn!'

Heresy! This couple of unbelievers were causing the faithful gathered in front of the great glass tank to begin muttering. Doubts were growing. Schism loomed!

To nip things in the bud I must tackle the precocious Doubting Thomas at once. Picking my words with Jesuitical care, I said loudly, 'Aha, sonny, but if you knew the giant red Pacific octopus like we know him, you would have learned that he is not given to dashing about his tank with the scatterbrained abandon of a guppy. He looks fine, to be sure.'

The boy was plainly unimpressed and wrinkled his nose. Mercifully the loudspeakers announced the beginning of the whale show and the crowd moved upstairs, including the boy and his father. When they had all gone out of sight I called Martin and dashed into the service area behind the octopus tank.

'Quick, get a pole,' I shouted. 'We must re-arrange our exhibit before that brat comes back.'

The ruddy corpse was not so co-operative this time. First it flopped over onto its back and lay looking very dead. I pushed and prodded frantically. When one tentacle did what I asked, the other seven lolled and drooped and snagged on stones. When I did manage to pose the creature in a suitable spot at the other side of the tank, the air tube secreted under its mantle released big bubbles that blooped noisily out of it and up to the surface.

'Looks like it's burping. It must be alive,' Martin grinned, keeping a wary eye open for intruders.

I groped about in the icy water with my sleeves rolled up. I was filled with uncharitable thoughts about the budding biologist, now no doubt casting a beady eye over Cuddles to make sure he was not a blown-up plastic dummy, and tried to get out of my head Sir Walter Scott's couplet about what a tangled web we weave, when first we practise to deceive.

At the exact moment that my fingers became blue and stopped functioning the octopus finally regained its composure, just as the crowd came pouring down the stairs again. The boy and the father appeared. I withdrew and watched. The boy looked puzzled, but he was a tenacious child. The afternoon drew on and during each whale show we moved the octopus about. The cunning child, with parent always in tow, popped back to the tank at unpredictable intervals. Martin and I sweated it out. It had become a battle between us and the boy, unspoken, undeclared but grim and determined. Then the boy switched the attack and appeared in the aquarium during a whale show. Martin countered neatly by innocently hosing down the concourse with a high-pressure spray. 'Sorry about this. It's the only chance I get of keeping things clean,' he explained to the couple as his powerful jet of water bouncing off the floor and walls kept them at bay long enough for me, behind the scenes, to work feverishly at moving the corpse yet again.

By the evening it was obvious we had won. The boy and his father made a final visit to the aquarium and then departed. The little fellow was looking somewhat chastened as they made their way to the coach park, and his parent was heard peevishly to remark, 'Clifford, you're not always right. Now damned well let the matter drop!'

The aquarium concourse had never looked so clean.

Martin and I paid for our duplicity when at the end of the bank holiday we removed the octopus and laid it decently to rest. Nothing, but nothing, smells more awful than a three-day dead giant octopus when it is out of its tank of water. Clifford would no doubt have been ecstatic if he had known that the experience put us off our food for the rest of the day.

Eleven

That summer was rich in fragrant, shimmering days. I saw my first adder basking on a rock on the moors above the Vale of Pickering. Evening skies were shimmering cyclamen. As the park's Chilean flamingoes seemed desperately in need of someone to give them fatherly chats about birds and bees and gooseberry bushes, I built some mud pies for them by the lake. They caught on, doubled the height of the mounds by adding more mud themselves, laid eggs on the uncomfortable tops of these spartan nests and hatched out a trio of fluffy grey chicks. I broke a rib trying to catch harbour porpoises off the Yorkshire coast, and discovered a marshy hollow where sundew plants grew wild and snapped up flies. An olive-green toad came to live in the long grass under my caravan; to save him the effort during the baking days and humid nights I brought him mealworms that I had taken from bush-babies' dinner plates. Purloining two mealworms from each of eight bush-babies did not harm them a bit but kept my toad plump and genial.

In early July, Rolf Rohwer telephoned from Rio Leon: it was time to collect the giraffe and two elephants from the defunct safari park near Madrid. Lloyd's of London were insuring the animals and insisted that a veterinarian was present while the animals were being transported, not least to tranquillise them if necessary. Yet again I found myself getting the jitters at the thought of doping a giraffe.

I flew over and met Rolf in Madrid, then we drove out to the safari park. When we arrived, a mobile crane and a brand new articulated lorry, which had been specially hired for the job, were waiting ready for the loading. The lorry was the entire fleet of a one-man firm whose sole proprietor, driver and driver's mate was standing proudly by the vehicle, pointing out to a knot of former would-be fox-lynchers the glories of the gleaming, yellow-painted, spotlessly clean monster. It was immensely long, but we saw at once that it was far too high: normally a low-loader is used for moving giraffes by road. But it had come all the four hundred miles from a village near Rio Leon and like it or not, we were going to have to use it.

I went to look at the giraffe, which had already been lured into a box whose sides reached up as high as her elbows. She was plainly very apprehensive and was beginning to strike with her hooves at the box walls. When anyone went close to her she started to stargaze, with her head and neck held in a straight line pointing up to the heavens or even tilting grotesquely back towards her tail. It was all frighteningly like poor Pedro. The crate was useless—she could vault out of it with ease—and to make a new one would take several days. Rolf made numerous phone calls and eventually arranged to borrow an old giraffe crate from the zoo in Madrid. It would arrive next day.

The first day had been wasted, but we found an isolated farmhouse where an old lady filled us with fresh bread, olive oil and tomatoes from her garden and cold, cloudy yellow wine from her cellar. Before dawn we were back in the safari park. The crate from Madrid had arrived. It was indeed old. The wood had been patched innumerable times, the leather padding of the interior had rotted into shreds, there was damp everywhere and rusty nails protruded dangerously in a hundred places. While the men set to work lining the box with hay-filled sacks and flattening the nails with hammers, we began loading the elephants onto the front of the open lorry.

The vehicle was brought alongside an earth bank and planks were placed to make a bridge. The elephants were let out of their house and we tried to tempt them on board with apples and bananas. Despite our proffered fruits, the nearby olive trees proved more attractive, and the two animals spent three hours squealing with delight as they rampaged through the groves, vandalising trees and scoffing foliage to their hearts' content. When we finally got them under control they settled down, walked up to the plank bridge and the first elephant put a tentative foot on it. The bridge gave slightly. That was enough. No great mammal with its wits about it is foolish enough to walk on unsteady ground. The elephants backed off and dug their heels in.

Another day was lost, and more of the old lady's victuals and yellow wine were called for. We had not gone a yard on our long journey towards Barcelona.

The third day started more promisingly. The elephants still distrusted profoundly the bridge onto the lorry, but with chains on their legs and an improvised winch we slowly hauled them on. Once they were in place side by side, looking out over the driver's cab, they seemed to relax and tucked in to a meal of fresh alfalfa and carrots. Now for the giraffe. The crate was ready and the crane stood poised to pick it up with steel cables. It was up to me: the insurance did not come into effect and the animal was not Rolf's until I gave the word to begin loading.

I walked round the old box. It had been repaired as much as possible, it seemed. The floor was the only doubtful part, but it looked strong enough.

I watched the giraffe nervously pacing her loose-box and wondered about tranquillising her. Pedro's sudden collapse had unnerved me—suppose this one fainted under the sedative or, like the Flamingo Park giraffe, had some physical condition which might combine with my drug to kill her. I made my decision. 'Get her into the crate with food,' I shouted. I was not going to give her a shot unless absolutely necessary.

I was surprised how quickly the gangling animal was

boxed, but once trapped in the wooden container she began to kick and her breathing rate increased tremendously. If anyone got within twenty feet of the box, she rattled round in a panic. It did not look good.

I gritted my teeth and gave the order to start loading. The giraffe was Rolf's from that moment. Back in pin-striped London EC3, underwriters with bowler hats and high blood-cholesterol levels would about now be leaving the Underground at Bank, unaware that I had just put them on risk to the tune of £3000.

When the crane's jib with its four cables swung out over her little prison, the giraffe became even more alarmed. She began stargazing again. I reached for the dart-gun and syringes—anything more and I would have no choice but to sedate her. Four of the Spaniards darted in and attached the cables. The crane took the strain. With much creaking and groaning, the crate started to rise. Soon the boxful of unwilling giraffe swung in the morning air ten feet above my head. The animal's long neck curved round the steel ropes as it waved its head from one side to the other. Bits of wood and puffs of dust fell from the crate. The jib reached maximum height and began to traverse steadily towards the lorry.

Suddenly there was a loud crack. The crate lurched and shuddered. A stout plank of wood whistled past my head and crashed to the ground. From the bottom of the box I could see the two hind feet of the giraffe protruding as far as the fetlocks. The floor of the old crate was breaking up. Any second, the whole one and a half tons of animal could come plummeting sickeningly down to the sunbaked ground.

'Move it, move it!' I yelled, dashing towards the crane driver's cabin. 'Lo mas rapido que posible! Fast as you bloody well can!'

The man understood at once. The crane accelerated, the jib swung over towards the lorry at full speed and the cables were begun on their descent simultaneously. Unceremoniously, the giraffe crate made a bumpy landing on the metal flooring behind the elephants. Chunks of rotten wood fell away. The animal reeled but remained upright as her feet were pushed back through the holes in the floor. She was aboard safely.

Rolf and I were both visibly shaken. Each of us could visualise the scene if the beast had gone through the crate bottom at that height. It would have been a surprise but nothing more for a tiger, maybe even a bear, but a giraffe's legs fracture if you no more than look at them: a stumble over a fist-sized rock can snap them. We had had a narrow escape, and neither of us dared think about how we were going to unload the beast.

'Let's have a word with the driver and then get going,' said Rolf, rolling his eyes. 'Mad onagers, fox-hangers, lousy crates—this place is bad medicine.'

The lorry driver was standing in front of the shining silver radiator grille, looking proudly down the length of his enormous vehicle. The elephants were calmly munching away at the front and the giraffe seemed less nervy now that the cables had been taken away. She blinked down at the assembled men gathered round the back of the lorry. The distance from the ground to the tips of her 'hat-pegs' was a daunting eight yards; it looked like an attempt at the altitude record in animal transporting. 'My right arm for a low-loader,' I muttered as I reflected on what our journey was going to be like. I did not know the roads we would be using, but I knew for certain that there would be a bunch of bridges, pipes, cables and other impedimenta strung across the road at just the right height to decapitate our lofty purchase.

'Now, Señor, about our trip,' Rolf was asking the driver. 'How long do you think it will take us to reach Rio Leon?'

The driver was a tubby man in his mid-thirties who sweated continually and who took a swig every few minutes from a litre bottle of red wine which he carried in his boiler-suit hip pocket. He looked at the sky, screwed up his face and scratched thoughtfully at his buttocks. After a few moments he replied, 'Mas o menos, around about a week, I guess.'

'A what?' I gasped. 'A week to do 350, maybe 400 miles? What's he talking about?'

The driver looked resentful and reached for his red wine again.

'The doctor's right,' said Rolf. 'How do you work that out?'

'Pero señores, the distance. The roads I must take. I have to obey the permisos. The authorities, the policia, the Madrid municipal office, the guardia civil, they have laid down the rules in the permisos.' He fumbled inside his shirt and pulled out a sticky sheaf of papers covered with the grandiose stamps and innumerable signatures of Spanish bureaucracy.

'What rules?' growled Rolf.

'Señor, there are so many. We cannot cross Madrid by day, there are some roads we must not use and under no circumstances must we travel on the bits of motorway between here and Rio Leon. Also I need to eat, siesta and sleep. So you see, we arrive no problem in one week, I think.'

'Balls to that!' I exclaimed angrily. 'I'm not having those animals up there for a week, unable to get them off for exercise. Let's get cracking and keep motoring. We'll run through the night, permisos or no permisos. One of us can take turns with him at the driving. If we're stopped we can blarney our way out of it. I've always found policemen intrigued by the novelty of big zoo animals on the move. I've never had any trouble bending the law in such matters.'

Rolf nodded. 'I agree. Bulldust baffles brains. We'll have to try it.' He turned to the driver again. 'Now then, Señor, we must get there quicker than one week. We must travel by day and by night if possible. I will arrange the permisos.'

The driver became agitated. 'But I can lose my licence just like that, pouf! I must obey the permisos.'

'Give me the permisos, my friend,' said Rolf. 'I'll carry

them and have them altered and stamped officially as we go along. Dr Taylor and I are going to be in the car driving directly behind your lorry. When we need to have a permiso changed, we'll overtake you, drive to the guardia or wher-ever and explain the problem.'

'But, Señor, the night driving! My siesta!'

'Don't worry. We'll relieve you. And there'll be a fat bonus for you in cash on top of our agreed price for the transport.'

Looking less than happy, the fat man agreed. We began loading bales of alfalfa onto the lorry and instructing the four fox-lynchers who were to travel on the back of the vehicle how to keep an eye on the animals. They cut tree branches with small forks at one end and put them on board; with these I hoped they would be able to lift and manoeuvre cables and wires in our path without themselves or, more importantly, the animals getting electrocuted. We did not forget buckets and two galvanized tubs, since in this heat the massive creatures would require frequent watering. At last we were ready. The lorry engine roared into life, the men clung to the vehicle sides as it began to judder forwards, and Rolf and I in the car took up our position three yards behind the sparkling yellow tailboard. We were off.

Rocking and reeling over the hard-baked uneven ground, we slowly approached the road outside the safari park. The elephants leaned for support on the yellow slats that ran along the sides of the lorry. The giraffe bumped and banged in its crate.

'She'll have swollen joints and deep abrasions before we've gone a mile at this rate,' I told Rolf gloomily. 'If things don't improve when we hit the road, I must call off the whole affair.'

As we went through the gateway onto the road, the heavy section of slatted metal on the left side gave way under the elephants' weight and crashed onto the tarmac. A moment later the right-hand section followed suit. They lay bent and chipped in the gutter. Everyone stopped. Rolf jumped up

566

and down on the metal to try and straighten it. I hammered at the distortions with the car jack. Yellow paint-flakes flew. The driver held his head. With wire and rope we fixed the bits of the lorry back into place, but a certain newness had already departed from the front half of the vehicle.

Under way again, the animals settled down remarkably. The giraffe seemed surprisingly soothed by the movement. She turned to face the front and became as quiet as a mouse. Perhaps it was the flow of air over her face that she enjoyed, or maybe it was the constantly changing scenery. As we entered clumps of overhanging foliage, I was delighted to see her take mouthfuls of buds and leaves, quickly coiling her tongue round twigs and letting her momentum rip the morsels away. On corners she balanced herself expertly, and she was no longer coming into contact with the sides of the crate.

The elephants, too, were interested in the abundance of herbage passing above, around and even below them. They used their trunks to grab bigger helpings than the giraffe behind them, and sizeable branches came toppling down into the lorry. The two elephants considered themselves to be off on a tour gastronomique. The first few miles were on a twisting road through forests of pine trees whose cones were fat with succulent kernels. Having tried some of these, the elephants found them to their tooth and began feasting happily. Little squeals of joy would greet another branch brought down with a hollow clang onto the roof of the driver's cab. More yellow flakes of paint were left behind us in the dust.

The animal keepers on the back of the lorry had, in the usual Spanish style, stocked up copious supplies of red wine for the journey. I had always been alarmed by the way in which Spanish keepers began a day working in the reserves with deadly and powerful wild animals by having a couple of large brandies for breakfast and then taking bottles of wine with them on the job. These would be consumed while guarding the gates of the tiger section or standing in a kiosk in the bear enclosure armed with something about as big and lethal as a walking stick. Our chaps on the lorry were true to form and more ominously we saw that the driver had apparently swallowed his private supply and was being passed more by one of his compatriots who squeezed past the elephants and handed a couple of bottles in through the cab window as the lorry bowled along.

By late afternoon we drove into the outskirts of Madrid and faced the first test of our permisos. The lorry driver pulled up and declared that he would not go a foot further unless Rolf did what he had said he could do: get the permits altered by the hundred and one civil servants who had signed, stamped, initialled and endorsed them. It was four o'clock and the offices were closed. Only the policia head-quarters was still open, so leaving the lorry by the roadside surrounded by whooping children and ancient ladies in black who stared incredulously, Rolf and I went to see the Chief of Police.

We sat for what seemed like hours in the corridor outside El Jefe's office, while the permits were inspected, shuttled back and forth by a bevy of minions and finally stacked on the big man's desk. When we were called to his presence, he went through the necessary rigmarole of 'being busy on other important matters', made some phone calls, sniffed, coughed and pulled faces as he thumbed listlessly through some papers and finally sat in ominous silence, staring out of the window at the view of a bleached brick wall. At last, when my kneecaps were beginning to protest their boredom painfully, the Chief spoke.

'No es posible,' he said. 'It can't be done. You must travel only by night. You cannot come through Madrid. I am sorry but the Mayor's office alone can alter that. You must see them tomorrow.'

Rolf started to argue, at first reasonably and then loudly, with an occasional daring thump on the Chief's table. Here

568

comes my first peek inside a Spanish dungeon, I thought.

'Dammit, it looks like we're going to have to push on and risk them grabbing us,' Rolf eventually murmured to me, exasperated. That is the snag of asking permission: if we were caught now, we could hardly plead ignorance or innocent mistake.

'I assume, Rolf,' I said loudly and clearly in simple Spanish, 'that you have explained to El Jefe the nature of the giraffe and two elephants?' Before he could begin to look puzzled I continued, staring him hard in the eyes, 'That these creatures for your safari park are travelling in exchange for a flight of Imperial eagles that you have obtained for Madrid, to be presented to El Caudillo, General Franco himself?'

Rolf shook his head solemnly.

'No, Doctor, I haven't,' he said, also in Spanish, 'but no matter what happens I shall feel obliged to keep my side of the bargain. The eagles will still be sent to the Generalissimo.'

As one we stood up, trying to look resigned and dignified in defeat. 'Muchas gracias y adiós, Jefe,' said Rolf.

The police chief began to cough loudly as we turned away. 'Er . . . uno momento, Señores,' he said sharply as we reached the door. 'I cannot promise what will happen beyond Madrid on the rest of your journey, but perhaps I can, just on this one occasion . . .'

Ten minutes later we were back at the lorry and showing the driver our amended permiso. 'Get going at once,' Rolf instructed, 'straight through the middle of the city. Rush hour, daylight, it don't matter a damn! Pedestrian precincts, Triumphal Arch if you have to—straight as an arrow! Let's clear the city and make some good mileage before we begin night driving.'

'B-but how?' stuttered the driver.

There was no need to answer. Six blue and white uniformed motor-cycle cops roared up to us on BMWs.

569

Their leader explained that they were the personal escort of the Chief, and were to see us safely through the capital and on the road to Guadalajara. With three of the cops in front and three behind, the lorry and our car charged through that delightful and bustling city at 5.30 pm. Sirens screaming and red lights flashing, we swept up the grand avenues, through traffic lights that were against us, across squares closed to traffic and down the normally choked back streets of the old city. Taxis and buses screeched to a halt, folk flattened themselves against walls around the Plaza Puerta del Sol, windows were flung open as we careered along. The giraffe carried herself with the poise of a Queen of Spain making a Royal Progress. With her two bulky grey equerries in place at her feet, her aristocratic features looked down upon the common herd that thronged the pavements.

On the far side of the city we stopped to thank our police escort, water the animals and do a general check. The sky was cloudless and the deep pink of a Cuban flamingo as our driver and the keepers disappeared into a bar to replenish their wine bottles. Climbing up onto her crate I found that the giraffe was now much more approachable and could actually be touched by hand without lashing out. Obviously travel was broadening her mind. Her legs were in good condition, with no rubs or abrasions, and she took alfalfa and water greedily. The elephants were still content, though the lorry was now carrying a fair load of elephant droppings, which steamed away on the once spotless yellow floor.

'What do you think about night driving?' Rolf asked. 'Not much trouble with wires so far, but it could get worse.'

Although the city run itself had been fast and furious, elsewhere we had already been brought to a slow crawl by all sorts of wires and cables that crossed the road. Unless you do move giraffes by road, I suspect you never really appreciate the vast numbers of cords, ropes, cables, wires and conduits that infest the landscape. They are like Father Brown's postman, invisible through being utterly commonplace.

570

Spain certainly must be well in the running for first place in the most wired-up country competition. Carrying electricity, telephone conversations and often, we came to suspect, nothing at all, the wires festoon poles and masts and lamp standards at all levels. We had to avoid them all if I did not want to handle my first case of electrocuted giraffe or have her garrotted in true Spanish style. On the other hand we were anxious to avoid bringing the whole of Spain between Madrid and Barcelona grinding to a halt by severing power and communications links along our way. Wine or no wine, the men with their forked poles had quickly become adept at judging which wires were likely to be too low, neatly intercepting them and lifting them up so that the giraffe's head passed underneath.

'Yes, the wire lifting is going well,' I agreed. 'It should be possible to do it at night as well as long as our headlights pick out the overhead cables.'

When we got rolling again I calculated our average speed. The escort in Madrid had been a great help, but still we were not doing much better than ten miles an hour. Barely had we picked up speed after lifting one wire before we had to slow down for another. What was more, we found that the wires were often laid across our path in fiendish groupings of six or seven at different heights, tensions and thicknesses; it was a sort of minefield in the air. Our men soon had little time for their wine. We were getting out into the dull, flat country of red earth that stretches north-east of Madrid. Little groups of houses dotted the roadside every few kilometres and they positively bristled with wire traps. Even an isolated half-ruined hut by the edge of a cornfield was likely to be wired up for some purpose.

The sun set and we continued to press on. The men were working fluidly, passing the overhead obstructions from one forked stick to another with considerable skill. If they were quick enough, it meant that our driver did not have to reduce the speed quite so agonisingly low. Twilight set in, and the

571

pink sky rapidly filled with smokey violet hues which deepened as the moon rose. We could still all see the wires sharply outlined against the cloudless sky. What we were slow to realise was that our sense of perspective was about to be lost. Slumped in the seats of our Seat Saloon, Rolf and I dawdled along at a snail's pace with our eyes fixed on the giraffe. Suddenly we saw her head snap back. A wire had caught her momentarily. I cursed, Rolf honked and we both shouted. Then it happened again, and again—nothing serious, just quick pluckings of the animal's head by a wire. There was no sign of spark or shock, just an occasional metallic twang. We had to face it: the twilight had destroyed our ability to estimate the distance and height of the wires as the lorry approached. At our slow speed I was not so much afraid of a serious neck wound as of the strand of metal damaging the large, delicate eyes of the animal.

A hundred yards ahead we could see a restaurant. 'Let's stop there,' I said. 'We must wait until it's completely dark and then see if our headlights and the moonlight change matters.'

We pulled in, parked the lorry under some trees where the animals could use self-service and, after watering them again, went in for beer and tortillas. After the meal we took the car on a short wire-hunt. It was useless. There was no reflection on overhead wires from our headlights or from the moon. Night travel was out. We prepared to camp.

Next morning when the grey-blue sky was just light enough for us to be able to see the wires and judge their height, we set off. It was tedious sitting behind the lorry, constantly moving up and down between second and third gear. The countryside was unspectacular as we approached Guadalajara and we were under a permanent, horn-blowing barrage from motorists behind who could not understand why we did not overtake the slow lorry.

The originally straight sides of the lorry were now grotes-

572

quely distorted. Our view from directly behind was one of a once sleek vehicle that had developed alarming bulges round its waistline. The elephants seemed to prefer leaning outwards into the slipstream. The metal sides did not fall off any more, they were simply buckled outwards.

Not long into the second day we encountered our first really low bridge. With some trepidation we crept up to it. Forked sticks would be no use now. The best we could do was to drive down the centre of the road and try somehow to persuade the giraffe to lower her head. We tried to get her mouth down to some tasty food, but alfalfa proved no attraction, so we offered apples, bananas and finally, under protest, the sugary buns which the men had bought for their mid-morning snacks but which Rolf ordered them to place before her. She licked them briefly but did not keep her head down for more than a second or two.

'Try tapping her very gently on her hat-pegs with one of your sticks,' I called up. One of the men tried it, but she calmly swung her head away from him.

Rolf sighed deeply. 'We'll just have to take a chance,' he muttered. 'There'll be lots more beside this one, I reckon. Roll on slow!'

The driver heard his shout and inched forwards. Closer and closer came the keystone of the archway. The giraffe was around two feet too high for the bridge. I held my breath. Then, as naturally as could be, when the stone was almost touching her, she ducked just enough and found herself under the bridge.

'God don't let her suddenly crack her head up onto the roof,' I said aloud. I had seen too many giraffes scalped by blows against their short, firmly fixed horns.

The lorry edged on. The giraffe stayed sensibly down, clear of the roof by three or four inches. Two minutes later we pulled out at the far side. The humans involved cheered with relief while the giraffe looked down benevolently, wondering what the dwarfs were making such a fuss about.

When we had gone through Guadalajara, where Rolf quickly avoided wrangles over permisos by passing out a bottle of vintage Osborne brandy to a policeman in a white helmet controlling traffic at a roundabout, the day became a succession of wires, cables and bridges. Past houses of red adobe, blood-red soil, fields of stubble stretching into the heat haze and hills of ugly, fractured, yellow rock, our strange caravan made its painstaking way. Old men in berets crossed themselves as we went by, frowning in doorways at glimpses of beasts they had never believed existed. Boys clambered up the sides of the lorry to touch elephant skin, and knots of blushing girls clutched one another when the giants gushed waterfalls of urine. Shopkeepers came out and offered bunches of radishes and artichokes for the animals to eat; to us they gave slices of Serrano ham and glasses of wine as we waited for some particularly intricate web of wire to be unravelled.

Approaching Zaragoza we found ourselves weaving down from the high plain along narrow rocky gorges dotted with scrub and sheets of scree. When we reached the first of a series of tunnels cut through the hillside, the giraffe showed once again how eminently sensible she was. Tunnels were just long bridges to her—head well down, turn your long-lashed eyes towards the glow of light at the far end and caramba! There's nothing to it. Not once did she touch rock or raise her head suddenly to scrape painfully against the ceiling.

Out of the final tunnel we found ourselves being waved down by a pair of green-uniformed Guardia Civil. This para-military organisation is built up of men who are tougher, brighter and often meaner than the average Spanish policeman. Our lorry driver was out of his cab and nervously hopping about the two Guardias when we walked up. We were on the right road at the right time and our permisos for this section up to Zaragoza should be in order. Rolf handed them over and the two unsmiling Guardias pored over them. They asked for everyone's driving licences, inspected registration plates and went through their usual routine, oblivious to the elephants which were clumping about above them and giving an impatient trumpet or two. Rolf gave them the patter about the amazing trip we were on, giraffe, elephants going all those miles, animal doctor from England in attendance, Rio Leon Safari Park—great place to go, would they like a couple of free tickets—and so on, but they continued humming and hawing, peering and cross-checking, without so much as a glance at the animals. Perhaps they thought we were Basque terrorists indulging in some fiendishly elaborate exploit using elephants as a distraction.

As the Guardias stood sternly by the side of the lorry, grunting and passing sheets of paper to one another, the elephants decided they had had enough of this waiting. If I had been a bit quicker I could have averted what happened next, but I was too busy wondering what, if anything, might be wrong with our papers. The rushing sound from above warned me too late, and a pungent, warm cascade of yellow liquid poured through the gap at the bottom of the lorry's side. To the elephants' relief and our horror, the two Guardias were drenched instantly in strong-smelling urine.

Swearing, they both staggered away from the lorry and began spitting furiously. Their faces were wet. Some had gone down inside their shirt-collars. Their holsters were dripping; I hoped their guns were waterproof. It was nobody's fault, although we apologised profusely. What else could we do? There was nothing we could wipe off them. They were just soaked through—and smelled awful.

'A million apologies, Señores,' said Rolf, with a face that was incredibly straight and sincere. 'If our papers are in order, then, may I offer you some advice? Even after washing with water and soap, the smell of elephant urine clings to the skin.' The two Guardias listened with misery written all over their brown faces. 'So to remove it, rub the damp used grains of coffee all over your body. I have found that this will remove the unpleasant odour. But be quick now, before it gets embedded deep.'

Thrusting a soggy collection of documents towards us, the two men swore some more and hurried away to their motor-bikes. With a kick and a roar they set off at speed in the direction of Zaragoza.

When we had stopped laughing so much that I gave myself cramp, I said, 'Can you imagine what their Captain will say when they report they've been peed on by elephants?'

'And when they start grabbing all the police-station coffee for an after-shower talc.'

'That bit about coffee grains. That wasn't just a leg-pull, was it? Does it work?'

Rolf grinned. 'It sure does. I've used it a hundred times in Zambia.'

He was right: the next time I had to rid myself of elephant essence after taking a urine sample at a circus, coffee grains proved a remarkable deodorant.

The lorry driver was obviously weary by now, but refused to let one of us take over. At each stop he would walk slowly round his vehicle, lugubriously taking note of its steady deterioration. The comfortably leaning elephants had now pushed a deep bulge into the slatted sections of metal on each side. The cab roof was dented and chipped as if raked by shrapnel, and it was becoming plain that a man with entrepreneurial flair might make a million by bottling elephant urine and selling it as the ultimate in paint removers; the yellow had vanished from the front of the lorry and the wondrous solvent was now making short work of the rust-coloured undercoat. The driver was having to travel and drink his wine in silence, for his radio aerial had been thrown away by one of the elephants doing a bit of tidying up during a boring stop while a cluster of particularly devilish sets of cables was outwitted.

576

Our growing expertise at wire-raising, coupled with the giraffe's impressive commonsense approach to each and every obstacle, had increased our average speed considerably. By the evening of the second day we were on the outskirts of Zaragoza city. Rolf and I went ahead and persuaded a small and impressionable traffic policeman in a blue uniform and white topee who was standing in the centre of a dusty plaza whistling and waving furiously and being totally ignored by a mêlée of motorists, to come with us and conduct us through the centre. He took one look at the lorry with its usual crowd of curious spectators and puffed up visibly. His dark eyes gleamed with excitement as he snapped his coat cuffs and pulled his white gloves tight. Then, pointing to the space between the two elephants just behind the cab, he proclaimed firmly, 'I will stand there.'

Inside with the driver would have been the sensible spot, but our policeman was having none of it. He obviously felt that a leader must be seen to lead, and had no qualms about standing so close to a pair of four-ton giants. I admired his style, but warned him about the dung on the floor, the possibility that he might have his official topee forcibly removed and eaten or that his uniform could be drooled on.

He was deaf to such cautions. 'I will stand there,' he repeated, 'and give directions to the driver. It is no problem, Señores.' He explained that by shouting and banging on the left or right side of the cab roof he would guide the man sitting below without any difficulty.

We watched as the policeman climbed up onto the lorry, squeezed into position and then stood with his elbows on the cab roof, looking proudly down at the crowd. It was a fine sight. Flanked by the two impassive beasts, his diminutive uniformed figure reminded me of the Viceroy of India in the days of the Raj turning out for a Durbar. To the cheers of the folk on the pavement the lorry set off, its big engine roaring. We heard the policeman starting to shout, we saw his gloved hands beat on the cab as the lorry pulled out into the

577

swarming traffic, then all was hidden behind a haze of exhaust fumes. We jumped into our car to catch them up.

Three hours later, we found them. It had taken innumerable calls to the police department and much driving to and fro and round and round the city by us, who were worried at losing a giraffe and two elephants, and by the police department, who eventually realised that they had lost an officer who was supposed to be on point duty.

They were run to earth finally on the road to Pamplona, ten miles north of the city and going steadfastly in the wrong direction. It was almost dark. At any moment the overhead wires would become invisible. The policeman was still in his cockpit, his topee was straight and unblemished, his gloves were intact and there was no ropy saliva on his blue coat. He climbed down to face the music. Two car-loads of his colleagues, Rolf and I, tired and worried, and a brace of Guardia Civil listened po-faced as he gave forth a torrent of words and gesticulated like Quixote's windmills. Apparently his communication system with the driver had been faulty from the start. His shouts had been drowned by the engine noise, and his banging had been confused by his elephantine companions hammering with their trunks. He had tried to get back to our men who were lifting wire busily from positions beside the giraffe crate, but he had been squashed and impeded repeatedly by the elephants. He ended his explanation with a shrug and a salute.

One of his superiors spoke for the first time. 'Mire! Look at your boots, Garcia,' he snarled, pointing downwards.

We all peered through the gloom at the unfortunate policeman's feet. Unlike the rest of him, they had not avoided trouble, and he was walking on two massive cakes of elephant manure that totally enveloped his regulation boots. Rolf's elephants seemed to be delighting in discomfiting the Spanish constabulary.

The matter was closed over several bottles of cognac which all of us, in and out of uniform, consumed in a nearby

578

inn. We also bivouacked there for the night, drawing the lorry up beside a tree-covered bank. The animals began browsing enthusiastically over the side.

Before turning in, I managed to get a phone call through to home. Shelagh was coping with worried owners of parrots and gerbils fretfully awaiting my return. She had passed a falcon with what sounded like severe respiratory trouble down to an eager Andrew at Cambridge University, put a stitch in a hedgehog and been over to Oldham to console a distraught old lady whose even more ancient Patas monkey had collapsed suddenly and died. There had been trouble with a bison at Belle Vue; she had asked my old partner in general practice, Norman Whittle, to go and see it. Flamingo Park was running smoothly.

'One of these days you're going to have to get a partner in the zoo business,' she said. 'What happens if there's a really serious emergency while you're off on one of your trips?'

It was good to know that she was looking after things, but she was right. Not only was the practice keeping me fully stretched, but at this rate there would soon be enough work for another partner, who could also cover for me when I was away and so take some of the pressure which at the moment I was unfairly loading onto Shelagh.

Next morning I was wakened before daybreak by a cacophony of extraordinary sounds. The elephants were making a fearsome din, trumpeting, bellowing and squealing. There was a clanging of metal and splintering of wood, men's shouts and the dull thudding of feet running across hard ground. Bleary-eyed, I went to the open window and looked out. Our men were scuttling excitedly round the lorry, but the dark bulks of the elephants were indistinguishable.

I ran downstairs, pulling on trousers and sweater against the early morning chill. It did not take long to find the cause of the bedlam: the two elephants were reeling drunk. They were smashed, sozzled, pie-eyed. Wobbly-legged and

579

droopy-faced, they staggered and stumbled against the lorry sides, making a thunderous noise. There were sections of twisted metal panel on the ground all around. Only the restraining chains on their hind legs, bolted into the steel flooring, kept them from blasting their riotous way to freedom. Like human drunkards they were maudlin one moment, genial the next and then again argumentative and ill-tempered. Their eyes rolled as mischievous jollity alternated with red-rimmed malevolence. Stroke one and it would rub dreamily against you for some time and then suddenly flail you irritably with its trunk.

I had seen the same thing before, not in zoos or circuses but in Africa, where at certain seasons of the year elephant herds will travel miles to have a week-long binge on the over-ripe, fermenting fruit of the so-called miracle tree. It is best to steer clear of such gargantuan bacchanalia, for there are always a few over-indulgers around with hangovers and long tusks. Here there were no miracle berries. I went over to the trees on which our elephants had been browsing. They were medlars. Fruit lay in the grass. As I picked some up and pulped it between my fingers, I caught the winey aroma. The elephants were high on medlars that had rotted so far that they were fermenting and producing alcohol. They would have the headaches today; I would have them tomorrow, when the inevitable diarrhoea ensued. For the first time on the trip I would have to give the animals an injection. I filled 60-cc syringes with vitamin B complex to speed the breaking down of the alcohol in the blood and smaller, 10-cc ones with a light sedative. Jabbing the haunches of the swaying sots, I started the drying-out process.

An hour later our troupe set off once more. All was silence on board the patched-up lorry. Two elephants lay drowsing and exhaling steamy, fruity fumes, while from on high the giraffe, who had apparently either eaten none of the alcoholic vegetation or possessed the liver of an Irish navvy, looked down with a faintly disapproving gaze.

580

Although forbidden to use the motorway on the last lap, we could not resist the thought of the time that it should save us. It took only a few furtive minutes to alter the wording on one of our permisos and to fudge up some imposing signatures. We joined the motorway but soon found that although it was free of overhead wires, there were far more bridges than on the older roads. Our average speed did not rise much, so forgery had yielded meagre rewards.

At last, at the end of the third day, we reached Rio Leon and prepared to unload at once in the light of car headlamps. First to be tackled was the giraffe. We had a crane ready for the crucial lift. Sheets of wood were dropped into the crate and pushed under the animal's legs to block the holes through which she might slip again. Rolf gave the order and the crate slowly moved upwards. The giraffe stayed put. The wooden walls had broken away from the floor. It looked slightly improper; as if the lady's wooden skirt was being ripped off. 'Down!' yelled Rolf, and the walls bumped back into place.

Whereas the elephants could be walked off onto a bank and then rounded up, the nervous, fragile giraffe could not be let loose that way. Eventually we hit on the idea of bringing another box onto the lorry, moving the giraffe into it and then, once she was secure, lifting the new, sound box off. It took all night for a suitable box to be found, modified and strengthened. As dawn broke on the fourth day, we at last freed the giraffe at the entrance to her new quarters. She walked sedately in to meet her new mate.

The two chastened boozers were no trouble to unload. Meekly they trooped off the lorry. Their sedatives had worn off and I had buckets of boiled rice and hay tea prepared to ward off any stomach upset following their celebrations. They swallowed their bland medicine politely. Both looked fit enough, although perhaps a little distant in the eye. I could imagine them wishing for a football-sized Alka-Seltzer. I sympathised and looked towards the lake at the valley bottom. 'I suggest, Rolf,' I said, 'that they do what you or I would do on the morning after the night before—have a refreshing shower.'

Minutes later the two animals were happily squirting cool water over themselves and dunking their foreheads with relief. I could relax; all the animals were safely delivered, and I had managed to avoid another confrontation with the need to dope a giraffe.

Twelve

In my office at Flamingo Park I was going through Andrew's dung list. While I was in Spain he had collected samples of droppings from every animal in the collection. With a microscope he had painstakingly searched for parasite eggs, identified them and calculated the actual number contained in every gramme of dung. Now complete and neatly tabulated, Andrew's figures gave a valuable run-down on the present status of everything from elephants to egrets. The complicated cycles of parasites passing through a variety of hosts, the ingenious methods they use to protect themselves and to find and enter their prey, their amazing reproduction rate and the subtle damage they can inflict deep inside the body are of crucial importance to zoo veterinarians. Andrew was providing valuable intelligence.

The telephone rang. It was the main gate. 'Someone to see you. Big car. Posh,' said the cashier. 'Urgent, they say.'

'Send them over, please.'

As I walked outside, a pre-war Daimler limousine, gleaming black with headlamps like frogs' eyes, drew up. A uniformed chauffeur leapt out, opened the rear door and stood smartly to attention. After some seconds a lady emerged. The chauffeur saluted crisply and closed the door behind her. My visitor was a tall, skinny woman of at least seventy years. She did not stoop, nor was her back hunched, but she somehow tilted the whole of her body forwards as if supported by invisible wires. I wondered why she did not fall flat on her face. The way she slanted, together with her scrawny long neck and aquiline features, reminded me strongly of an Egyptian vulture. She was wearing a big black straw hat and a long green velvet dress that smelled of camphor, eau de Cologne and mentholated vapour rub. Deep-set behind curtains and palisades of waxy flesh, two lizard eyes fixed me.

'Dr Taylor? How do you do. I'm Philomena Rind, from Harrogate.' Harrogate is the spa town near Leeds where the woollen merchants and others who, as they say in the North, 'think they're no cat muck' dwell in stone mansions behind thick privet and rhododendrons.

As I showed the old lady into my room, I wondered what animal she had got wrapped in a blanket on the floor of the Daimler. Animals resemble owners in my experience, and I weighed up the possibilities. Hardly a vulture or condor, despite the strong resemblance. Macaw? A strong possibility. Monkey? No, Miss Rind was not one of the distinctive monkey-owning types. Hawk or falcon? No: once upon a time maybe, but not now with her powdered throat and fingernails as long as a mandarin's. Her vibrations were of something quite different. Reptilian? Yes, that was it. She was going to send for the chauffeur in a moment and he would bear in a dyspeptic alligator or some such.

'An urgent matter, I believe, Miss Rind,' I said.

She sat clutching a large velvet handbag and scrutinising me intently with the lizard eyes. 'Yes, indeed, Doctor. It's Hugo.' She unclasped the handbag and put a hand inside. 'Hugo, my dear old friend.' Her hand emerged from the bag and carefully set something on my desk top.

It was a terrapin, as big as a saucer and with handsome striped head and red flashes behind the eyes. It began to row its way clumsily over the surface of my blotter.

Hugo's owner leaned even further towards me and spoke again in confidential tones. 'Do you see his eyes, Doctor, how they're becoming sore? And he's not eating a thing. That's why I've come to see you.' Her voice became a whisper. 'Mr Lawrence sent me.'

I picked the terrapin up and looked at it closely. The under-shell was softer than normal, yielding easily to finger pressure. The eyes were indeed inflamed and oozing cloudy tears. It was typical terrapin trouble—a deficiency of vitamin A and probably vitamin D and minerals too, most likely brought on by a diet of too much raw meat and no nourishing pond snails with their livers rich in the essential vitamins. Under that dark green shell there would be a pair of kidneys starting to pack up. An injection of vitamin A in oil might be just in time. It is an irreversible and lethal disease once it is well established.

'Mr Lawrence?' I remarked. The name was not familiar to me. 'Is he your vet in Harrogate?'

Miss Rind sat back and looked miffed. 'Dear me, no. Certainly not.' She seemed to soften slightly and leaned forwards once more. 'Doctor, do you know D. H. Lawrence?'

'D. H. Lawrence? The writer? *Sons and Lovers*, you mean? I thought he died years ago.'

'Yes, passed on. Have you never read his poetry? He wrote beautiful poems about tortoises.'

Oh Lord, I thought, a time-wasting crank. Poetry— what next? Anyway I never realised that Lawrence wrote poetry, let alone anything about tortoises. This must be a batty old bird with more money than she knows what to do with.

'I'm afraid I haven't,' I said coldly. 'I thought sexy gamekeepers were more in his line. Now, about this terrapin, the problem undoubtedly is . . .'

Miss Rind stood up abruptly and loomed over me. 'I haven't come for a diagnosis on Hugo, Doctor,' she interrupted with a boom. 'All I want is what Mr Lawrence instructs—Balm of Micomicon.'

I was totally at a loss. I had better start from the beginning, slowly. 'Please do sit down, Miss Rind. Just tell me the whole story.'

She lowered herself into the chair and started whispering

585

again. 'Are you a believer, Doctor? In the after-life, the world beyond?'

'Well, er, yes. I suppose so.'

'Good. You wouldn't be one of us, I suppose—a spiritualist?'

'Afraid not.'

Hugo was snuffling about the plastic sachets containing Andrew's dung samples. He did not appear to be paying any attention to the conversation. Was he supposed to be a spiritualist, I wondered.

'Well, I am a believer, Doctor,' Miss Rind went on. 'I'm not fortunate enough to have been gifted with clairvoyant powers myself, but I have been greatly helped and uplifted by Mr Pickersgill.'

'Mr Pickersgill?'

'Our wonderful leader at Otley Road Spiritualist Church. A most talented medium.'

'And Hugo?' I interposed quickly.

Hugo had just recklessly launched himself over the edge of my desk when Miss Rind shot out an arm that looked like a flamingo's leg and took the catch in mid-air.

'Hugo here became ill, like he is now, about two weeks ago,' continued the old lady placidly, as though nothing happened. 'Mr Pickersgill held a wonderful séance shortly after Hugo stopped eating, and that's when Mr Lawrence came through.'

'Came through?'

'He's on the other side now but still interested in animals—tortoises and things. He wrote so beautifully about tortoises when he was among us. "You draw your head forward, slowly, from your little wimple . . ." That's from his poem, "Baby Tortoise". Odd you've never read it, someone like you.'

I was losing the thread again. 'I'm sorry, Miss Rind, but I still don't understand.'

For the first time, the old lady smiled. 'No, of course,

586

Doctor. Anyway, Mr Pickersgill suddenly found that Mr Lawrence was coming through, trying to communicate a message. And it was for me. I'd spoken on previous occasions to my father and to a Red Indian chief called Fire Mountain, but here was a famous writer concerning himself with me!'

It was interesting, but I must get back to being a zoo vet. Again I said, 'And Hugo?'

'That's who the message was about. Mr Lawrence said he knew Hugo was ill, that his eyes were diseased and that there would be no difficulty in curing him if I anointed them with—and he was quite clear about the name—Balm of Micomicon.'

'I'm afraid I've never heard of the stuff,' I said.

Miss Rind sighed heavily and flapped her arms. 'Just what the vets and doctors and chemists in Harrogate and Leeds all say. They've never heard of it and have no suggestions to make. That's why I came to you, knowing you have so many reptiles under your care.'

'But perhaps the name's wrong, garbled. If it's not in the drug lists, maybe it doesn't exist, unless it's some obscure old herbal remedy.'

'Dr Taylor!' She stood up again. 'I hope you're not suggesting that one who's passed into the Greater Awareness would lie. Mr Lawrence was quite specific. What's more, we used the ouija board afterwards and it spelled out Balm of Micomicon for all to see!'

I fetched a dictionary. There was no mention of Micomicon or anything like it.

'I'm sorry,' I said finally. 'I can't help with this balm, but I do know what's wrong with the terrapin. An injection is needed. Eye drops and ointments aren't the way to treat what is in fact a general deficiency.'

There was a long silence. Miss Rind sat motionless with her eyes glued on the reptile in her lap. Bubbles of liquid came out of Hugo's nostrils. He looked as if he had a rotten head cold, but he was far sicker than that.

'I don't know what Mr Lawrence will say, nor how Mr Pickersgill will take it,' she murmured eventually. 'They were so adamant, and said nothing about injecting the little mite.'

'It would be wise, I can assure you. If you like, I'll make you up a balm to apply to his eyes. It's the best I can do. Not this Micomicon, of course, but something soothing.' Then, like a sycophantic prig, I heard myself add, 'Mr Lawrence might understand the substitution in the light of our failure to locate the precise thing he prescribed.' Lord, I'll be spouting ectoplasm before long, I thought.

That did it. The old lady nodded. I prepared an injection and mixed a little chloramphenicol cream with a teaspoonful of colloidal silver. I jabbed Hugo in his groin and showed his owner how to apply the quasi-Balm of Micomicon.

Then, with the terrapin back in her handbag, Miss Rind thanked me, said she would let me know how Mr Pickersgill and others took things, stuffed a ten-pound note in my top pocket and swept out to the limousine.

Ten days later there came a phone call from Harrogate. Hugo was fighting fit, eating again and no longer having trouble with his eyes. 'Mr Lawrence says he's very pleased with you, Doctor,' Miss Rind purred. 'He came through again last Sunday. He thought your concoction was an admirable second-best.'

I put the receiver down and had an interesting thought: maybe if I ever got to Heaven I could swap my harp for a microscope and syringe and find plenty of work as a zoo vet?

Cuddles, the corsair of the oceans with a computer for a brain and the lethal power of a wolf-pack submarine, was like a lamb, as gushily soft as a Liberace with water wings. Martin Padley and I and the others working in the dolphinarium knew that; the public did not. The very name, killer whale, the vague recollection of stories by polar explorers of how these creatures had lunged up onto ice floes in pursuit of human prey, the way whaling fleets detested marauders who blatantly freebooted among the coveted blue and fin whale herds, memories of old seafarers who had seen the sea turn red as packs of the distinctively marked assassins slaughtered whole dolphin schools just for the hell of it; all this patchwork of myth and reminiscence and folk memory made a reputation for his kind of which Cuddles, as he basked in his pool with love in his heart and his belly full of prime herring, was quite unaware. He liked people and seemed to try to reach out mentally towards them. People got delicious goose-pimples as they looked down at him. They thrilled and admired and shrank back. There was a chasm of incomprehension between the whale in the water and the primates with smaller brains that gibbered on the pool-side.

Martin and I did not include ourselves among these landlubbers. With much delight and more than a touch of exhibitionism we continued to swim daily with the whale. The crowds thought us ever so daring. In fact, I had never felt safer. Not noted for intrepid acts of derring-do, a fair to middling swimmer only, and with a concern to preserve my own skin from the attentions of nature red in tooth and claw, I nevertheless felt at home with the whale from the very beginning. I had been frightened by horses that lashed out with both hind feet at the slightest touch—not to mention a mad onager—cornered by hysterical Alsatians that made me sweat, and forced to back down by bloody-minded alligators. But Cuddles I knew instinctively to be benevolent. It was in his eyes, the carefully measured pressure of his jaws on my hand or leg, the squeeze of his flippers round my trunk, his very presence, We had our lingua franca of squeaks and whistles. Like making love to a girl from Venus, it was the way things were said and done rather than the actual meaning of the words exchanged that mattered. Looking through the literature, I could find no authenticated cases where killer whales had been proved to attack humans. The polar explorers' story of the animals breaking a pathway through ice to reach them did not end in actual assault and was, I believe, more probably just sheer curiosity on the whales' part. Americans had already swum among schools of wild killers and come to no harm. Eskimo lore contained no hard evidence, only tales of hunters paddling their kayaks into a fog-bank, never to be seen again and presumed taken by one of the 'Lords of the Sea'.

Scientifically, we were convinced that unlike the dim-witted and primitive shark which will snap at anything, even its own entrails after being disembowelled, the highly sophisticated whale does not do anything without thinking first with fine precision. It is equipped with sonar that can not only judge ranges but identify the nature of objects with a precision far beyond the capabilities of man-made devices: in pitch-black water it can distinguish between one kind of fish and another and even read the emotions of another of its species by 'looking' into the skull sinuses to detect internal blushing. It has an intricate communications system that uses unjammable codes so far uncracked, and eyes that see well above and below the surface. It seizes only what it wants to seize, never attacks blindly. And whereas it counts dolphins, seals, walruses, fish, diving birds, jellyfish, squid and, no doubt, ships as familiar inhabitants of its environment to be eaten, hunted, ignored or avoided in the natural order of things, free-swimming, awkward humans are outsiders, objects merely of curiosity and of less significance than a clump of floating seaweed. Killer whales do not waste time on seaweed, so we romped with Cuddles in the water during his first year without qualms. My own children did it. Nude model girls did it. The whale treated each and every playmate considerately and benignly.

I had overlooked one very important fact. Bright as they are, killer whales are not omniscient. Wise in the ways of the deep waters, of hurricanes that madden the breakers above and of the fire-jewelled shrimps that troll the abyss below, they know nothing of fellow mammals who stayed on land when they, aeons ago, went back to the seas. They assume that creatures plying their trade in the ocean can survive in a liquid world. Watching, touching, tasting me, Cuddles must have assumed too much. I imagine he was amused by my inelegant paddling around and impressed by the way in which so clumsy a beast could evidently hunt. This flailing pink ape had a knack of somehow coming up with an inexhaustible supply of fast-running fish like herring and mackerel. In my bathing trunks I showed no sign of possessing much in the way of weapons and my feet seemed very inferior to flippers and flukes. Still, the proof of the pudding was in the eating, and I appeared good at catching fish.

The crunch came when Cuddles assumed that I was good at something else. Killers can hold their breath underwater for more than a quarter of an hour. While it is true that a man has stayed under without special gear for $13\frac{3}{4}$ minutes, most homo sapiens, including pearl divers, have a far lower limit of endurance. Cuddles could not be expected to know such statistics when we began a new game one rainy morning in late summer after I had dived into his pool for our regular daily mixture of fun and veterinary checks while Martin and his trainers prepared the whale's food downstairs in the fish kitchen.

It all developed out of something we had enjoyed many times before. Cuddles would push me round his pool with the point of his snout stuck in my navel. I was expected to tickle his throat with my toes as he propelled me backwards through the water. Sometimes he would angle me down a bit and we would take a quick swoop towards the pool bottom, then up he would soar, balancing me perfectly as I crashed through the surface in a welter of foam. This morning Cuddles decided on a further variation. He would push me as usual, then he would stop abruptly. I quickly caught on that I was supposed to flounder away, escape him even, and when I was a few yards off he would come after me and gently pick me up once more on the tip of his snout. It was a sort of tag. Cuddles enjoyed the competitive aspect of the new game immensely. He would roll slightly to one side and, with one syrupy eye held well above the water, watch me make off. There was the glint of an excited puppy in the eye.

I did quite well and on the odd occasion almost managed to sideslip when he took up the pursuit, which is not to be sniffed at when you realise that killers can turn on a sixpence and use their great tail-flukes to brake to a dead halt from sixty miles per hour in a second. I tried rolling under him; that worked quite often. The pink ape was learning. Cuddles thought it was all a marvellous wheeze but unlike a dog or cat, that will repeatedly make the same error at ball-games where humans are involved such as 'pig-in-the-middle', Cuddles used his vast expanse of grey matter to neutralise my evasion tactics. He began to come in twisting like a snake so that I could not see him for foam, or climbing up like a fighter plane to intercept me at my blind spot, below and behind. Always his final attack was gentle; I felt the round, warm smoothness of his muzzle press into me and I knew I had been caught again.

Next I tried deflecting his muzzle at the last moment rugby-style by pushing him off with a hand so that he cruised by me. Full marks to me. That, and a kick back with one foot pressed against his side, and I was away. Cuddles squealed contentedly and turned to follow me. I raised a hand to deflect him again. Before my fingers could touch him, he stopped dead, sank vertically a few inches and zoomed in for my stomach. With consummate ease he made contact, and to secure his hold dived slowly at a shallow angle. Holding my breath I went down, expecting any second to be taken up to the surface as usual for the next round.

But no. With a soft thwack, my back was flattened against the wall of the pool. Not painfully—Cuddles was far too careful with folk to act roughly, even in the heat of a good game. He simply pressed me against the concrete. I could

592

almost hear him clicking through the water, 'Now, old friend, gotcha! Get out of this one if you can!' All of which was fine, good, clean, healthy fun—except that we were four feet under water. He could hold his breath for fifteen minutes and I knew it. I might manage no more than two at a pinch, and he did *not* know it.

I pushed. Cuddles increased the pressure just enough by the minutest vibration of his tail fluke. I wriggled, tried to squeeze sideways, thumped on his fat-filled forehead. Cuddles did just enough to make sure I was fixed. My wriggles and thumps no doubt showed how much I was enjoying myself. Cuddles liked being thumped.

Fear swept through me. My lungs were ready to explode. I must breathe, even if it was only one last inhalation of sparkling blue water. I remember the resentment I felt at dying accidentally, the ridiculousness of it all. It seemed absurd to be drowning in fun instead of dying in a rational, professional manner under the fury of a badly tranquillised polar bear, lanced unexpectedly by an oryx or even from some virus picked up at an autopsy. As my fear turned to terror and my resentment to despair, Cuddles remained motionless but transfixing me as surely as a pin holds a butterfly in its glass case.

The haze of green and blue, the dancing white bubbles, the black fuzz of the whale's head were beginning to spin when I heard through the rising roar in my ears a far-off whistle. Instantly the pressure on my stomach disappeared and I felt my hair grabbed and pulled painfully. The next moment my head was above water and I was pulling in chest-fulls of precious air. Martin was kneeling on the pool-side, holding me up by my hair while the rest of me dangled like a string of frog-spawn. Cuddles was floating a few feet away with his mouth open and his eyes fixed on the gleaming bucket by Martin's side. By good fortune the head trainer had come up with the first fish of the day at exactly the right moment. He had taken in the situation immediately and blown his whistle to give the 'come and get it' signal to the whale, who had at once left our deadly game and gone to breakfast.

Martin helped me out. When I had got my nerves under control I issued an instruction that no-one was to swim alone with Cuddles ever again. Killers may not attack human beings but I knew now how easily they could kill accidentally.

Things were never the same again. Children and model girls were no longer invited to have a dip with the genial giant. When we went in, there was always someone on the side with a whistle and a bucket of fish, just in case. About that time we found out that some of the American marine-lands always had a baseball bat on hand when their killers were being ridden. They did not like talking about it, but it was plain that other folk had had their doubts about the safety of these whales.

Before long it was Martin's turn to revise his ideas about our cuddly Cuddles. 'I can't put my finger on it,' he said to me one day after a session swimming with the whale, 'but I don't feel as secure with him any more.'

We discussed it, but could not arrive at any precise reason for his apprehension. Perhaps it was Martin's knowledge of my experience. Certainly Cuddles was playing games with greater gusto than ever, but he was still good-natured and cheerful all day long.

Then Cuddles developed a fetish for rubber flippers. First he started refusing to release the grip of his teeth on the black, webbed footwear of a diver in his pool. Quickly this worsened to the point where he was obsessed with the things and, with a jerk of his head, would wrench the flipper off the wearer's foot. A pink and white unclad human foot, complete with toes, was of no interest; Cuddles was just kinky about frogman's gear. His pursuit of a man wearing the flippers became doubly keen to the point where he would surge up and snatch them off as the swimmer scrambled over the pool edge. The first Achilles tendon sprains appeared. Martin's fears deepened, but we decided to continue swimming with the whale whenever necessary for veterinary inspections and for cleaning and maintaining the pool.

The next stage was more serious. Like an underwater commando, Cuddles would neatly break the air-pipe of a diver's scuba gear, forcing him to surface rapidly. The latter was not so easy if the attack then turned, as usual, to the flippers. We stopped the use of scuba gear unless absolutely essential and made do with masks and snorkels. Cuddles soon found he could rip the masks off, breaking the rubber retaining bands with ease.

Finally, Martin walked dripping into my office with his wet-suit in tatters. There were blue weals on his skin below long tears that had shredded the rubber in half a dozen places. He looked pale and grim.

'I went in to seal a leaking window,' he said, shivering. 'Cuddles came up like an express train and tried to rip my suit off. His teeth bruised me for the first time. I can tell you, I was bloody scared.'

So our salad days were over and swimming with Cuddles came to an end. On special occasions when we had to go into the water, we wore bathing trunks and hung protective nylon netting between us and him. I believe that the wet-suits were the key to the problem. In them men became sealions. Sleek and shiny, with a changed outline and a different, more facile movement through the water, maybe these mermen awakened memories in Cuddles' subconscious of those fin-footed creatures like seals which, while of the ocean, have not totally forsaken their ancient home on land and which, while able to dart like arrows through the dark water, are not able to out-think or out-manoeuvre the killers who find them such tasty morsels.

Thirteen

Once the busy spring and summer holiday periods at Flamingo Park were over, I decided to go on one of what I called my 'walkabouts'—a wander around places abroad where things of zoological interest were to be found. Increasingly, I was combining pleasure, work and study in such a tour: my list of clients overseas was growing, and most of them were in places like the Côte d'Azur, the Spanish coasts, Switzerland or the German Rhineland. In such places blood samples, vaccinations and hysterectomies could be neatly blended with sunshine, sea, old cities or mountain villages. After the wrestling with gorillas or gnus came the opportunity for wines of Rüdesheim or Cariñena, for fruits de mer, chorizo or rum topf. A good example was, and still is, my association with the river Rhine. I could not get away from the charms of the greatest of all Europe's rivers, and on its banks from its sources in the Swiss mountains, down through southern and then northern Germany to where it reaches the sea in Holland, I found myself dealing with all sorts of exotic creatures and getting the chance to taste the variety of cultural styles through which the dark water runs.

At its head, near the Bodensee, there was a tiny hamlet, just a church, a post office, an inn and a farmhouse. In a quiet meadow behind the farmhouse was an old wooden barn, the inside of which had been converted by a travelling flipper show into a miniature dolphinarium, the winter quarters for a bunch of porpoises under my care. Visits there meant staying in the most cosy yet sumptuous hotel rooms I have ever seen, at the Drachenburg in Gottlieben, with wild boar and morels for dinner, with excellent Swiss wine, and afterwards riotous dancing with the Yodelling Club, a form of music that elsewhere I utterly detest.

Further on, where the quiet Alpine stream has become broad and busy with barges, the Rhine passes by the vine-yards and orchards of the German Pfalz region. Beyond the woods and farmland that surround the ancient four-towered cathedral at Speyer is a holiday park with more very un-German animals—sealions, flamingoes and chimpanzees. After sunset, with my patients settled down for the night, my samples labelled and my instruments cleaned, here I could sit in the scented air beneath lime trees, drinking cold golden beer and watching the inn-keeper roasting his kasseler, smoked loin of pork.

More dolphins were to be found near the Rhine at Bonn, and at Duisburg is the zoo with another sort of marine animal that was on my list of patients, a beluga whale. There was always time after emergencies had passed to walk round Cologne Cathedral, sample hot wurst from kerbside stalls and rubberneck around the Eros Centres.

On its last miles, slipping strong, flat and oily by Dutch water meadows, the Rhine passes close to the gates of Rhenen Zoo, where I actually watched for the first time a baby hippopotamus being born, and where an eland antelope bull I was treating fatally impaled its keeper on its horns in one terrifying, unexpected sweep of its head. In winter, when all the animals had been checked at one of my routine visits, Henni Ouwehands, the director's wife, would warm us with steaming plates of boerenkool-met-wurst. In summer I tried to make my visits to Rhenen coincide with the town's street market, where green herrings and onions were sold. The succulent slivers of raw fish were washed down by cold Genever gin and Amstel beer and the evenings spent at the shooting club in Wageningen.

I was not finished with the river until it actually swirled

under the keels of ocean-going vessels in Rotterdam. Even there, dolphins from Florida swam in a floating dolphinarium made from four converted Dutch barges and moored to the quayside. Rotterdam meant Indonesian rijstafel and gossip in harbour bars, with salt in my hair and lanolin under my fingernails after unloading and checking a couple of new arrivals.

One way and another the Rhine is a very zoological sort of waterway for me, but on this particular 'walkabout' I decided to go far away from the Rhine, up to the edge of the quite Teutoburger forests of Westphalia. I would have a look at the animals in a safari park on the edge of Bielefeld, which oddly enough is Rochdale's twin town. There the Wurms family had cleared a vast area of pine trees on the sandy soil of a village named Stukenbrock and turned it into a place where lions, tigers, elephants, antelopes and ostriches roamed. There were the usual gastronomic and other attractions: the district teems with trout farms and little gasthofs that serve the fish fresh in a dozen different ways, and it is an easy drive to places like the famous Hamelin, with the church whose carillon and moving figures I find eerily compelling, or Karlshafen, where the carp in the river chomp with audible, lip-smacking noises at bread thrown to them by folk like me. Nothing in the world is more satisfying than watching a hungry animal obviously enjoying its food.

It was a typical early autumn evening as I drove up to Stukenbrock. Flags of grey mist were hanging from the trees, and the road through the forest glistened with sticky condensation. The visitors had all gone. In the lowering gloom I could just make out the upper halves of yaks and Watusi cattle standing silently, black, featureless torsoes floating on a sea of eddying vapour. Fritz Wurms, the director, whom I had never met before, invited me to his office for a glass of schnapps. By the time we came out it was fully dark. The mist had turned into a dense fog that was biting cold.

'The new tigers should be all bedded down by now,' said

598

Wurms. 'Come and look at them. We have the finest tiger sleeping-quarters in Germany.'

With the director leading the way we set off on foot into the foggy night. I was walking in a cloud of eye-stinging mist. The torch held by my companion cut a narrow beam in front of him for a yard or so and then was swallowed by the fog. I could see my knees if I looked down, but my feet were invisible. Fortunately Herr Wurms knew his way. We went through a wooden gate and began to trudge across a flat expanse of what felt like grassland. From time to time I would wrench my ankle in a rabbit hole bored into the sandy soil.

'We're in the main reserve,' my companion told me. 'We'll have to watch out for the lake-side. Careful with the tree trunks.'

He told me that after hundreds of trees had been cleared for the safari park, their stumps had been left projecting a few inches above ground level. It was like stumbling through a minefield. Unable to see the low obstructions, we advanced cautiously.

'What animals are out at night in this reserve?' I asked, stubbing my toe and staggering awkwardly as my feet found my first stump.

'Oh, yak, Watusi, ostrich, zebra. Nothing troublesome.'

We plodded on. I heard the dull thud of hooved feet nearby. The dark mist billowed and something snorted its way past me. I could smell animal. Was it a yak, or a sweating zebra? I could not tell. Wurms' feeble torch beam lit for an instant on a dark flank of hair. It quickly dissolved into dripping wreaths of black cloud. 'Watusi bull,' said the director. He was right. I felt my foot sink into a warm pile of sour-smelling droppings.

'A bit to the left here and we should be at the gate to the tiger reserve.' Wurms stopped and fumbled in his pocket. In the light of his torch I saw he held a small walkie-talkie. He spoke into the transmitter. 'Hallo, hallo. Ulli, bitte melden—please report. Are all big cats in compound?'

The walkie-talkie crackled and a voice confirmed that the lions and tigers had been called in for their dinner of cooked tripes. Reluctant diners are rounded up by rangers in Land Rovers. I wondered how they would have fared, chasing lions and tigers in this pea-souper of an evening.

'Good. Ulli says we can go into the reserve.' Wurms put the walkie-talkie back into his pocket and pulled out another device. It was a box the size of a cigarette packet bearing two buttons, one red and one green. He pressed the red button and I heard a humming noise. Flicking up the beam of light, the director picked out the steel gate of the tiger reserve. It was opening after receiving a signal from his remote control device. As soon as we had moved through, Wurms pressed the green button on his box and the gate began to close behind us. After a couple of steps we were once more cocooned in dank and chilly steam. I could smell cat now. The acrid stink of tiger excrement and urine hung in the clinging vapour all around us.

'Only a hundred metres to go,' came the voice from in front. Any moment now and the torchlight should give way to the glow from the big cats' warm and well-lit night-houses.

Wurms walked carefully on, swinging the light beam from side to side to avoid stepping into a drinking pond. I stuck close behind him. All at once he stiffened and stopped dead in his tracks. I blundered into him and very nearly brought us both down.

'Scheisse, look at that,' he hissed.

I looked down the short beam of milky light. It ended in two shimmering orange discs. That was all—two glowing coins, newly minted from red gold, were suspended on invisible strings. They hung steadily in the coiling mist. Beyond them was impenetrable darkness. There was no doubt what they were. They were the clever, light-reflecting, starlight-gathering devices that nature invented millions of years before human snipers were equipped with night-sights and image-intensifiers. They were the layers of scintillating cells behind the retinas of the eyes of certain animals. Such as tigers.

'It's a tiger,' I whispered lamely. I was astounded to find myself smiling. This was ridiculous. Even in horror films they did not come up with scenarios as bizarre as this: two unarmed fellows on foot in the fog, finding themselves face to face with a tiger. It was like a horrible mismating between a Victorian gaslight melodrama and *The Jungle Book*. Except it was really happening.

'Hold the torch just as it is, straight in the eyes,' Wurms said without turning his head. 'I'll call that verdammte Ulli again.'

Carefully I took over the torch. I looked at the unblinking eyes. I tried to distinguish other features, nose, ears, whiskers, but they were invisible. Somewhere I had read that attacks from big cats are not particularly agonising, the damage is so severe and shock numbs sensation so quickly. But could anyone be sure? What were those reports of humans who had survived attacks? Was Cecil Rhodes one? Or was it Teddy Roosevelt? At that moment these seemed the most important things in the world to remember. My mind shuffled thoughts frenziedly.

Then Wurms' voice was rasping into the transmitter. 'Ulli, du Idiot! How many tigers did you count in, man?'

There was silence for a while and then I heard Ulli's voice, worried, explaining, excusing. Ulli was feeling as bad if not worse than we did at that moment. There were numbers I recognised: 'Zehn . . . neun . . . nebel (the word for mist) . . . schwer' (difficult).

'Come on,' I said aloud. 'The fellow's going to talk us into our graves if he goes on any longer.'

'It's Rajah, a male, one of the most dangerous,' Wurms whispered presently. 'Let's start moving towards the house but keeping the light in his eyes. Go carefully sideways'.

We began to edge away. The gold coins remained hung on

the end of the torch beam. When we had travelled seven or eight paces they had not dimmed or changed their size.

'He's coming with us,' said my companion.

'And he's not had a meal since yesterday.'

'Worse than that, I'm afraid. Yesterday was the weekly fasting day. He's not had a bite for almost forty-eight hours.'

My stomach went into intricate contortions.

I had always enjoyed talking to tigers. It does not matter if you have not been formally introduced or never met before; just make a lip-flapping imitation of a tiger purr and nine times out of ten the animals will answer back with friendly civility. I tried it: 'Prr-prr-pch, prr-prr-pch.' It sounded louder than usual and echoed faintly in the oppressive fog. No answering purr or chirrup. I tried again. The gleaming eyes were still there but not a sound came in reply. To my dismay I saw that the light beam was now no longer white but a feebler yellow and did not reach into the gloom as far as before.

We continued in a nervous, slow-motion pirouette. Somewhere in the gloom there was the sound of an engine starting up. Ulli was coming to get us. A minute more, his headlights would cut through to us and we would be OK.

Wurms stopped suddenly again. 'Dr Taylor, with all this turning in the fog I've lost my bearings. I'm afraid I can't be sure we're still going towards the night-house. We'd better go in a straight line and try to make for one of the fences.'

I was cold and frightened. The thick water vapour was searing my lungs. I cursed my decision to go walkabout. Next time, blockhead, I said to myself, an end-of-season laze-around at Reid's Hotel, Madeira—if you get out of this.

The torch battery was definitely on its last legs. The light began to flicker. Suddenly the tiger eyes vanished.

'He's gone,' I whispered. My tongue was dry and made speaking difficult.

The German must have been holding his breath, for he

exhaled explosively between clenched teeth. 'Stand back to back,' he muttered. 'Let's wait for Ulli.'

There was the sound of a revving motor and the harsh grind of gears off to our right. It was difficult to judge the distance. Wurms waved the torch and spat some words into the walkie-talkie. The engine noise became distinctly louder. I strained to see the first glow of the lights. 'Come on, Ulli,' I prayed. Wurms began to shout at the top of his voice, 'Over here, here, here, here!'

Somewhere in the spongy darkness a tiger, lord of the jungle, crouched listening. The sweat of man-fear permeated the dripping darkness. The tiger's sensitive nose was at that moment telling him loud and clear that the two humans were terrified, and with a puny, two-legged, ill-defended scrap of a beast like the human being, terror meant that the battle was half won. But did the great cat want to do battle? The one thing on our side was that tigers are as unaccustomed to hunting in dense fog as we are. Still, I could not forget what Wurms had said about yesterday having been fasting day.

Suddenly there was a thunderous crash. It was followed by some yelling and the frantic revving of an engine to screaming pitch. There was the roar of spinning tyres and then silence. The walkie-talkie crackled with voices. Ulli had gone over the edge of one of the drinking pools. He was stuck, with the Land Rover's exhaust pipe submerged.

Contrary to what is written in books and films in the English language, annoyed and exasperated Germans at moments of crisis do not say 'Gott in Himmel!', 'Schweinhund!' or even 'Donner und Blitzen!' What Herr Wurms uttered as he fired the unfortunate Ulli by walkie-talkie was unprinted and unprintable.

All we could do was to go on again in a straight line, hoping to find a wire fence sooner or later.

Every sense alert, we linked arms and began the twisting, turning, laboriously slow dance. The torch penetrated only a foot or two by now but it was our best hope of locating the tiger eyes should they re-appear. Our complicated footwork made keeping a straight course extremely difficult. After what seemed like half an hour but could have been only minutes, we were relieved to find ourselves with our noses up against the wire fence. Then we realised its mesh was too small to provide footholds.

'Shall we walk round the fence until we come to a gate?' I asked.

'I'm not sure where we are, and the length of fencing in this reserve is as much as three hundred metres between gates. We're perhaps more likely to meet the tiger near the fence, too.'

As in most big cat compounds, the tigers liked to pace the boundaries of their territory. There was a well-beaten track just inside the fencing. No doubt every few yards there would be invisible 'markers', where the animals had sprayed urine to lay claim to their patch.

'What shall we do, then?' I was shivering more than ever.

'Try to get over the top, Doctor,' said Wurms. 'Stand on my shoulders. With your height, maybe you can reach the top and scramble over. Find one of my men and tell him to fetch Poludniak, the curator, and to make sure Poludniak brings the guns.'

He clasped his hands into a stirrup and I climbed onto his broad shoulders. Taking a hold on the wire mesh and unceremoniously putting all my weight on one foot planted on his head, I strained to reach the top of the fence. I was feeling around blindly. Jagged twists of wire cut my hands. Then my heart sank; the top twelve inches of fencing was angled inwards. A baboon might have got over it with ease but I had no chance. I thudded back down onto the ground beside Wurms.

At that moment there was a shout from nearby and a dark shape loomed up out of the fog on the other side of the wire. 'Herr Wurms, Herr Doktor!' called the shadowy figure.

'It's Poludniak. He's found us.' Wurms gave a relieved

laugh. 'Over here, Poludniak,' he called. 'Got the guns? Good man.'

The curator levered open a gap in the wire with the steel barrels of one of the two shotguns he was carrying and pushed both weapons through. Things were improving. We were armed, although with the fog as dense as ever we might not get a chance to pull the trigger in self-defence.

'Hold on a moment,' I said. 'It still isn't safe to walk towards the gate. How far is the nearest one, Herr Poludniak?'

'150 metres, I reckon.'

'That tiger could be anywhere and on us without warning. Get back to the drug cabinet as quick as you can and fetch a bottle of ammonia and two 20-cc syringes.'

The curator disappeared at once.

'Let's stand back to back and keep moving the torch around,' I said.

Twelve-bores at the ready with their safety catches off, we must have looked, if only we had not been shrouded in fog, like Custer's Last Stand. The first barrel contained a blank charge. The second held a lethal cluster of elephant-shot. One flash of a golden eye and I was ready to let fly. Apart from destroying dogs when I was a student with the bloody, ear-shattering but humane captive-bolt pistol, I have never shot any sort of animal in my life. Clutching the shotgun and seeing phantoms swirling in the mist, my dislike of firearms was as strong as ever.

Poludniak lumbered up out of the cloud. He passed a bottle and two syringes through the wire.

'Now we are safe, Herr Wurms,' I said, as I filled the syringes with the pungent ammonia. 'We take one syringe each and spray a little of the liquid around us as we move towards the gate. No tiger will come through ammonia vapour.'

We began to spray and walk along the fence line. The chemical hung in the thick air and caught our breaths. We coughed but kept moving. If it was irritating our nostrils six feet up, it would be even more obnoxious and repellent to anything stalking us closer to the ground. Matt Kelly at Belle Vue had introduced me to the defensive uses of ammonia when in a tight spot—only orang-utans would keep coming through showers of the stuff.

The torch battery gave up the ghost just as we reached the gate. One final burst of ammonia, a press of the button on the director's remote control box and we were out. As the gate clanked to behind us, I leaned up against the fence and laughed with relief until my ribs ached. The tension drained away and my legs felt like soft rubber.

All at once a piercing pain shot through my backside. I yelled, fell away from the fence and crashed to the ground. The curator shone his torch on my offended rear parts. There was a V-shaped tear in the seat of my pants and blood was welling out. 'Was ist?' gasped Wurms, and swung the light onto the fence.

There, wreathed in smoky haze, was the tiger, one paw pressed hard against the wire and each scimitar-shaped claw extended and glistening white. He had got me after all—just.

Next morning the telephone rang early in my hotel. I had not finished with the Stukenbrock tigers, it seemed. One of them was apparently choking on a lump of meat; would I go round at once. I jumped into my hired car. This walkabout was becoming anything but a relaxed toddle round Europe's beauty spots. And my bum was sore.

Back at the safari park I found everyone in the tiger house gathered round a year-old tiger that was obviously in serious trouble. It was fighting for air, heaving desperately with its mouth agape. Its gums and tongue were a delicate and sinister violet shade. Despite its frantic efforts to breathe, only a faint squeak came from its throat.

'It must be a chunk of the tripe from last night. You can feel it in the throat, Doctor.' The tiger was too agonised

606

to object as Wurms poked a finger at a lump in its neck.

I dropped to my knees and examined the animal's throat. As so often happens, the 'lump' was the perfectly normal Adam's apple or larynx. The tiger did not care as I thrust my fingers down its throat and probed rapidly round his tonsils and epiglottis. I ran a hand down its neck. Nothing. I could find no evidence of an obstructing foreign body. The larynx was not swollen. Maybe something was lodged well down in the windpipe. I decided to do a tracheotomy straight away. There was no time for skin-shaving, asepsis or carefully balanced anaesthesia.

'Get the oxygen from your welding equipment in the workshop,' I ordered. 'I'm going to open the windpipe.'

I reached in my bag for a scalpel. No time to sterilise it. Fixing the gristly cartilage rings of the trachea with two fingers, I stabbed a hole low down in the centre of the underneath surface of the neck. The tiger was groaning and completely oblivious to me. I twisted the scalpel blade in the incision to open up the hole in the windpipe. Bubbles of froth emerged but the tiger's breathing did not ease noticeably. I needed a tube to keep the hole open. Grabbing a 2-cc plastic hypodermic, I sliced off the front half with my blade. That would fit nicely and the plastic finger grips should stop it slipping completely into the trachea. As I started to insert the tube into the hole in the neck, the tiger gave a strangled cry that sent shudders through me. It stopped breathing. I pumped its chest furiously, massaged its heart, got three men to hold it vertically by the hind legs and swing it, jabbed a shot of theophylline into its tongue vein. When the oxygen cylinder arrived I stuck the welding head down the end of the improvised tracheotomy tube and turned the tap on gently. Nothing worked. I felt the pulse in the animal's groin fade, flicker and finally become imperceptible. The tiger was dead.

'I'll do an autopsy at once,' I said. 'Let's have him in the hospital.'

There is something troubling about doing a post-mortem on a newly dead animal. The body is warm, fresh and vital. Muscles still flicker. Cells still truly live. What is the dividing line between life and death? I sometimes feel like an intruder irreverently rooting round the remains where dignity still lingers. Yet in cases like this, and indeed in post-mortem work in general, the fresher the material the more the knowledge that can be obtained.

No piece of tripe was jammed in the windpipe. The body was that of a plump adolescent tiger in first-class condition, except that the cause of death was as plain as a pikestaff. The animal had literally drowned. Every nook and cranny of both lungs was filled with water.

'Drowned? But how? In his sleeping place with a small automatic water bowl on the wall?' Herr Wurms looked incredulous.

Drowned the tiger certainly had, but not in water from outside. Somehow it had produced the water itself. It had seeped rapidly and in vast quantities out of the lungs' blood vessels and had filled up the essential air spaces.

There was no sign of inflammation, no pneumonia, and indeed the whole course of the tiger's suffering had been witnessed and seemed too rapid for infection of any sort that was known to occur in cats. The keeper cleaning the house early in the morning had actually seen the animal begin to behave strangely, to breathe heavily and finally to collapse, fighting for air. The entire course of the attack before I arrived was no more than thirty minutes. I was mystified. I went with Wurms and Poludniak back to the tiger house to check on the others. Surely, I thought to myself, this must be a one-off, sudden dropsy of the lung caused by allergy, as can happen when sensitive folk are stung by bees. Allergic reactions are often extremely speedy; I was to find this out when a year later I unaccountably became sensitive to zebra and horse blood and nearly got jammed inside a zebra's womb when foaling it. My arm swelled up as if inflated by air.

If, as seemed likely, the tiger was an odd case of allergy, the others would not be at risk. No doubt it was something in the cooked tripes that had triggered off the trouble. It was odd, though, that it should happen this morning when the last feed had been the night before.

The three of us walked slowly up and down the passage-way in front of the tiger cages. It is a fine building with perfect heating, ventilation and lighting. Each tiger has a comfortable bedroom, fitted with all 'mod cons' including a soft straw mattress. I had slept myself in worse places in Spain and the Far East.

'Everything looks OK with these others,' I said as the big cats yawned and stretched at the beginning of another day. 'Prr-prr-pch,' I went.

'Prr-prr-pch,' responded each tiger, including a sleepy-looking Rajah, who after frightening the life out of us the previous evening had eventually been lured by hunger into the night-house.

'Allergy', I declared confidently. 'Something in the food or possibly the straw. We'll do microscopic tests of course, but I don't think there's any likelihood of a recurrence.'

We walked towards the door. Just then I heard a soft noise. It was a faint, hoarse wheeze and it was repeated regularly. I looked round. A magnificent young female stood looking at me from behind the bars. Each time she breathed out she made the noise.

'Prr-prr-pch,' I purred. The tigress blinked at me calmly but did not answer.

'She's eating fine. No problem,' Wurms told me. 'Maybe she's always been a little thick in the wind and we've not noticed it.'

It was certainly nothing very dramatic. Perhaps I was wrong. But . . .

'I tell you what,' I said. 'Get a pole or something and chase her about in the cage. I don't like to do it. Just enough to make her move.'

Poludniak got a brush handle and poked it through the bars. He rattled it against the metal and waved it up and down. Annoyed, the tigress snarled and ran up and down at the back of her cage, well out of reach.

'Good. Now stop,' I said after a minute. 'Let her settle again.' I wanted to see what effect the slight exertion, running perhaps a hundred yards, had had on the cat's breathing.

Poludniak withdrew his brush handle and we watched. The tigress slumped onto the straw as if exhausted. Ribs heaving, mouth dribbling foam and tongue protruding, she puffed and panted like a chronic asthmatic. We were stunned. The faint hoarseness was now a bubbling, rasping torrent of sound.

Within five minutes the tigress was dead. Once again the lungs were bursting with water.

The whole complexion of things had changed. I considered the possibility that we were faced with some new form of virus, perhaps a vicious mutant of the bug that causes influenza in domestic cats. I prepared for the worst.

'A twenty-four hour watch on the animals. The welding oxygen to be kept in the house. Change the food and the bedding. Shoot all stray cats that are found scavenging for food round the park,' were my orders.

For hours on end, Wurms and I walked along the line of cages, listening intently for the first signs of hoarseness. We were not long in finding number three; again it was a healthy-looking one-year-old. As its breathing worsened, number four appeared: Rajah. I injected all the cats with anti-allergic drugs, but unfortunately it had to be done by dart-pistol, which excited the beasts and did not help their respiration. Numbers five and six were revealed by the darting process. Within twenty-four hours I had seven gasping, groaning tigers on my hands. Only an undersized runt of a cub, the weakest of the bunch which had been retarded in its growth by bowel trouble months before, and all the lions were unaffected. Antibiotics did not appear to make any inroads into the disease, but if it was a virus that was to be expected.

By dashing up and down with the oxygen we managed to keep the air-hungry creatures alive, but there was no sign of improvement and the strain on the animals' hearts was becoming severe. I wracked my brains. Why not the lions? Although in a separate house, they had been given the same food of tripes. There was nothing else with which the cats had come into contact, except the bedding and the reserve outside. Could it really be a virus that selected only tigers? I wandered over the grass and round the tree-stumps, now warmed by autumn sunshine. There were rabbit droppings, pine cones, mosses—all manner of objects that conceivably could cause allergy, but nothing that I saw was a serious possibility. Anyway, the lion reserve was identical.

I turned my attention to the bedding. 'Where does the straw come from?' I asked the director as I filled a batch of syringes with cortisone to see whether this potent drug could reverse the deadly accumulation of water in the tigers' lungs.

'A local farm, Müllers. It's stored in our barn in bales.'

I tackled the keeper who bedded the tigers down. 'Show me exactly what you do when you put new straw down for the tigers each night,' I asked, 'right from the beginning.'

He showed me the neat stacks of bales in the barn. 'I take two of these each afternoon, load them on the cart and make up the tigers' beds with them before the animals come in in the evening.'

'And the lion keeper does the same?'

'Yes. We both use the same bales.'

'On the night before all this began you did nothing different?'

'No, I don't think so. I took my two bales from down there.'

I walked over to where he pointed. There was a pool of water on the barn floor where a broken roof panel had let

611

rain in, and a few bales at the bottom of the stack had soaked up the moisture. Bending down, I saw that they were becoming mouldy.

'You might have picked up a bottom bale, then?' I asked the tiger keeper.

'Very possibly. As long as it was dry I didn't mind a bit of mould; tigers don't eat straw.'

Light was beginning to dawn. I went to the lion keeper and questioned him. Yes, he knew the damp spot in the barn. He had never drawn bales from there. The old straw from the beginning of the outbreak was now all steaming away on the manure heap and there was no point in rooting about in that. But no matter how I looked at things, the only significant difference between the tigers and the lions was the bedding quality. This must indeed be a rare outbreak of allergy to mould fungus spores, an acute form of a disease that in humans is called Farmer's Lung. The tigers were drowning because of musty bedding. Why the retarded tiger remained unaffected we shall never know.

The cortisone injections produced a perceptible improvement, but the tiger house remained a grim place full of loud wheezes, hoarse rattles and tortured breathing. Much more cortisone, and the animals' ability to fight off penumonia germs might be affected. Before long the bacteria would be joining in on the act. What I needed was a drug that acted similarly to cortisone in some ways but did not reduce the body's resistance. There was one available—phenylbutazone, a preparation normally used in treating rheumatism and arthritis in old humans and show-jumping horses. What its effect on drowning tigers would be I had no idea. I decided to try it anyway, darting small doses of the chemical into the seven tigers' rumps.

It was not turning out much of a fun trip to Stockenbrock: I had not worked so hard for years. But with the phenyl-butazone injected, there was nothing to do but sweat it out over beer and frankfurters.

612

Two hours after the injections, the tiger keeper came into the restaurant where I sat with the director to say that the animals were looking distinctly easier. We went over immediately. It was true. The tigers were more relaxed, breathing less laboriously and even sniffing at their food trays.

Next day there was no doubt. The tigers were all on the mend. Everyone was still breathing hard but there were no more groans. Dishes had been licked clean and I was given the odd 'Prr-prr-pch'.

Progress continued dramatically, and at the end of a week I was able to leave seven bouncing tigers behind and drive down to Dusseldorf for the plane back to England. The tigers, or at least old Rajah, had left me a souvenir, but I had been too preoccupied to worry about my clawed posterior. Now, inspecting the wound awkwardly in a Viscount wash-room while flying to Manchester, I discovered that it had gone septic.

'Physician, heal thyself,' said Shelagh, laughing as she swabbed the claw-hole and I knelt, trouserless, in an undignified position on the bathroom floor.

Fourteen

The following summer was exceptionally busy. It was the height of the craze to open safari parks, following the lead of places like Woburn and Longleat. Every duke, earl or impoverished fellow who fancied he had a teaspoonful of blue blood in his veins, and who was certain of the jaundiced tinge to the Inland Revenue inspector's eye whenever the stately pile cropped up in conversation, was scattering lions and giraffes around the Nash terraces and along the rose-walks. Capability Brown was turning in his grave and being dug up to make room for dolphin pools.

The safari parks undoubtedly saved a number of aristocratic residences from having to be taken over by the National Trust and contributed a great deal to our knowledge of keeping wild animals in captivity. Jimmy Chipperfield showed at Longleat, Woburn and elsewhere that properly acclimatised tropical mammals, with their built-in heat-regulating systems, could prosper in the depths of an English winter without fancy heated housing. Town folk got a taste of the African bush without driving far from London or Liverpool. Species such as the cheetah, notoriously difficult to breed in traditional zoos, began to reproduce at an increasing rate.

There were problems, however. The wide open, grassy spaces of the parks, with an abundance of food lying around, encouraged rodents and other pests to move in, join the fun and import troublesome diseases. Parasites thrived comfortably in the semi-natural terrain. Animals were not as easily inspected and handled as in the closer confines of a zoo.

614

Not all of the problems were purely veterinary ones. The controlling of social groups of creatures like lions, zebras and baboons in extensive parkland presented many challenges for the pioneers. I found myself one of those pioneers when, through my connections with the Smart circus family, I became involved in helping them to set up a safari park at one of the finest sites in Britain, on a hillside looking towards the Royal castle at Windsor.

Baboon reserves are one of the commonest and certainly one of the most entertaining features of a safari park, and the baboons were some of the first animals to take up residence at Windsor. They, and their cousins in other parks, gave us a heap of headaches in the early days, mainly because of their obsession with escape. Compared to baboons, prisoners of war with their wooden horses and other feats of mental and physical ingenuity were mere beginners. If they could talk, some of the baboons I know and respect, with names that sound like hoods in a Cagney film—'Scarface', 'Tin-Ribs', 'Wart' and 'Squint'—could confidently drawl, just like Cagney, 'The jail hasn't been built that can hold me!' and mean it. At Windsor the baboons were originally corralled, or so we fondly thought, by a high wire fence with a sheet of smooth, slippery plastic on the top. The idea was that they could not get a grip on the plastic; that was what was going to keep them in. The baboons solved this minor problem by climbing up the wire until they reached the bottom of the plastic sheet and then, like a troupe of circus acrobats, forming a baboon pyramid to by-pass the puerile device. Sitting on the top edge of the fence, the first escapers would then reach down, if necessary with someone holding their ankles, and give a hand up to their mates who had been the sturdy-shouldered base of the pyramid.

To make the baboon pyramids unstable and unworkable, we stepped the plastic sheet inwards a foot or so from the fence. Back went the baboons to the secret drawing-board. The next schemes involved either unpicking the slippery green sheet with the persistent patience of a few dozen Counts of Monte Cristo or mounting diversionary attacks on the Alsatian dog that guarded the gate to the reserve whilst the main bunch of escapers slipped out on his blind side.

In the end the Windsor baboons opted for a peaceful life within their compound, mainly because their successful break-outs led either into the tiger reserve, where they got the fright of their lives and quickly 'escaped back in', or into less lethal parts of the park where meal tickets were hard to come by; meals in their reserve were plentiful and tooth-some. Also there were lots of fun things to do inside, like dismantling cars. The baboons could take the trimmings off a moving car far quicker than any automobile worker on the production line could put them on. As I discovered to my cost when I first drove my own car into the Windsor baboon reserve to visit a patient, Citroën saloons were bristling with lamps, bits of chrome and other trimmings that French workmanship had neglected to make monkey-proof. Having dealt with my sick baboon, I returned to the car to find the exterior denuded of everything portable. Aerial, screen wip-ers, lamp glasses—all gone. It was not as if the animals wanted to do anything useful with the articles that they stole. Like their human counterparts with birds' eggs, butterflies or beer mats, they just collected them for collecting's sake.

I at least knew where I might find the looted bits of my car in a day or two. Along with the baboons in the reserve at Windsor lived a lugubrious coven of Egyptian vultures. These harpies never caused anybody any trouble and were remarkably diligent in building nests, not nests of twigs and sticks in the manner approved by the ornithological rule-books but jazzy, glittering, pop-art bowers, comfortable lattice-work constructions made from screen wipers and radio aerials gathered from the ground after the baboons had knocked off for the day.

At a safari park which I visited in Spain, the wire fence of the baboon reserve was topped not by slippery plastic but by a strand of electrified wire of the sort used to corral cattle. Here the baboon POWs adopted a method of escape which might have been copied from the way soldiers are supposed to deal with barbed-wire barricades. One individual would fling himself onto the wire and lie there, twitching and jerking, whilst the others would quickly scurry over the bridge made by his gallant little body. When all had gone, he would drop back exhausted. It would be his turn to go out with the next batch, when someone else would act as the insulator.

Unlike the prisoners of Colditz, the baboons did not need to fudge the numbers at roll call to give fugitive comrades valuable time to get well clear of the camp. Keepers and curators do make regular checks of the stock list, but by their very nature the shifting, fidgety bands of baboons in a spacious reserve are as uncountable as a flock of sparrows. So some who 'make it' are not missed for a long time and their disappearance can remain permanently undiscovered or forgotten as numbers are built up by breeding or as the keeping staff change. I know one deep wood of birch and fir trees, fringed with palisades of brambles and wild roses that are heavy with juicy hips and blackberries in the late summer. Its inner fastnesses are carpeted from June with succulent red-cap boletus mushrooms, and edible blewits can be found even in the first frosts. White truffles sleep just below the beech mast. There are breaks in the trees where the grass grows tall and is speckled with vetches. Shallow, reedy pools tremble as water beetles, caddis-flies, water snails and frogs go about their business. In the depths of that wood live at least three baboons with long and glossy coats. They supplement the harvest of food, which each season naturally brings and which hunger, curiosity and intelligence revealed to them, with occasional forays for eggs, vegetables and discarded goodies from the gardens of cottages just outside the wood.

There was another baboon, a female, in the fugitive band

but she was caught in an illegal gin-trap and died miserably. I was brought her emaciated and multilated corpse. At autopsy I found the pieces of insect carapaces, seed husks, toadstool stems and bone fragments from small creatures that revealed how she and her comrades feasted in their woodland territory. And there is an abandoned badger sett, which I found at last after days of searching, where the gang holes up, dry and snug, during the dripping chill of winter.

I would not reveal the location of these English baboons for a king's ransom; unlikely to be able to trap them, but fearing claims for damages from folk who have been relieved of a few apples or radishes, their former owners would send in the shotguns. Like slaves in ancient Rome, these doughty creatures have earned their freedom; they have been on the run for more than a year and a day.

One of the first parks I visited in Europe was the superbly designed and beautiful zoo at Kolmården, on the Baltic coast of Sweden. I was there to study, among other things, their well-built baboon compound. High fences with their top sections angled inwards, deep foundations to thwart tunnellers, electrified mats at the exits and entrances—this was surely a maximum security unit. But they said that about Colditz.

Beyond the baboon compound was a lovely wooded reserve of pine trees in which a number of bears ambled about. The ground was covered with delicious pine kernels. The baboons could see and smell the tantalising morsels through the wire, but how were they to get at them? The 'goon squad' of keepers at the gates was very alert. The first attempts were not up to the expected standard: they tried stowing away on the roofs of coaches or sneaking along beside a car, keeping the vehicle between themselves and the guards and then, as the car reached the electrified mat, jumping up, holding onto a door handle and keeping their feet clear of the ground until they were safely through. Using a pair of guards, one at each side of the mat, soon put a stop

618

to that. The Escape Committee had to put their heads together. It took time but in the end they came up with the answer. As a coach approached the exit gate, the baboons would nip smartly between its wheels and with both hands and both feet latch onto the chassis. Best of all, on some models they could pull themselves up into secluded recesses in the bodywork or behind the mudguards. Out went the coach with its stowaways, who dropped from the undercarriage like autumn leaves when they reached the pine trees. The answer to that one was to equip the guards with angled mirrors on the end of long poles. Before each coach left the reserve they inspected its underside carefully for contraband apes, just like the stony-faced East German border guards at Checkpoint Charlie.

Baboons are a hardy breed, and the group at Belle Vue needed my attentions only once in about eight years. Manchester air and the carefully planned diet agreed with them and they, a peaceful, well-balanced social group, agreed among themselves. At the safari parks, on the other hand, I was kept busy patching up the bruises, cuts and knocked-out teeth of the day-to-day squabbles which regularly arose from disputes over marital and territorial matters, from greed, jealousy and the eternal clash between youth and age. To watch them at it reinforced my opinion that the naked ape in New York, London, Ulster or Moscow is barely a step ahead of his simian cousins in the evolutionary race.

Although my baboon friends did not pose any exceptional veterinary problems for me, I did meet a certain baboon, named Wunn, who had had a whole bundle of surgical problems heaped on his little shoulders by mankind. Wunn was an experimental baboon in a University laboratory involved in advanced transplant research. After being captured as a youngster in Africa, he knew no home other than the small galvanised box with a metal grille at the front, one of many identical one-man cells that stood in rows in the antiseptic, green-tiled room. He grew well enough on a scientifically perfect but unutterably boring diet of monkey pellets with the occasional half-orange and, when his turn came around, was experimented upon. Bits were taken out and put back in, plastic tubes were inserted to replace portions of his natural ones, miniature electronic gadgets were buried in his flesh to record this and that and always, always he was being sampled—a biopsy today, blood tomorrow, urine catheter the day after. For years Wunn bore it all stoically and displayed a gentle and warm nature towards the laboratory staff. Eventually the series of experiments came to an end. The men and women in white coats were pleased, and moved on to tinker with other baboons that Wunn could not see but only smell and hear.

Wunn had made his contribution to medical science. Now, instead of an OBE, there was only one remaining thing: death. According to the strict vivisection laws which operate in Great Britain, a laboratory animal which has played its part in a series of experiments must be put to sleep. There are no exceptions, no question of finding it a good home like a retired greyhound or redundant pit pony. The Home Office is adamant.

The girl laboratory technicians who had worked all along with Wunn had become particularly attached to the sweet-natured baboon. With the tacit approval of the surgeons involved, and with even the august head of research turning a Nelson's eye, they contacted me. Could I find a zoo where, without any chance of Government snoopers finding out, Wunn might for the first time in his life rattle about with a troupe of other baboons just like baboons are supposed to do? I was all for it. The secret of the bionic baboon would never be leaked to the Government but there was one possible snag: baboons live in strictly organised social communities where everyone knows his place. Singleton strangers are rarely tolerated and at worst are beaten up and driven off or killed.

Windsor Safari Park agreed to acccept Wunn, and we decided to put him first in the baboon reserve in a cage normally used by nursing mothers. Wunn could see and be seen by the other animals but was protected from them by the wire. They became used to his presence and his smell. But what would happen when the newcomer was eventually let out into the main bunch? When should we try it? It was my decision, and I knew that if I saw Wunn at the receiving end of a lot of punishment from the other adult males, I would have to dart him and put him painlessly to sleep.

After Wunn had spent three weeks in his separate cage, during which time he had aroused a certain but not inordinate amount of curiosity from a few of the other baboons, I decided to release him. My heart was in my mouth as a keeper opened the cage door and Wunn shuffled out into the grassy reserve. Now for it, I thought. My dart-gun was ready and loaded in case of a mugging. Wunn went a few yards, sat down and blinked towards the sunlight. He picked idly at this funny but tasty green matting all around him. His eyes followed a great grey and white cloud moving gently across the blue sky and then flicked across to where the cloud was suddenly pierced by a 707 climbing out of Heathrow airport. Slowly, nonchalantly, the baboons began to gather round him. To my surprise, instead of marching up to him and demanding to see his credentials, or beating up the stranger first and asking questions afterwards, they drifted up in twos and threes diffidently and almost respectfully. As would happen were a white explorer to stumble into the camp of a band of nomadic tribesmen, the first individuals to come right up to Wunn were the children. Within minutes, one or two of the smallest baboons were climbing over his hairy mane as if he were their long-lost favourite uncle.

We were overjoyed. So far, so very good. After the kids, one of the dominant male baboons cautiously approached the stranger, sniffed at him from a couple of feet away and then walked off unconcernedly. Wunn gazed benignly after him. I had already noticed that Wunn's testicles were abnormally small, probably because of his lifetime of acting as a surgical swap-shop. Perhaps he did not give off enough of the masculine scent to provoke the males; if so, I thanked God he was so poorly endowed. A few of the females came closer, emboldened by the first male's display of disdain. They gave Wunn the once-over, but from their reaction it did not seem as if the baboon equivalent of Richard Burton had arrived. It was all going far better than I could ever have hoped. The main group moved off and carried on with their foraging, feuding and courting. Wunn was left peacefully alone to begin doing amazing, novel things like sticking a finger into the soil or finding his first discarded screen wiper.

Not once in the days that followed did we see Wunn get into trouble. The kids liked him and a gang of them were constantly in attendance on him. The women continued not to be turned on by his charm, but then there was obviously more of the philosopher than the philanderer in his sage countenance. And the bellicose, butch leaders of the pack ignored him; the newcomer, they had concluded, was not going to make any waves. Gradually, as the months passed, Wunn was absorbed smoothly into the troupe. He seemed, and still seems, one apart, a member of the society but with no precise place in the hierarchy. The important thing is that he enjoys the sunshine and the rain, chasing the vultures, climbing over the rocks, taking handfuls of warm meat and vegetable stew in the winter and riding round the reserve on car bonnets during the summer. Two recent events have given me the utmost pleasure: Wunn has acquired a timid and devoted lady companion who grooms him whenever he feels lordly; and I have watched him deftly steal the chromium-plated wheel-trim from a coach—a coach carrying a visiting party of eminent surgeons.

It was at Windsor that summer that I was approached by 'Mac' McNab, the head keeper there, a plump, genial individual and a dead ringer for film comedian Oliver Hardy. 'We're going wallaby catching,' he announced. 'Do you know much about them?'

The honest answer was 'No'; I had already found these mini-kangaroos from down under to be unco-operative in responding to the medical ministrations of a Pommy veterinarian. With the aid of a certain brand of mint which these animals adore, a tip that I had picked up from my professor of surgery whilst at university and the only piece of exotic animal know-how I had been given as an undergraduate, I had been able to come into close contact with the timid marsupials from time to time but had found the early diagnosis and effective treatment of their ailments difficult. They are particularly prone to infection by a germ called actinomyces, which is carried into the jawbone and later to deeper parts by the tiny, barbed awns of grass on which they graze. The awns get jammed between their teeth and gradually work their way down into the gums. It was not an easy condition to tackle: the wallabies' struggles while they were injected often overstrained their hearts fatally and the surgical attempts I had made to cut out diseased areas of bone had been dogged for many years by the animals' unpredictable reactions to the only anaesthetics available.

'Not really, Mac,' I told him, 'but I'd dearly love to come on the catching.'

'Right,' he replied. 'We're going down to Hampshire. Leonard's Leap, a private estate, has a surplus of the little beauties. We've got to grab them ourselves, though. It'd be best if you came along in case they need doping.'

Although McNab's words made it sound as if I were a key member of the hunting team, I had a feeling that I was being invited for the sake of appearances, more as a professional scapegoat than as an insurance against mishap. My old partner, Norman Whittle, had warned me early in our days together of how often the zoo vet finds himself playing this role.

With an assortment of wooden crates and three vehicles we set out from Windsor and drove down to Hampshire. Leonard's Leap is buried deep in the countryside and is to be found by strangers only with much difficulty after wending through a maze of leafy, un-signposted lanes that fork a hundred times. Not only that, but wallabies at the time were hard to come by, yet the owner of Leonard's Leap, a gentleman apparently quite unaware of the going rate in the zoological business, was asking a ridiculously low price for his animals. No wonder McNab, a wily Scotsman, went to great pains to keep the source of the bouncing bargains a close secret. The keepers who drove the vans carrying us and the crates were given maps in case the convoy became split up. The maps had been carefully drawn by the head keeper and bore only the barest details necessary for arriving at our destination. When all three vehicles finally reached the estate, a network of small valleys thickly scattered with large rhododendron bushes, McNab dashed round retrieving the maps from the drivers and put a match to them. It was all rather melodramatic but to this day, although I have got the name right, live within forty miles of the place and have occasionally driven around on a summer Sunday trying to find it, I have never been able to locate the hidden haunt of the wallabies. McNab is an ex-gamekeeper and knows a thing or two.

The rhododendron bushes at Leonard's Leap have dry and hollow centres where the wallabies could be found, snugly holed up and proof against the elements. All that McNab, I and the keepers on the expedition had to do was to chase the wallabies out of their rhododendron hideaways and into a funnel-shaped trap which the estate gardeners had made with wire-netting at the head of one valley. This was the athletic side of a zoo vet's life. All through that hot afternoon we panted and puffed, running up and down the grassy slopes, crashing headlong through bushes and hurling ourselves in futile rugby tackles at the lithe, grey-brown bundles of fur that sprang silently over the ground as we approached. By late afternoon we had at last bagged our quota. Although not as winded and worn out as we were, the wallabies had begun to pant and their heart rates were almost too rapid to count. I decided to give each animal a shot of tranquilliser before crating it so that it would be able to relax on the long journey home.

McNab held the wallabies by the base of the tail while I gave the injection and checked to see how many of the females were carrying babies or 'joeys'. Of the twelve wallabies we had caught, ten were females and eight of them had sausage-sized infants firmly attached to the milk teats in their warm pouches. Safely on board the vans, the animals settled down quickly and without fuss in their boxes. I felt confident that I had done a good job in helping to catch the wallabies, and that my little drop of tranquilliser had set a seal of professionalism on the proceedings. McNab had told me that previously wallabies had been captured and moved without drugs being used. Sometimes an animal or two had died, probably of heart failure. Get this load back alive and well and McNab would undoubtedly appreciate the superior virtues of modern veterinary science in the zoo field. We set off home, map-less, following our noses towards a main road.

Back at Windsor, as the light began to fade, the wallabies were released into their grassy paddock. Ten, eleven, twelve: I counted them out. They were all alive and looking fit, and immediately began jumping uncertainly around their new compound. They bounced nervously along the perimeter and glanced with darting dark eyes at all the strange surroundings, at the humans peering through the fence and at the giraffes strutting in the adjoining paddock. They cocked their heads to listen to the sound of roaring lions, the screeching of bus brakes on the road outside and the thunder of jetliners making their final approach into London. McNab and I watched them, but suddenly he cursed and leaned forward. As the wallabies hopped, wriggling pink lumps of what looked like denuded mice fell onto the ground from the pouches of some of them. Within a minute or two, eight helpless baby wallabies, still with the foetal appearance of marsupial young, who are normally ejected from the womb to spend the latter half of 'pregnancy' in the pouch, were blindly writhing on the grass.

'Jeez, will ye look at that!' exclaimed McNab. 'Every mother's lost her young 'un!'

Quickly but carefully, we began to collect the hairless infants. They felt red-hot in the palm of my hand.

'Why, why d'you think that could have happened?' mused the head keeper as we stood looking at the adults springing quietly around us.

Suddenly the answer came to me: my wretched tranquilliser. It had done the trick all right on the mothers during the journey, but a proportion of it must have passed from their blood into their milk. Taken in by the babies, it had made them slightly drowsy and, when their parents were released at the park and began to leap about, they had lost their hold on the teat in the pouch and had been thrown out. I had given them each an indirect Mickey Finn.

I explained my theory to McNab, who nodded grimly. 'Hrrumph. Never did like the idea of all these new-fangled chemicals. Too much of it. Far too much of it,' he growled.

His opinions had been confirmed, but there was no time for further recriminations. Something had to be done—fast. The awful thing was that all the babies looked alike in their shiny, frail nondescriptness and so did all the mums. There was just no way we could tell which infant fell from which pouch, but back into someone's pouch each would have to go. McNab called in some keepers and the job of re-catching the wallabies began. Carefully, and with fervent silent entreaties to the gods to forestall what might turn into a joey holocaust, I stuck a couple of fingers into the pouch of each female. If I found a damp teat from which a drop of milk could be drawn, I plugged on one of the rudely evicted innocents.

Back in the security of a pouch, each joey latched firmly onto its allotted teat and snuggled down, but the chances that I had paired the right mother and offspring in each of the eight cases was something like one in five thousand. What if wallabies were like many other mammals and identified their own babies by scent, rejecting all imposters? In that case there would be de-pouched youngsters on the ground again in a little while and the deadly game of snap, using flesh and blood creatures instead of cards, would have to be played over and over again. Please God, let them be like caribou cows who willingly accept infants not their own, I prayed.

'Let's put them all in the night-house now,' I suggested to McNab. 'That way, at least they won't be bouncing around and it will give more time for any tranquilliser still in their systems to wear off.'

He agreed, and we released the nursing mothers into their indoor quarters. Now there was nothing more to be done except to leave them in peace for a few hours and hope that St Francis was listening. There was no point in saying anything to Shelagh about the affair when I telephoned her that night. I felt wretched enough as it was, without re-hashing everything. Nothing even she might have said could have provided any mental loophole through which I could wriggle away from the brutal fact that I had put the joeys' lives at great risk.

After a sleepless night I went down to the safari park early. It was seven o'clock. McNab and the rest of the staff would not be in for another hour. My heart was bounding as I went to the wallaby night-house and opened the sliding door an inch. Peeping in with my stomach anxiously churning, I scanned the sawdusted floor. There was no sign of any still, pink sausages. I went over every square inch again, straining my eyes till their muscles ached: not a joey in sight.

Only then did I raise my head a little to look at the crouching wallabies. All twelve of them seemed in good order, but there was no way of knowing how things were going in their pouches. Maybe the flattened corpse of a joey was underneath one of them or hidden under a layer of bedding. I pulled the door right open and gently shooed the animals out onto the grass. Nothing fell out of them as they hopped off into the morning sunlight. On hands and knees I meticulously picked through the sawdust, the bedding and the droppings, sweeping clear every inch of the floor with my bare hands. Saints be praised! Not one single baby could I find.

I went outside and watched the wallabies moving about, busily cropping the short grass. All seemed perfect. I hurried off to see if McNab was in yet and to give him the good news. In the days that followed, frequent inspections by McNab and his keepers turned up no evidence that any of the willy-nilly adoptions had failed. To my delight, it gradually became obvious that all eight babies were none the worse for mum-swapping; after a few more weeks furry brown heads began to peep out of the pouches on sunny days.

'Well, Mac,' I said, when it was clear that the wallabies were out of danger, 'it seems that they must be very civilised and tolerant creatures. One kid's as good as the next to those little ladies.'

'Yes,' he murmured, 'but no thanks to your tranquillisers, David. How many millions of years have wallabies been happily bringing up their young without 'em?'

He had a point, and a good one, but it struck me then how generally accepted on the zoo scene the veterinarian had become. Of course some of the old prejudices still lingered on, and calamities like the wallaby affair did not help, but most zoo men appreciated well enough how veterinary science could make their jobs easier and raise the standard of zoo care by—and this was the fundamental and important thing—improving the health, diet, handling, breeding and day-to-day welfare of the animals. I thought back to my early days at Belle Vue, when I despaired of my medical knowledge ever matching the wisdom and experience of Matt Kelly, or of showing him that modern drugs and other developments could go hand in hand with his innate animal-craft. Now even old hands like Kelly and McNab would grudgingly admit that perhaps my potions, flying darts, autopsies and analysing did have something to offer. That battle was all but won at last, I felt, and it would be together that we would tackle the numberless problems that lay ahead.

Fifteen

Andrew Greenwood spent less time with me during that summer. He was on the run-up to his final examinations. Nevertheless, he took time off to come up to Flamingo Park when he heard that one of Cuddles' regular blood samplings was due. He had asked me over the phone if it would be OK for him to take a biopsy of the whale's skin. Professor Harrison at Cambridge was working on the curious problem of why dolphins and whales can swim so fast with such little expenditure of energy and without setting up turbulence. The secret, he suspected and was later to discover, lay in the skin itself. I had given the go-ahead until Andrew arrived at the park with a fearsome kit of biopsy instruments like miniature apple-corers. Science or no science, I was as proud as Punch of Cuddles' billiard-ball-smooth skin and I worried over every little nick and pimple it developed. I chickened out of having him sampled like a cheese at a gourmets' gathering and sent Andrew back empty-handed and, I fancy, rather niggled.

I was a trifle embarrassed by my change of mind, but I had come a fair way since my early days of reckless post-graduate enthusiasm, when I would dash into major, complex surgery at the drop of a hat, stick needles into and take innumerable samples from every long-suffering patient that came my way. With the benefit of time, that precious, unteachable, elusive thing, clinical judgement, had grown, as it does in all medical practitioners. Leave well alone was its cardinal maxim: if in doubt, do nowt, as the Lancashire farmers would say. Cuddles was a big responsibility, and I was not prepared to risk the slightest chance of anything going wrong with him because of interference that did not contribute directly to his well-being. The question of how these creatures slip through water so easily was fascinating, but not important to Cuddles and me. As essentially a clinician, though now working with unusual and glamorous animals, I have often had to dowse with iced water the enthusiasm of academics for the advancement of pure scientific knowledge. I had learned this as a student, when a bunch of keen young anaesthetists from the Manchester Medical School had been let loose to experiment on some lions at Belle Vue. They had dashed joyously back to their laboratories and seminar rooms—while Matt Kelly had had to arrange the disposal of several overdosed cadavers.

No, I stand for the animal. If not me, who else? I am happy to think of myself as nothing more than the family doctor, but to a dumb family of extraordinary folk.

In June, Andrew telephoned to say that he had qualified. He was now a fully fledged Member of the Royal College of Veterinary Surgeons. After congratulating him, I asked about the future.

'I'm going to stay on in Professor Harrison's department at Cambridge and do some research in diving animals.'

'You're still keen on exotic creatures, then?'

'Most certainly. I'll be able to help out, do locums when you're away, that sort of thing.'

I was at least glad about that, but once the mill that grinds out PhD's had swallowed him, I feared he would be lost to the real world of animals with aches and pains and pestilences.

'What diving animals will you be working on?' I asked. 'Seals, dolphins?'

'Nothing so grand,' came the reply. 'I've got a research grant from the Royal Navy and they do their diving experiments with far more prosaic species.'

'Such as what?'

'Would you believe, goats? Goats that get the "bends".'

Over dinner that evening I said to Shelagh, 'Pity about Andrew. What a waste of a good man. Research! Goats! And I thought he had the makings of a first-class zoo vet.' Thoughtfully, I stabbed at a potato.

My visits to cases outside Flamingo Park had meanwhile become steadily more frequent. Pentland Hick was very patient; sometimes I would be gone for two weeks at a time. I was driving 70,000 miles a year, flying four times as far and becoming accustomed to sleeping by the roadside in my car. Rochdale to Stirling to London and back to Rochdale all in one day by road was nothing abnormal: 850 miles virtually non-stop except for fuel between a sick dolphin in Scotland and a dying sealion in southern England. I existed on a diet of peanuts, Haydn and Bach from my cassette player and the banter of the girl operators who manned the car radio telephone transmitters round the clock. It was a cracking pace that was required, manning a practice that had grown to be almost a thousand miles square.

I saw Rochdale and my family less and less and I formed the opinion which I still hold: that being a peripatetic, single-handed zoo vet is ideally work for a bachelor. I sympathised with Shelagh when I rang her from a hotel bar in San Diego or Nassau. She was at home, running this one-horse practice, bringing up the girls and keeping the house together in the rainy north-west, while I was grumbling about being delayed for an extra day on Grand Bahama Island by airline foul-ups, or about the indolence of a laboratory in Venice which meant that I must pass yet another salmon-skied evening watching the world turn round the Piazza San Marco. I could not see any obvious solution. One thing I was certain of: nothing, but nothing, would tear me away from exotic animals in a million years. Cats, dogs, pigs and sheep were things I seemed barely able to remember.

After a year and a half at Flamingo Park, I decided the time had come to return to full independence: there was an abundance of cases and little likelihood that I might have to sit in the office at home, waiting for the telephone to ring. I was not sorry to leave. Pentland Hick had sold his zoo empire out of the blue and, as happened in so many similar cases around that time, the big public company moved in. Anxious to diversify into what they believed to be a lucrative sector, these experts in bingo, casinos, catering and discos looked at animal collections and assessed them like banks of one-armed bandits or seats in the dress circle. Animals became units. Targets, budgets, productivity were words bandied about when animal diets were adjusted to suit the changing seasons or repairs to houses had to be made. The dead hand of the Accountant lay on the beasts' backs and the Public Relations Officer held sway over all.

Cuddles the whale suffered a grave attack of intestinal ulceration with massive bleeding, but after intensive treatment he rallied and pulled round.* Against my advice, the animal was moved shortly afterwards to Dudley Zoo in Worcestershire, where he was put on show in a hurriedly adapted pool. He proved a great attraction, but the writing was indelibly on the wall. From now on, commercial considerations took pride of place, even where the health of a very valuable animal was at stake. I continued to act as Cuddles' doctor until 1973. Then, whilst I was on a visit to Communist China, he mysteriously broke a rib, developed an abscess at the site of the fracture which sent seeds to infect his brain, and died within three or four days of falling ill. Having been in at his beginning, I was heart-broken not to have been on hand when he was finally up against it. But I was pleased that Andrew did the autopsy and that I, half a world away, could not.

*See *Zoovet*

My life as a medical carpetbagger, a vagrant veterinarian-in-a-suitcase, here today and gone tomorrow when a gorilla hiccupped in Paris or Port of Spain, suited me, except for three things. First, I was seeing Shelagh and the girls but rarely; second, I was abusing my digestion in motorway cafés; and third, I still had this 'thing', this blue funk about doping giraffes. After the Belle Vue specimens with hypothermia, after Pedro, after the Flamingo Park giraffe which had died under my hands, giraffes gave me the jitters. I consoled myself with the thought that with a little bit of luck I might be able to keep dodging the issue. Deep down, I knew that there was no hope of things always going as smoothly as they had with the Rio Leon specimen. One day, probably soon, I was going to have to anaesthetise another giraffe.

So the familiar butterfly sensation started in my stomach when Matt Kelly telephoned from Belle Vue, where I was still veterinarian and which still provided a good proportion of my cases. The Irish head keeper sounded concerned but hardly panicky. 'Oi've got a giraffe with a tomato stuck in its gob,' he told me. 'Strange thing is, she's still eating foine. Not causin' her trouble. Mebbe it's caught on a tooth. The keeper thinks he got a glimpse of it two days ago.'

If it was a tomato, it should not take long before the squashy fruit disintegrated without causing any further trouble. Still, it sounded a rum story and I promised to go straight over, though I reckoned it unlikely that I would have to do much else but mutter a few reassuring words and let time do the rest.

Molly was a lovely specimen of Masai giraffe and had already produced three healthy calves. Standing looking up at her, I could see what Matt was talking about: a red sphere that protruded from the right-hand corner of her lips. It was smooth and shiny and about one and a half inches in diameter. It looked at first glance like a tomato but, encapsulated in a fold of gum tissue that had at last grown big enough to flop out of the animal's mouth, the spherical object was without doubt either a cyst or a tumour. The giraffe would not be able to feel any pain from the lump and it had not grown enough to interfere seriously with her feeding.

'What d'ye think, Doctor?' asked Matt after giving me a few minutes to ruminate while the butterflies in my stomach become bat-sized.

'A growth, Matt. It's probably been hidden in there for quite a while, but it's not causing problems yet. Let's wait and see first.'

There were two chances that I might be really lucky. If it was a saliva-duct cyst it might burst or subside spontaneously. If it was a papilloma, it might drop off like the related wart on a human hand or leg. 'I'll have a look at it in a couple of weeks,' I said as we went out of the house.

Two weeks later, the tomato had grown into an apple. Its presence was beginning to irritate the giraffe as she ate. There was not the slightest sign of bursting or separation, in fact the lump looked to be blooming with health and well supplied with blood vessels. I stood on stepladders to try and touch the thing, but Molly swung her head as I approached and sent me tumbling down onto the straw.

Picking myself up, I said the words that sounded in my head like a death warrant. 'There's nothing for it. I'll have to take it off—under general anaesthesia.'

I arranged the operation for the next day. Andrew was still messing about with goats. He was always ready and eager to do work for me when asked. I gave him a call and explained the position.

'We'll put her under,' I said, 'then I'll get the surgical side over as quick as possible while you keep an eye on her system reactions. Then we'll pull out all the stops to reverse her.'

We talked for a long time about what drugs to use and how we might approach the difficulties that we felt sure were associated with the giraffe's peculiar blood circulation to the head and neck.

'This fainting under tranquillising is the problem,' said

Andrew. 'If they do that, everybody rushes around trying to hold their massive heads up in a "normal" posture; it strikes me that's just the wrong thing to do. The beast should be laid flat and given deeper anaesthetic at such times.'

It made sense physiologically, I saw, although I had made the Belle Vue keepers hold Pedro's head up when he fainted. We would try it Andrew's way and, as well as using etorphine and xylazine, would experiment with Dopram, a new American drug that counteracts the respiratory depression caused by narcotics. Our armoury of drugs was increasing every day. We had not used Dopram on giraffes before and decided it would be best to base the dosage on human requirements. Molly weighed as much as eight adults, so we agreed on 500 milligrams. The animal would not be allowed up onto her feet until any chance of fainting had gone.

Next morning we all assembled at Belle Vue. Andrew had driven up from Cambridge overnight. Matt was organising his keepers and looking very apprehensive. The giraffe keeper was truculent and pale-faced. I tried not to let my own trepidation show, but I suspect I failed.

When everything was ready we began. First a small dose of xylazine was injected into Molly's shoulder then, when she went drowsy after a quarter of an hour, I jabbed the etorphine into her jugular vein. She went down onto the thick bed of straw and, while Andrew was still attaching the electrocardiograph leads and administering the Dopram, I splashed iodine over the operation site and grabbed the lump. A glance showed me that it was a benign tumour. My mind empty of thoughts, all my attention fixed on the cold, silver edge of my scalpel blade as it swept round the base of the tumour, I worked as if it were a small time-bomb. It fell free. Blood welled up. I staunched hard with a gauze swab punched into the wound and then clipped off the main blood vessel. One, two, three, four—I slapped in the sutures and knotted them furiously. Swab again. No blood ooze. Done. It had taken about two minutes.

636

'Right, Andrew,' I said, louder than I intended. 'Bring her round.'

Andrew moved to the animal's neck and shot the syringeful of blue antidote, cyprenorphine, into her vein. Almost at once, Molly gave a great sigh and blinked. She was coming round. If we were in for trouble, this was where we would run into it.

'Keep her head down at all costs until we give the word,' I instructed our helpers.

Andrew gave Molly more Dopram. He pressed the button on the electrocardiograph and more coils of paper bearing the characteristic tracings were spewed out. He disconnected the leads and bent over the giraffe's heaving chest with his stethoscope.

'How's it going?' I asked.

He gave me the thumbs-up.

I took two keepers to sit on her head and neck. When she struggled I added a third. Andrew stayed at her chest. I looked at my watch. After five minutes, Molly was obviously very conscious and wondering why she had the heavy bottoms of three men pressing down on her. I slipped a final two millilitres of cyprenorphine under her skin to guard against any anaesthetic that had still not been neutralised.

At last I took the bit between my teeth.

'Everybody off,' I shouted. 'Stand clear!'

The men jumped to their feet and we all moved smartly back. Molly lifted her neck, looked round at us and slowly fanned those long, glamorous eyelashes. Effortlessly, she gathered her legs under her and stood up.

I bit my lower lip till it bled. Molly walked slowly over to her feed-trough high on the wall. Was that a slight flicker of the muscles in her haunches? She caught one hoof in a twist of straw: was it a stumble, the first before she keeled over? Molly looked into her trough and cast a liquid eye over the pile of fresh fruit, corn and fresh celery that Matt had prepared. Then she curled out her grey tongue and began to eat avidly.

We all stood as the minutes went by. No-one spoke until a quarter of an hour had passed. Molly had cleared the trough and was looking round for dessert.

I cleared my throat and licked my now sore lip. 'Er, I think, gentlemen, she's going to be OK. Thank you very much. One stays with her. The rest come and have a beer.'

Andrew grinned. 'We've cracked it,' he said.

It certainly looked so. 'Look here,' I said to him as we walked over to the dispensary to wash up, 'why don't you pack up this research business and come into partnership with me? Do some real work.'

He answered immediately. 'Of course I will. I wondered when you were going to suggest it.'

Molly was to be the last case I treated as a solo zoo vet. We were on our way.